EXPLORING THE INTERFACE BETWEEN THE PHILOSOPHY AND DISCIPLINE OF HOLISTIC NURSING: MODELING AND ROLE-MODELING AT WORK

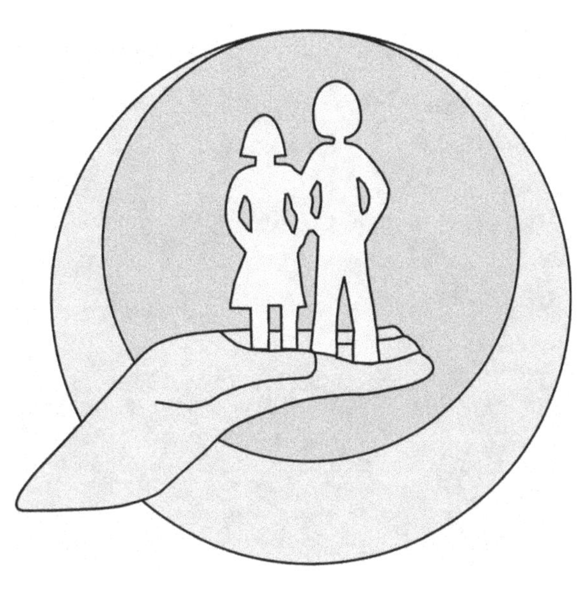

EXPLORING THE INTERFACE BETWEEN THE PHILOSOPHY AND DISCIPLINE OF HOLISTIC NURSING: MODELING AND ROLE-MODELING AT WORK

Helen L. Erickson, PhD, RN, AHN-BC, FAAN
Editor

Unicorns Unlimited
Cedar Park, Texas

MRM Logo Reprinted with Permission of EST Co.

Library of Congress Cataloging-in-Publication Data

Exploring the Interface Between the Philosophy and Discipline of Holistic Nursing: Modeling and Role-Modeling at Work

Helen L. Erickson (1936-), Editor

Includes bibliographic references and index.

ISBN: 978-1451511734

1) Holistic nursing 2) Discovery-Learning 3) Ways-of-Knowing
4) Modeling and Role-Modeling 5) Teaching-learning

Copy Editor: Geeta Erickson, MA
Graphics and Interior Design: Lance Erickson, MA

Published by
Unicorns Unlimited
406, Trail Ridge Dr.
Cedar Park, TX 78613
Unicornsunlimited.com
unicornsunlimitedbooks@yahoo.com

TABLE OF CONTENTS

CONTRIBUTING AUTHORS

Linda Baas, PhD, RN, ACNP
Professor and Director of Nursing Research, University of Cincinnati College of Nursing, The Christ Hospital;
Cincinnati, OH
linda.baas@uc.edu

Susan S. Bowman, PhD, RN
Professor Emeritus,
Humboldt State University;
Arcata, CA
susan.bowman@humboldt.ed

Da'Lynn Kay Clayton, PhD, RN
Imagine Nursing Consultant;
Associate Professor, Associate Dean of Nursing, Harding University;
Searcy, AR
dclayton@harding.edu

Helen L. Erickson, PhD, RN, AHN-BC, FAAN
Professor Emeritus, The University of Texas at Austin;
Cedar Park, TX
helenerickson@mail.utexas.edu

Margaret E. Erickson, PhD, RN, AHN-BC
Executive Director, The American Holistic Nurses Certification Corporation;
Cedar Park, TX
ahncc@flash.net

Judith E. Hertz, PhD, RN, FNGNA
Associate Professor, School of Nursing & Health Studies, Northern Illinois University;
DeKalb, IL
jhertz@niu.edu

Christi A. Holland, PhD, RN, FNP
Adjunct Faculty, The University of Texas at Austin; President and CEO, Contemporary Healthcare;
Austin, TX
info@chcaustin.com

Barbara L. Irvin, PhD, RN
Professor Emeritus, Oregon Health & Science University School of Nursing, Ashland Campus;
Ashland, OR
birvin433@charter.net

Christopher Johns, PhD, RN, PACT
Professor of Nursing, University of Bedfordshire, 76 Goldington Avenue
Bedford, MK40 3DA
chris.johns5@btinternet.com

Carolyn Kinney, PhD, RN, AHN-BC
Integrated Health Care Therapist and Wellness Consultant;
Austin, TX
ckkinney@aol.com

Sharon Rogers PhD, RN
Healthcare Solutions Consulting,
Georgetown, TX;
shari.rogers@suddenlink.net

Ellen Schultz, PhD, RN, CHTP
Professor, Metropolitan State University;
St. Paul, MN
ellendschultz@comcast.net

Lynn Smith, MSN, RN, CCRN, CMC, CCNS
Clinical Nurse Specialist, Critical Care
St. Elizabeth Healthcare;
Edgewood, KY
lynnwsmith@hotmail.com

Acknowledgements

Persons whom I wish to acknowledge for this work can be classified in three ways: First, are those who inspired the work; second, are those who did the work; and third, are those who supported us, so we could do it. Together, these three groups of individuals have created the energy field necessary to bring this work to fruition.

The first group includes personal mentors who have shaped our thinking through the years; students and colleagues who have helped us clarify our beliefs and premises; and the authors of many magnificent writings that have led the way, encouraging nurses to stretch their minds and imagine a better world for Nursing and for the consumers of our professional practice.

The second group includes those who completed the tasks that made this book a reality. This group includes, first and foremost, the authors of the chapters herein. I have been inspired by their work, encouraged by their dedication, and will be forever grateful for their contributions.

Equally important are Lance and Geeta Erickson, the two people who have worked night and day, weekends, vacations, and every moment possible to put our work together; to create graphics, format, change, revise, clarify thoughts, and just be there when needed. Without their work, this book would not be here today.

Finally, the third group, those who have supported us, include all the members of the Society for Modeling and Role-Modeling who have insisted that they wanted this product; and those who have encouraged each of us individually, to continue writing, even when we think that what we are saying makes no sense.

And last, but not the least, our families and friends who have been there to inspire and support us as we have struggled to articulate what we know. On behalf of the authors of this book, I wish to thank each of you for your priceless contribution to this work.

Dedication

On May 26, 1873, Florence Nightingale asked nurses to think about what it would be like in 1999 and then went on to say that it would be what we have made it. Nightingale, F. (1873). A subnote of interrogation. *Fraser's Magazine*, 567-577.

Today, March 1, 2010, we dedicate this book to the holistic nurses who aim to change healthcare, to proactively create a more compassionate, caring healthcare environment, build a knowledge base that will inform holistic nursing practice, and inspire colleagues to fully embrace the core values of holistic nursing.

I also wish to dedicate this work to Mary Ann Swain, my mentor, colleague and friend, who believed in me when others viewed me as just another student.

FOREWORD

I have been a nurse for 40 years, and have worn a variety of hats as "nurse educator" for over 30 of them! However, it is only for the past 20 plus years, (half my career as a nurse), that I have understood my personal beliefs and philosophy of Nursing.

In 1988, while in doctoral study, I walked into an Adult Health Nursing class. Dr. Helen Erickson was teaching the class, and I had "heard about" the Modeling and Role-Modeling (MRM) Nursing theory. I initially dismissed the theory because my understanding of "modeling" and "role-modeling" was quite different from the meaning in this paradigm. In fact, I recall picking up the book in the campus bookstore and putting it back on the shelf; a few days later, I went back and purchased it.

At that time, I was planning for my dissertation research and knew exactly what I wanted to study. Nevertheless, I struggled to convey my ideas to faculty—ideas that were not yet based in a theory. To compound the problem, I could not find a Chair for my dissertation committee. Nonetheless, I did not give up on my ideas. During that semester, I thought about my philosophy of nursing and wrote about my beliefs; after all, this was a required assignment. Then, one day, I opened the MRM book; the "aha" moment occurred! The MRM paradigm was congruent with my philosophy of nursing.

Of course, Dr. Erickson agreed to help me find a committee and, eventually, agreed to chair it. However, as part of the process and before everything fell into place, I needed to read more widely than I had in the past and reflect on all I had learned, and to "know" in a very focused and purposeful way. Since that time, my understanding of my beliefs and philosophy has deepened. They are part of my being and explain much not only about the aspects of my Nursing career that have felt "right," but also those that have been uncomfortable.

I have always been open to walking through doors of opportunity when they appear; writing this Foreword has been one of those opportunities! All nurses who espouse Holistic Nursing and who want to act on their belief that nurses care for persons as holistic beings must read this book. Even nurses who are skeptical about "holistic nursing" should read this book.

First, it is aptly titled! *It is an exploration* of the multiple facets of holistic nursing, and of the linkages between beliefs about nursing and how the discipline of Nursing is taught and practiced. The first chapters provide the context for Nursing as we know it today. The content presented is founded in classic and current writings, including the original book on the MRM theory and paradigm (Erickson, Tomlin, & Swain, 1983/2009). Although the lingo and buzzwords have changed (e.g., the Doctorate of Nursing Practice degree [DNP] rather than Doctorate of Nursing degree [DN], learning outcomes, rather than learning objectives, etc.), the past provides the context for the present and future of Nursing.

Linkages between the nurse's personal beliefs (i.e., philosophy) regarding persons, health, environment and nursing practice are presented in the introductory chapters and reinforced throughout the book. Accordingly, the perspective that belief systems permeate and drive practice is often overlooked in the literature. This book makes a contribution to Nursing as an art and science—an unfilled gap in the literature. The overall tone is to encourage nurses to be *compassionate* and *proactive* for the purpose of improving the health, well-being and growth of the client.

The authors of chapters in the second section build on the initial thought-provoking questions raised, either implicitly or explicitly, in Section 1. For example,

"Do nurses care for the persons or the problems that persons might exhibit?"

"Who benefits from the nurse-client relationship and whose needs are being met?"

"Is there a difference between what we do and what we think?"

"Why does there often seem to be a lack of connection between what nurses are taught during their education and what they do in nursing practice?"

"Why do nurses often discount as 'irrelevant' the subjective view of what clients tell them?"

"Why is reflective practice important?"

The content of the book most definitely provides ample food for thought and reflection. Besides being thought-stimulating, the book tackles other important issues rarely addressed in Nursing. The ideas of Evidence-Based Nursing, Evidence-Based Practice (EBP) and advanced nursing practice are not new. However, descriptions of how to integrate evidence into nursing practice and define advanced practice, threaded throughout the chapters (including one chapter devoted entirely to this topic), are new. Another common thread seems to be sociopolitical influences on Nursing. The reader is frequently reminded to balance nursing practice (in whatever role one holds), with the realities of the sociopolitical climate. This, too, is often overlooked in publications.

The important responsibility of educators in teaching the essence of Nursing and preparing nurses for current and future practice—presented in a logical, integrated, well-thought-out fashion—is emphasized from various perspectives. Nurse educators have an obligation to society to do this. The content regarding curriculum development (in all settings) and its relationship to philosophies cannot be overemphasized. In addition to serving as a guidebook, the chapters promote self-reflection about what drives the nurse educator's practice with Nursing students as clients.

Teaching strategies and techniques abound in the book. Storytelling is used as a strategy to illustrate points, demonstrating good teaching practices. Additionally, the tips for working with students in clinical settings with the aim of promoting their growth and learning are outstanding. The recommendations for providing evaluative feedback to students made me pause, examine my own practices and plan for changes, so that I can be more focused on facilitating their learning and growth!

The final chapter by Christi Holland clearly sums up and ties together all previous chapters as she reflects upon finding her Soul work. Her work serves as a strong impetus for others to self-reflect on their practice, wherever that may take place. From my perspective as a nurse educator, the book should be renamed and subtitled, "A Guide for Nurse Educators to Walk the Talk," or "Where the Tires Hit the Road for Nurse Educators!" I strongly recommend that all new Nursing faculty read this book. It should also be required reading for faculty serving on curriculum committees, and for faculties prior to developing or revising a Nursing curriculum. I would also recommend this book to all graduate students in Nursing programs, and mandatory reading for those preparing for roles as nurse educators, or other advanced practice roles in Nursing.

Finally, from the perspective of a nurse who is a believer in the MRM paradigm and embraces this Nursing theory as the key to true person-centered nursing, this book has been long-anticipated and is a welcome addition to my library. The information presented builds on the foundational publication of MRM's philosophical base, theory, concepts and related propositions (Erickson, et al., 1983/2009), and on the 2006 book (H. Erickson, (Ed.)) which was expanded to include concepts such as energy fields, spirituality, and Soul work. Many of us embrace and practice (i.e., teach) in systems that do not embrace or endorse MRM. Ideas and guidelines for how to include elements of MRM theory in various aspects of teaching and practice are welcomed. Most can be applied to either individuals or the whole system/organization. In addition, many of these "pearls of wisdom" are presented with recommendations on how to do this when one is practicing "alone."

This thought-provoking book fills several gaps in the literature, and makes a valuable contribution to the Nursing discipline. The content is pertinent to nurses in general, and to holistic nurses, nurse educators, and nurses who embrace the MRM paradigm. It is enlightening to read what many others have learned through MRM-based and true person-centered interactions. Readers will want to read and re-read this book.

Judith Hertz, PhD, RN, FNGNA
February 23, 2010

INTRODUCTION

> *A* profession *is an occupation whose core element is work based upon the mastery of a complex body of knowledge and skills. It is a vocation in which knowledge of some department of science or learning or the practice of an art founded upon it is used in the service of others. Its members are governed by codes of ethics and profess a commitment to competence, integrity and morality, altruism, and the promotion of the public good within their domain. These commitments form the basis of a social contract between a profession and society, which in return grants the profession a monopoly over the use of its knowledge base, the right to considerable autonomy in practice and the privilege of self-regulation. Professions and their members are accountable to those served and to society.* (Cruess, S. R., Johnston, S., & Cruess, R. L., 2004, p. 75)

The definition of a profession, clarified by Cruess, et al. (2004), implies that each professional group is actively involved in the development of a complex body of knowledge that can be used by its members to guide their practice. Driving these activities is the profession's societal responsibility to serve a specific role. Implicit is the belief that knowledge and practice are interactive, each contributing to the advancement of the other. Also implicit is the belief that Nursing's role in society can be clearly delineated by understanding how knowledge and practice interface.

While nurses have worked for years to clarify Nursing's unique role in society, there still appears to be confusion. One reason is that we still have a gap between what we know and what we do. That is, there is a gap between knowledge and practice.

Work such as *Teaching Medical Professionalism* (Cruess, S. R., Cruess, R. L., & Steinert, 2008) and *Work and Integrity: The Crisis and Promise of Professionalism in America* (Sullivan, & Shulman, 2004), and others, have provided some insights for members of the medical profession. At the same time, work such as *Curriculum Development in Nursing Education* (Iwasiw, Goldenberg, & Andrusyszyn, 2009) has helped those who needed direction on implementing a curriculum, and *A Contemporary Nursing Process: The (Un)Bearable Weight of Knowing in Nursing* (Locsin & Purnell, 2009) has helped educators rethink the nature of the nursing process. Yet, little has been published that addresses key Nursing issues.

We need to explore why this state of affairs is so persistent. Specifically, leaders in the profession need to ask questions such as,

1) *How do we advance the discipline of Nursing so that we can close the gap between knowledge and practice?*

2) How can we prepare novices of our profession so that they are not only competent, ethical practitioners, but also assertive, altruistic members of the profession, able to utilize Nursing's knowledge base?
3) What can we do, as educators, to facilitate nurses to become integrated holistic professionals?

This book is designed to offer some direction for nurse leaders interested in advancing Holistic Nursing, with a particular focus on the use of Modeling and Role-Modeling. Designed for all nurse educators in the academic or clinical setting, it is based on a few important premises including:

•Nursing is a person-centered profession.
•In order to be useful, the expansion of the Nursing discipline must be accomplished within the context of the philosophy of the profession.
•The philosophy of the profession is clear, but implications for the development of the discipline are not.
•The Nursing discipline includes multiple types of knowledge, not just empirical knowledge.
•Generally, when we use the term *knowledge*, we refer to the discipline of Nursing or multiple types of knowledge.
•Our personal philosophy impacts our thoughts and actions; therefore, it impacts our use of knowledge and how we practice professional nursing.
•Until we address these issues, we cannot close the gap between research and practice, a preliminary step in linking knowledge and practice.

Section One (Chapters 1-5) presents a background discussion of the relationships among Nursing as a unique profession within the context of healthcare, and Nursing's philosophy and discipline. It proposes a split in paradigms, curriculum development implications, and a model for facilitating the growth of students through discovery learning methods. The goal for this section is to challenge readers to think about the relationships among philosophy, discipline and professional activities. Premises for each of the chapters, stated and restated, include: Nursing is a person-centered profession; it exists because society needs the services Nursing provides; it resides within a larger system. Thus, there are driving and restraining forces which constantly impact its evolution.

Section Two (Chapters 6-12) presents more specific information about the teaching-learning processes. It is designed to provide readers with selected thoughts regarding selected factors that are needed to teach Holistic Nursing with an emphasis for those who base their curriculum in the Modeling and Role-

Modeling theory and paradigm. It is not intended to be inclusive, but addresses some of the more common concerns encountered by nurse educators in any setting. It focuses on selected issues relevant to the teaching-learning process and aims to stimulate discussion among colleagues.

Section Three includes three chapters, designed to provide a perspective on students' learning experiences often overlooked by faculty and other educators. First, we offer a discussion about the holistic nature of students and novice colleagues, including their vulnerability and human needs. We propose that, as humans, students are on a journey, seeking ways to accomplish their life purpose. Their interactions with educators and other nurse leaders have the potential to either facilitate them to find meaning in their lives, or to create distractions and confusion. We suggest story-telling and reflective practice as strategies that will facilitate their holistic growth. This is followed by a chapter on reflective practice, and includes models to guide nurses in the process. The final chapter of the book provides the reader with an inside-view of one life-journey. We hope that it will encourage educators to revisit or rediscover their own journey, and maybe, in the process, their life-purpose.

All chapters in Sections II and III are written within the context of the *holistic paradigm*. Some address specific concerns for those who facilitate students to learn Modeling and Role-Modeling (MRM), but not all. Nevertheless, those interested in MRM will find all the chapters relevant to their work.

SECTION 1

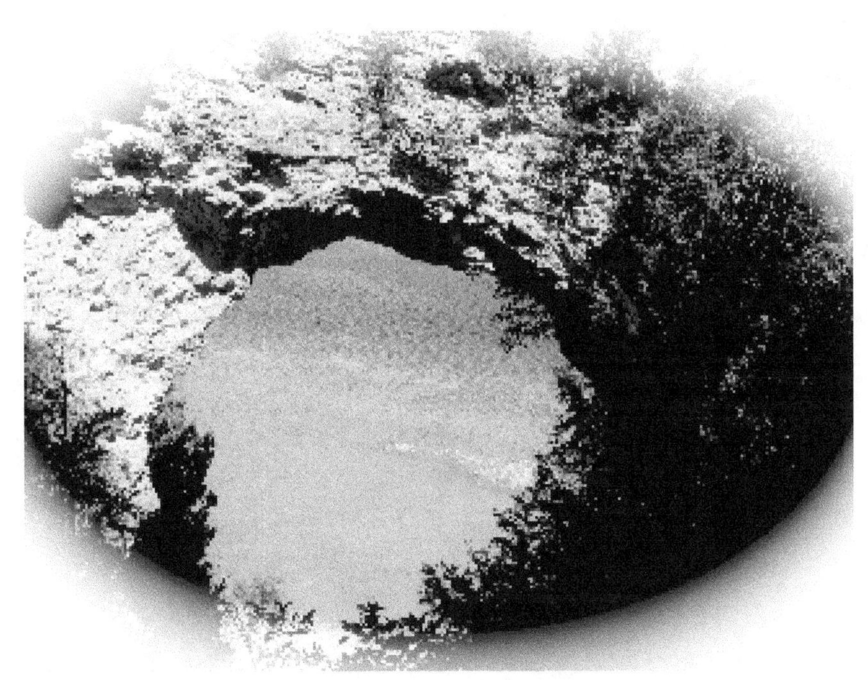

SECTION I

DEFINING THE PARAMETERS

How do we advance the discipline of Nursing so that we can close the gap between knowledge and practice?

This section presents a number of factors that educators need to consider as they plan nursing programs, curriculum development, course preparation, and teaching strategies for holistic nurses. *The specific intent is to explore factors that either facilitate or impede closing the gap between knowledge and practice.*

Chapter One revisits a time from the past when I was asked to address the question, "*What will it take to advance a model of communal, compassionate caring?*" It provides a brief overview of Nursing as part of the larger healthcare system, identifying driving and restraining forces that either facilitate or impede movements toward holistic nursing. It concludes with an argument that advancements in Nursing are impeded by a lack of cohesion in the profession caused by a split in belief systems or paradigms.

Chapter Two addresses Nursing's Metaparadigm and briefly discusses the forces that have influenced the split in paradigms. A table illustrating the two paradigms is presented along with implications for each of the two philosophical orientations. Chapter Three discusses the Ways-of-Knowing that guide our discipline. We propose a matrix model illustrating the convergence of the Metaparadigm and Nursing's Ways-of-Knowing.

Chapter Four discusses the process of curriculum development and focuses on the importance of recognizing the faculty's underlying paradigm choice. An expanded version of the matrix model presented in Chapter 3, illustrating the use of Modeling and Role-Modeling as a holistic nursing theory, is provided.

Chapter Five presents Bruner's Discovery-Learning Methods as a teaching model which helps students learn to learn, and jump the gap from learning to thinking.

CHAPTER 1

A VOICE FROM THE PAST: FACTORS THAT IMPACT PROFESSIONAL BEHAVIORS

Helen L. Erickson

"Those who cannot remember the past are condemned to repeat it."
George Santayana (1905-6)

OVERVIEW

About 25 years ago, I was asked to speak at a conference at Loyola University in Chicago. The conference was titled, A Call to Create, and the goal was to discuss how we could go beyond ourselves and move toward a healthcare model where nurses provided compassionate care. Our general objective was to identify aspects of transcendence and social consciousness as they relate to communal compassion. In other words, the objective was to identify factors that affected the nurse's ability to embrace a healthcare model based on compassion. My assignment was to address political aspects of compassionate care.

I presented this paper in first person, speaking directly to nurses then, just as I choose to speak to you today. I offer the entire paper here, followed by a discussion of the relevancy of my thoughts in 1984 to the work presented in this book. I start with a discussion of systems theory. This is because I believe that we cannot address how we practice or what we practice, until we first consider the context or environment in which we practice. I also believe that our practice varies, depending on the role(s) we choose within the Nursing system. Some choose the role of clinician; others choose to be educators, lawyers, administrators, coordinators, etc. In all cases, we are practicing our profession as long as we practice within the parameters of the discipline of the profession. I will discuss this further in Chapter 2. First, let's revisit my thoughts of 25 years ago.

A VOICE FROM THE PAST: POLITICAL CONSIDERATIONS OF COMPASSIONATE CARING

Good Afternoon. I am honored to be here today to address several questions [shown in Table 1.1].

Table 1.1 Questions for contemplation.

1.	Nurses spend a great deal of time in direct contact with patients and witness patients struggle to come to grips with their illness, suffering, and for some, their impending death. All these factors are highly charged with spiritual/religious meaning. Why is it that nurses are so reluctant or avoid involvements with patients, relative this dimension?
2.	What can we do, as nurses that would assist us in fostering a communal and compassionate approach in the provision of direct patient care?
3.	What would be the political impact of the nurse's communal and compassionate response in administering direct patient care? In other words, what kind of changes might result for patients, family members, professional peers, and administration if nurses were to respond in this manner?

Question one implies that consumers or clients constitute one of the systems embedded in the suprasystem;[1] *Nursing, Medicine, payment groups (such as insurance companies), etc., each constitute other systems within the same context. Question two addresses strategies that nurses might use to change the dynamics of the Nursing system. And question three addresses the potential impact changes in Nursing could have on the healthcare suprasystem.*

These questions, taken as a whole, imply that Nursing is an institution which interacts with other institutions in such a way that a change in one will impact the others. Or stated in another way, Nursing is one of many systems that, together, create a suprasystem. If changes occur in Nursing, these changes have the potential to effect changes in the other systems. Thus, changes in Nursing have the potential to affect the dynamics of the suprasystem. The suprasystem is healthcare. The environment in which health care is provided creates the context of the suprasystem, i.e., healthcare.

When Barbara[2] *invited me to participate in this conference, I experienced several feelings. I was deeply honored—not sure why I was*

---

[1] A suprasystem is a multiple system network which shares a common function. In the case of the healthcare suprasystem, the function is supposed to be the well-being of society. While each of the individual systems (or subsystems) has unique functions, as a group, they create a context unique to the suprasystem.

[2] Barbara's last name is Kennison. I met her during her doctoral study at The University of Michigan.

invited, but very pleased and privileged to be asked to participate. I also felt excitement—I was eager to see Barbara again, challenged by the invitation and excited about meeting new friends. I was also a little anxious—how could I possibly describe what I felt while talking about what I thought?

As I pondered these reactions, I realized that my anxiety was related to my desire to articulate my comments in a way that would neither, by omission or commission, point fingers or find fault with colleagues in healthcare. I thought about my undergraduate students who come to us with great enthusiasm and eagerness, ready to learn how to administer compassionate, holistic care. They don't know how, but they have a desire to be compassionate nurses. I've never seen one who didn't start out wanting to help people. And then, I thought about some of my nurse colleagues who had that same enthusiasm a few years ago, and today seem discouraged, disappointed, and sometimes, detached.

As I struggled with my thoughts and feelings, I concluded that the only way I could put it all in perspective in such a short time was to address my topic within the context of the healthcare system. This would enable me to think about change within the system and the forces that influence the behaviors of nurses. I do not plan to talk about how we got to this point. I want to merely discuss my perception of our status quo. I will ask you to draw upon your knowledge of systems theories to enrich the limited comments I will make.

I will not pretend to present an in-depth review of systems theory in this discussion. I hope merely to provide an overview of the major characteristics of a system and hope that this will provide us with a foundation for discussion of the potential impact of change within the system. But before I can talk about characteristics of a system, we need to have a common understanding of what I mean when I use the word system.

Systems Theory

Various definitions of systems have been developed over the past several years. Some say that a system can be conceptualized as "complexes of elements standing in interaction" (Ludwig von Bertalanffy, 1968, p.33), or as a "whole with interrelated parts, in which the parts have a function and the system as a totality has a function" (Auger, 1976, p. 21). Others define a system as "a set of objects together with relationships between the objects and between their attributes" (Hall & Fagen, 1968, p. 81) or as a "group of interrelated but separate elements working toward a common objective" (Duncan, 1978, p. 76).

While these definitions differ, they also share a commonality. All definitions state that a system is a set of entities that are interrelated and impact one another. The major difference among these definitions relates to the system's function. Most argue that the elements work together toward a common goal. On the other hand, Hall and Fagen (1968) state that the elements have interrelationships that tie the system together [as shown in Figure 1.1]. *It will be important for us to keep these perspectives in mind as we discuss the potential impact of a system change.*

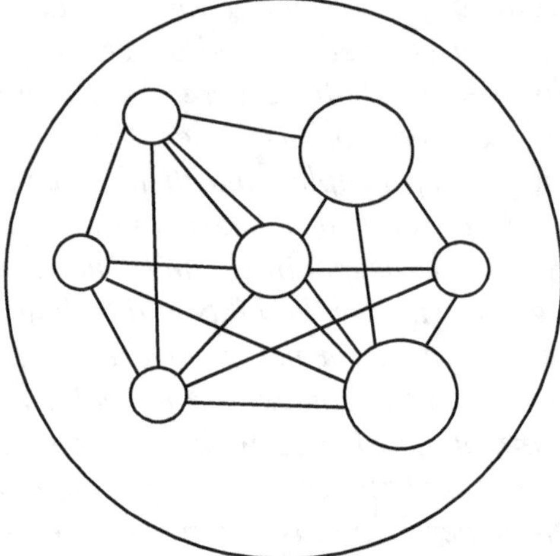

Figure 1.1 Relations among multiple systems included in the healthcare suprasystem.

System Characteristics

Structure

The structure of a system is the arrangement of its parts. Generally speaking, systems are arranged in a hierarchical manner with subsystems maintained within the framework of the larger system. Thus, within the framework of the healthcare system, there are several subsystems with some hierarchical order. Medicine, hospital administration, Nursing and Clients (or consumers) are examples of subsystems within the healthcare system. The hierarchical order of these subsystems is not absolute although most of us would agree that Nursing and Clients are probably near the bottom of this particular list.

The way in which subsystems interface with one another is known as the function within the system. When subsystems share a common goal, the system functions so smoothly that it is difficult to discriminate the function of one subsystem from that of another. On the other hand, when the goals of the subsystems differ, imbalance and inefficiency can occur.

Degree of Openness

Systems are thought of in terms of their openness to interaction with their environment. Usually, they are considered closed or open. A closed system is one that exchanges nothing with the environment, while an open system has a free exchange with the environment. Both closed and open systems attempt to maintain a steady-state or state of equilibrium. That is, systems tend to resist change.

Hall and Fagen (1968) defined the environment as a "set of all objects a change in whose attributes affect the system, and also those objects whose attributes are changed by the behavior of the system" (p. 83). Thus, a change in the environment would change the system, and vice-versa, changes within the elements (or subsystems) would impact the environment. Figure 1.1 [above] *shows how subsystems (within the parameters of a system) might be connected with one another. In this figure, each circle represents a subsystem within the framework of the healthcare suprasystem.*

You can also see how the suprasystem itself is organized within an environment. Not shown in this figure is the potential for other systems to interact with any given system, depending on one's view. When we look at it from a micro perspective, you would see multiple subsystems within each circle. When studied from a macro perspective, it would be possible to add hundreds, perhaps thousands, of other systems that would impact the healthcare suprasystem. Obviously, as we move from the micro perspective to the macro perspective, what is considered a system at one point becomes a subsystem at another. That is, if all things are connected, then the use of the terms system and subsystem become artificial boundaries used to define a specific entity.

Boundaries

The area that separates the system from the environment is the boundary of the system. Boundaries can be real or artificial, and in both cases, they regulate the exchange that occurs between the system and the environment. Subsystems have boundaries within the parameters of the whole system. The degree of porosity of the boundary determines the degree of exchange that occurs between and among the subsystems or systems. The greater the porosity the less stable the system. That is, the greater the porosity of the boundary, the more input the system receives from its environment.

Frequently, there is an interface between two systems or subsystems, so their boundaries cross. While the boundary generally serves as the filter for each system, separating the system from its environment, the interface between two systems is the overlap between two systems. The interface between two systems is different from a link between the two systems. The link is the person or persons assigned the responsibility for making contacts between systems. For example, within an organized system such as a hospital, there is an interface between Nursing and Medicine; members of administration and client care serve to link the two. Figure 1.2 shows these relations.

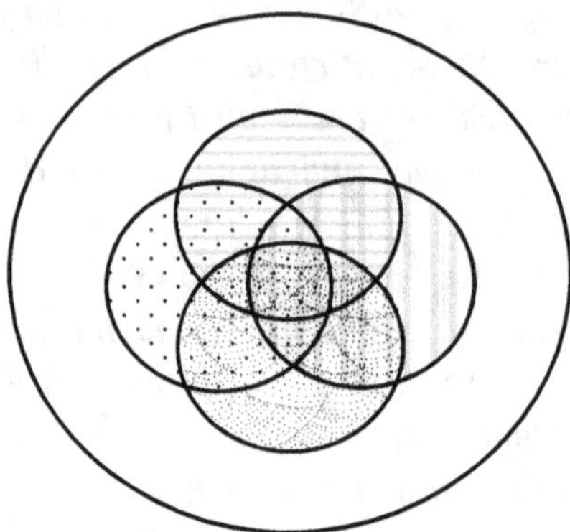

Figure 1.2 Overlap among the multiple systems included in the healthcare suprasystem.

Input-Transformation-Output

Systems constantly take in resources, transform these resources, and subsequently provide output to the environment. There are two types of input: human and natural resources. Human resources consist of the people in the system who contribute time, energy, cognitive perspectives, and so forth. Natural resources are the nonhuman resources that impact the system. Most important among these are funding sources.

***Feedback** is the process whereby "output at one stage of systems' operation is returned to the system in the form of input for a successive stage" (Duncan, 1978, p. 79). Feedback is essential for an open, evolving system since it provides input to the system regarding the way it is perceived outside system boundaries. Figure 1.3 shows this process.*

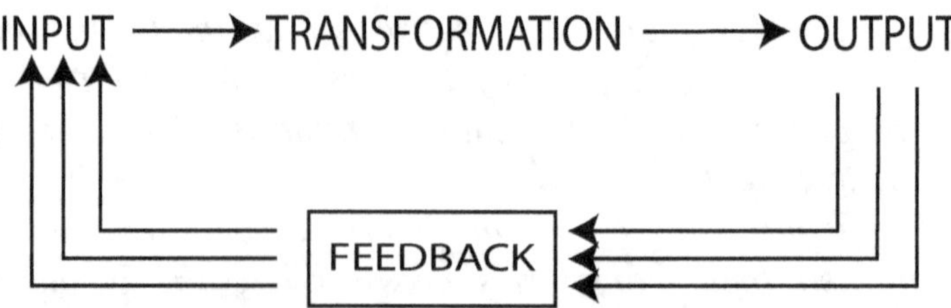

Figure 1.3 Feedback loops found in system dynamics.

Disorganization and Equilibrium

Systems, as a whole, strive toward balance or a steady-state among the parts. Thus, when there are changes within a subsystem, the other connected subsystems must change in order to maintain a steady-state or state of equilibrium. Furthermore, when there are changes in the environment that impact either the whole system or parts of the system, changes must occur in order to regain equilibrium. For example, if the power base within one subsystem should change, the power bases within the other subsystems would also have to change in order to compensate for the change in the first. The alternative—disorganization in the system—is, generally, not an acceptable choice.

These stabilizing relationships become particularly vital for the system as a whole when change in one subsystem occurs at the point where it interfaces with another. Without sufficient compensation, a system crisis can occur. For example, if Nursing were to change so that it impacts Medicine at the point of interface, unless Medicine accepts the changes and accommodates, disequilibrium can occur in the Medical subsystem. This would force the suprasystem (i.e. the healthcare system) to reorganize in order to regain equilibrium.

Power Bases

Within the suprasystem, power is distributed among the subsystems. Power is determined by a subsystem's ability to impact other subsystems and to maintain equilibrium within the suprasystem. Power is held by persons or groups within the subsystems, and is recognized by members of the other subsystems due to their need to maintain a steady state with the suprasystem. Power bases are generally defined in terms of five basic types: legitimate, reward, coercive, expert, and referent.

***Legitimate power** is the authority derived from the position or role held within the system. This authority must be recognized by other members of the subsystem as a formal type of power.*

***Reward power** is derived from the power holder's use of positive sanctioning. Such sanctioning can include anything perceived by the recipient as positive and can range from a compliment to monetary remuneration for behaviors. Reward power is sometimes called positive social-emotional power.*

***Coercive power** is the opposite of reward power since it is derived from the power holder's ability to either withhold positive sanctioning or, in more extreme cases, to use negative rewards such as threats or punishment.*

Expert power *is derived from others perceiving that the power holder has a base of valid knowledge, skills or information needed by the system, subsystem, or members within them. It is not sufficient for the system member to have knowledge for expert power to be present; other system members must perceive that the member has this knowledge.*

Referent power *is the subtle power derived from personal attraction of one system member or group for another. Appearance and personal characteristics constitute referent power. While the above forms of power are usually considered the main types, there is another that is important to our discussion, i.e., associative power. Associative power is derived from being associated with someone or some group that holds one or more power bases.*

Power bases are both within the system as a whole (therefore, within the subsystems) and within the environment that surrounds the system. That is, outside any given suprasystem, but within the suprasystem's environment, multiple other systems exist. Power bases exist in all these systems. This is important, since there is a constant exchange between the system and the environment. Environmental power bases can be very powerful; in fact, they can force change in strong, resilient systems. We'll discuss this later when we talk about the potential impact of compassionate care on the entire healthcare system.

Closely associated with power bases is the communication structure within a system (or subsystem). While this paper is not intended to discuss communication theory or go into detail, it is important for the reader to know that communication between subsystems can alter members' perceptions. When members perceive that other members do or do not have power, these perceptions have the potential to influence change within the subsystems. When group members perceive that other members have power, they tend to seek more interactions with them, and are more easily influenced by their use of such power, whether intentional or not. The feedback that occurs under these circumstances tends to help the first group build their power base, even when it isn't legitimate or expert power. [See Table 1.2 for a summary of these System Characteristics.]

Table 1.2 System characteristics, definitions, and implications.

Characteristics	Definitions	Implications
Structure	Arrangement of the parts of the system or suprasystem.	•Interrelation among the parts is the function. •There is a quasi- hierarchy among subsystems within the larger system.
Openness	Degree of interaction with the environment (and other systems within the environment).	•Usually open or closed, or some variation of the two. •Tend to resist change to become more or less open.
Boundaries	Area that separates the system from the environment (and other systems in the environment).	•Can be real or artificial. •Regulate the exchange among systems in a suprasystem. •Degree of boundary/porosity determines the exchange among the systems. •The greater the porosity, the less stable the system and vice-versa.
Input-transformation-output	The processes whereby systems take in resources, transform them, and produce output. Feedback is when the output at one stage serves as input at another.	•Types of resources: human and natural. •Human resources provide time, energy, thought, etc. •Natural resources are all others that impact the system; funding sources are very important.
Disorganization and Equilibrium	Occurs when changes in a given system or within the environmental systems result in an imbalance in resources.	•Changes in power bases can affect equilibrium. •Extended or excessive disequilibrium can result in disorganization. •Disorganization produces a crisis. •Disorganization is not acceptable and will be resisted as long as possible.
Power bases	Determined by the system's ability to impact another system. Power is held by persons or groups of persons within given systems.	•Five types of power: legitimate, reward, coercive, expert, and referent. •Power is impacted by the communication structure within the system and among the systems of a suprasystem.

System Change

Change within a system can be discussed given its characteristics [described above]. *The more open the system, the greater the chance for change, and vice-versa. The more closed the system, the less likely that external factors will influence the system. Since the healthcare system (a suprasystem), is composed of several smaller systems (or subsystems, depending on how you view it), change in one will automatically effect change in others. However, since there is a major force to maintain equilibrium in the larger system, change in the subsystems is generally met by resistant forces from others. Power bases within a subsystem provide forces for and against change within the whole system. These forces can be described as driving or restraining forces. The more power a subsystem has, the greater the potential influence the driving and restraining forces will have on system change.*

Driving Forces

There are several driving forces that support change in the healthcare system. One that warrants consideration is the Prospective Payment System, a federal model for financing health care that is regularly discussed today. While the creation of the PPS results in driving forces that will have considerable impact on the healthcare suprasystem, it is very possible that the affected changes could move the entire system toward dehumanized care rather than toward compassionate care. On the other hand, merely knowing that this potential exists can provide incentive for nurses to work to achieve what is needed to provide compassionate care. That is, this environmental driving force might result in nurses organizing to form a communal counter-force toward compassionate care.

This is similar to the balancing forces described by Naisbitt who predicts the hi-tech, hi-touch megatrends in the 1980s and 1990s. If nurses make the decision to purposefully offset this negative force, they will need to aggregate the driving forces that are directed toward compassionate care and synthesize them into a more powerful force that will impact the system, resulting in change.

Some of the more powerful driving forces already existing in the healthcare system and its environment that can be built upon are shown in Table 1.3. They include the following:

Nurses' intuitive knowledge of clients' needs. *Maslow (1968) stated that all humans have basic needs that motivate our behavior. These are arranged in a quasi-hierarchy with physiological needs first, followed by safety and security needs, love and belonging needs, and, finally, esteem and self-esteem needs, respectively. Nurses have historically addressed the first two levels of needs as a function of their professional activities. That is, they have focused on physiological and safety needs. Many have intuitively, and with compassion, addressed the remaining levels of needs as well. As some nurses state, they seem to "just know what our clients need to help them cope." Others state that they want to treat their clients as they would like to be treated under similar circumstances. In either case, some nurses are identified as "natural nurses." This* *characteristic is attributed to these nurses based on their intuitive responses to people.*[3]

Table 1.3 Driving forces that enhance nurses' ability to impact the type of health care provided in the US.

Driving Forces	**Characteristics of Specific Driving Forces**
PPS: Model of healthcare funding	Provides opportunities for nurses to practice and/or coordinate person-centered, compassionate primary care.
Nurses' intuitive knowledge	Many nurses practice compassionate care based on clients' perceived needs.
Positive reinforcement for compassionate care	Supports and encourages compassionate behaviors and increases communication.
Nurses as humans	Positive reinforcement meets nurses' needs for esteem, enhancing Nursing's power bases.
Being-love motivation	Being-love empowers nurses' behaviors.
Professional education	Nurses prepared from a holistic model adopt knowledge and skills related to compassionate care.
Society's demand for change	Consumer demand enhances the power of those who provide such care.
Proactive nurses	Nurses able to provide compassionate care can articulate and operationalize it.

These interpersonal interactions by these "natural nurses" create a driving force toward compassionate care that can be reinforced and strengthened. Generally, these interactions result in clients attributing their nurse with legitimate, expert, and referent power. On occasion, nursing colleagues share these perceptions and also attribute their colleagues with these power bases. Under these circumstances, these nurses also take on associative power.

Reinforcement for compassionate care. *As nurses respond to their clientele with compassion, they receive positive feedback from their clients and sometimes from colleagues. Such feedback reinforces their behavior, thus providing stimuli for repeating the behaviors. As the process evolves, the reinforcement can offset system-restraining forces that impede*

[3] During a recent interaction with Christopher Johns, I concluded that this is very similar to what he says is a Way-of-Knowing and defines as knowing used in moment-to-moment practice or the core of being.

communal and compassionate care. Clients want personalized, compassionate care and are becoming increasingly vocal about their needs. Such continuous, internal pressure provides a driving force that can also be used to change the system.

Nurses as humans. *When nurses receive feedback from their clients and colleagues who support their compassionate behaviors, they perceive satisfaction of their own basic love and belonging, and esteem/self-esteem needs. Many also experience satisfaction of growth needs. Since nurses, like all other humans, have basic needs that motivate their behaviors, satisfaction of these needs is a prerequisite to meeting the needs of others. Thus, satisfaction of both basic and growth needs reinforces the driving forces described above. These first three driving forces work together as an "input-throughput-output-feedback" process. In this respect, nurses and clients interface within the system and therefore, impact one another, as well as the whole system.*

Being-love versus Deficit-love. *According to Maslow, there are two kinds of love. Those whose basic needs are repeatedly met require little for need satisfaction. These individuals experience a form of love defined as Being-love. Those who repeatedly have need deficits (or unmet needs) experience Deficit-love. The essential difference between these two forms of love is the impact that one's type of love has on his or her attraction with others. Those who are motivated from Being-love aim toward meeting the needs of others in order to help the other grow, become independent, and achieve self-actualization. On the contrary, those motivated from Deficit-love aim to meet their own needs. Many nurses are motivated by Being-love; Being-love is a powerful driving force.*

Professional education. *The educational background of professional Nurses is an additional driving force toward compassionate care. In recent years, educators have refocused the educational process, so the aim of nursing is person-centered (rather than disease-oriented), holistic (rather than reductionist), and health-oriented (rather than disease-oriented). Nurses educated within the context of these concepts are prepared to identify, label, and articulate the phenomenon of compassionate care. They are also prepared to plan purposeful, systematic interventions that meet the basic and growth needs of their clients. Professional education of this type provides a powerful driving force toward both communal and compassionate care.*

Society's demands for change. *Probably, the most important driving force in today's health care system is the demand from the consumers of health care for personalized, holistic, health-oriented care.*

Our consumers have become increasingly vocal in stating their needs and demanding responses from providers. These demands have come from clients within the system and from consumer groups in the environment such as labor unions and congressmen who are proposing legislative changes that support change. Others, such as management in the auto industry are further supporting this movement by requesting health care that aims to prevent health problems rather than merely responding to the conditions caused by disease. These changes in the system and environment are extremely important driving forces for compassionate care.

Proactive nurses. *Many nurses are learning how to be assertive, how to negotiate leadership roles for themselves in the healthcare system, and how to clearly conceptualize and operationalize Nursing as a compassionate profession. These nurses are proactively supporting changes in the healthcare system which are not totally understood by their Nursing and medical colleagues. Some are aligning themselves with the consumers who are demanding such changes. These nurses provide another driving force that could be reinforced and built upon.*

Restraining Forces

While the above discussion presented several driving forces that have the potential to influence the desired change, there are also several restraining forces that interfere with changes in the healthcare system. These forces, shown in Table 1.4, can be related to the power based within the subsystems of the suprasystem. The first three restraining forces described involve all healthcare subsystems. The remaining restraining forces address issues unique to individual nurses.

Learned behaviors. *Many health care providers and consumers have learned to be concerned primarily with disease-oriented care. Thus, they place special emphasis on controlling, curing, or arresting the disease process. These behaviors have been reinforced by the explosion in technology that has occurred since the sixties. That is, most technological advancements related to health care have been developed in order to diagnose or treat a disease. This emphasis encourages health care providers to focus on the pathology, rather than the person who has the problem. Individuals with this orientation create a significant resistant force to change.*

Table 1.4 Restraining forces that impede nurses' ability to impact the type of health care provided in the US.

Restraining Forces	**Characteristics of Specific Restraining Forces**
PPS: model of healthcare funding	Without careful regulations and oversight, PPS has potential to effect dehumanized care.
Learned behaviors	Nurses' socialization may over-ride intuitive knowledge, resulting in dehumanized care.
Reinforcements for efficient, disease- or problem-oriented care.	Some nurses are disciplined or rebuked by colleagues for "getting too involved" or "wasting time" with compassionate care.
Nurses' personal perspective	Holistic nurses, unable to articulate their philosophy, may get negative reinforcement from those who don't understand their intent.
Deficit-love motivation	Nurses motivated with deficit-love motivation may seek power for the nurses' benefit, and see change as threatening.
Nursing education	Diversity in faculty philosophy may lead to divergent views of Nursing being taught, leading to a lack of common language.
Definition of Nursing	Consumers, unclear about what they can expect from Nursing, confuse the nurse's role with the doctor's.
Reactive nurses	Nurses who see change as a threat may react, create resistance, and impede changes.

System reinforcements. *While health care providers have learned behaviors secondary to the expansion in technology, many of these behaviors are reinforced by the system. Nurses in intensive care units have been paid higher salaries, have been told that they are the "best nurses", and have been encouraged to consider themselves equal partners of the team. However, the team's function is to diagnose, cure, or arrest a medical problem. Such reinforcement encourages nurses to discount their intuitive knowledge, and in some cases their professional education and socialization. Since it is possible to get their own needs met by working closely with physicians and/or managing the technical aspects of care, these nurses often support these system forces.*

To further compound the problem, many nurses who are person-oriented and try to give compassionate care have been told that they are "too involved", "unable to behave professionally," or "don't have time" to give such care. Such forces within the system reinforce disease-oriented care. They also create restraining forces for those nurses who want to transcend the system and provide person-centered care, and for others who are trying to build cohesion among nurses. Since these reinforcements generally come from system members who have the greatest power, nurses affected directly often have difficulty if they do not support these views.

System structure. *The structure of the system is another major restraining force for communal, compassionate care. While I can't address all the issues, there are few that must be considered. First, health care financing by third party payers has focused on care of the disease. While it is not essential for care providers to address only the disease aspect of the problem, it is difficult for them to provide holistic, person-centered care. For example, nurses are often not provided time to practice holistic care because the system is structured around the care of the disease process. Patient classifications are generally based on pathology, not holistic needs. Even nursing diagnoses often reflect this orientation. Thus, budgets are most often determined based on medical diagnoses and the related pathology.*

Power bases. *Another major factor that relates to system structure is the power base attributed to medicine by administrators, consumers, and the law. Most agency administrators still perceive the physician as the primary power-base and decision-maker. The related legal and ethical questions are enormous. While I don't want to elaborate on this point, it must be considered as a restraining force in the system. Since power is generally attributed by others based on their perceptions of one's ability to influence, the perceptions of administrators are very important to Nursing.*

Nursing education as a factor. *Finally, we must recognize that the different levels of Nursing education create confusion in the suprasystem, and within the Nursing subsystem. Confusion creates a restraining force since it interferes with nurses building a cohesive base with common goals. Consumers and interdisciplinary colleagues have difficulty understanding our goals. Their confusion is reinforced by the large number of nurses who are unable themselves to explain the role of Nursing or describe the phenomenon of Nursing care. The greatest problem is that nurses themselves often have difficulty supporting one another. Instead, nurses often look to other system members to offer and receive support, thus building power bases in subsystems other than Nursing. Over the last few days this issue has been raised repeatedly. I think that the real question of support emerges when nurses attempt to be* *different or take an advocacy role. It is at this time that they are often not supported by colleagues.*

Philosophical perspectives of nurses. *There are many nurses who have not taken the time to examine and clarify their own philosophical beliefs about the nature of man or the goals of Nursing. In some cases, this state of affairs does not influence their care-giving; in others, it does. While some of these nurses believe that Nursing is a profession of compassionate caring, they have not clarified their own values or explored the written philosophy of Nursing, so they aren't able to articulate how these values are related to compassionate, person-centered care. Thus, while it is contradictory to their intuitive nature, these nurses often succumb to the pressures of the system. Sometimes they "burn out" and leave Nursing since they are in constant conflict between what they feel and what they do.*

There are other nurses who philosophically disagree with the notion of "compassionate, person-centered care." They tend to have a different perspective about the nature of mankind and the role of nurses in helping people. Sometimes these nurses personalize client behavior, thus perceiving anger (for example) as being directed toward them, rather than as an expression of unmet needs. These nurses do not believe that compassionate care will alter untoward behavior from clients and are therefore, not inclined to change their views or support changes.

Definition of Nursing. *Nurses do not seem to share a common definition for the profession. While the ANA Social Policy Statement (1980) defines Nursing as the diagnosing and treating of human responses to actual or potential health problems (not the problems themselves), many nurses have failed to operationalize their care in this respect. Instead, many continue to focus on pathology and associated phenomena. Paradoxically, many of these nurses argue that they have operationalized the ANA Social Policy Statement. However, when analyzed, they have only done this in terms of human responses related to pathological processes, rather than holistic responses that relate to the multi-system, spiritual human being. Without a common definition of Nursing, we have difficulty developing a common language. Without a common language, we cannot achieve cohesion, a prerequisite to building a strong power base.*

Deficit-love motivation. *Nurses who function from a deficit-love motivation base constitute another restraining force for change toward a more holistic, compassionate model. While these individuals might be interested in increasing cohesion among nurses, their aim is to increase the power base for nurses in order to benefit the nurses, not the clients. That is, their goal is need-satisfaction for themselves, not their clients.*

Since growth of the client is not a motivating force, it is, therefore, not very satisfying to provide care that has as its focus, the growth and well being of their clients. Generally, nurses who are motivated by deficit-love do not have the resources needed to reach out and provide care without an expectation of a return. They themselves are frozen spiritually.

Reactive nurses. *The last restraining force I'd like to address I've labeled as reactive nurses. There are many people who tend to respond to change reactively rather than proactively. Since these individuals perceive change as threatening, people often describe them as negative. They tend to support system stability and therefore, do not support movements that will change the system. This attitude differs from those who attempt to proactively change the system.*

Since most nurses are women, and women have generally been socialized to be submissive rather than assertive, proactivity creates cognitive dissonance in many. This dissonance, in itself, creates a restraining force for change in a system that is hierarchically ordered.

Previously, I discussed a number of factors that create either driving or restraining forces for healthcare reform. Now, I hope to address these issues within the context of the questions posed in the introduction.

1. Why are nurses so reluctant to avoid involvement with patients relative to the spiritual/religious dimension?

First, we need to address the language, spiritual/religious dimension. While many might view these words as interchangeable, from my perspective, they are not. I perceive the spiritual dimension to be a dimension of the human being, connected to one's inner Self, one's inner knowing. One's Self is the core or essence of who we are; it is what connects us to a higher power which is usually defined as God by most of us here today. Religion, on the other hand, is a set of symbols, traditions, practices, and beliefs that vary by culture, and are designed to help us get in touch with our spiritual self, and although very different at face value, often lead to the same outcome, but not always. Since most religious practices are impacted by how they are interpreted by the practitioners, they can serve either as a driving force or restraining force for humans seeking higher understanding of self, spirit, and God. However, for the purpose of this discussion, I will address this question as though the two words were synonymous, each referring to that dimension of the human being that connects us with our soul and an understanding of our life purpose. Given this delineation of these two words, spiritual and religious, let's return to the question at large: Why are nurses so reluctant to avoid involvement with patients relative to their spiritual dimension?

Let's first consider the nursing process, what nurses are taught to "think", and how they are socialized to process information. Many nurses are not educated to listen to their client's perspective, to understand what they are hearing, to interpret and analyze these concepts within the context of a holistic theory base. Many nurses perceive spiritual needs as something that should be attended to by other professionals (such as chaplains); others believe that a person's spiritual needs are not relevant to the immediate problem. These nurses fail to understand that spiritual needs are linked to the core or the essence of the human being—that they are prerequisite to fulfilling any other needs.

Coupled with this state of affairs is the fact that many nurses continue to treat people from a wholistic rather than a holistic perspective. Wholism, where the whole is equal to the sum of the parts, allows the nurse to reduce the individual to a biophysical subsystem. This differs markedly from the holism perspective where the whole is greater than the sum of the parts. When nurses practice from a holistic perspective, they must consider all aspects of the individual, with a primary consideration for the client's view of the relationships among the parts.

While some nurses respond to their clients intuitively, without a cognitive understanding of the holistic relationships among the phenomena of the individual's perspective of his/her basic need deficits and potential for attaining holistic health, these nurses tend to discount the subjective aspect of clients' statements. Instead, they focus on the physical needs that can be concretely observed.

This state of affairs is compounded by the multiple restraining forces within the system, such as negative reinforcement for compassionate care and positive reinforcement for technological expertise. The situation is further aggravated by the number of nurses who are unclear about their own professional beliefs, the role of professional nurses, the profession's goals, and/or are motivated by Deficit-love. Clearly, nurses cannot repeatedly reach out with compassion when they themselves experience need deficits. This is particularly true when nurses are not positively reinforced by colleagues for their efforts, creating yet another restraining force.

Two final thoughts regarding these issues: First, nurses who have not explored their own belief system often get confused about the difference between helping people live a quality life (until the last breath is taken) and helping people overcome a disease or stay alive as long as possible. Without a clear understanding of the difference between these two, nurses tend to feel helpless and sometimes hopeless when they are unable to see satisfying results from their efforts. The major problem in this case is that these nurses are looking for the wrong results. They seek evidence of curing or controlling the disease or pathology rather than evidence of holistic wellness and spiritual well-being.

The last issue to consider as we try to understand why nurses have difficulty relating to clients relative to their spiritual need concerns the nurses' ability to find appropriate mentors. Many beginning nurses are at the age and stage in life where they are trying to sort out their own role in society, without consideration of their professional role. As these young nurses enter systems, they seek mentors to help them adjust to the system and system demands. If nurse leaders are lacking in the system, these nurses naturally seek other mentors. They naturally link with those who have attributed power. Associative power becomes extremely important at this point in one's career path. Thus, young nurses seeking assistance in the system-entry process and in the related socialization processes seek out those who they perceive have the power base. These nurses learn from their mentors and over time, many adopt their ways of thinking, doing, and being. Mentors who are reactive and/or disease-oriented teach inexperienced nurses about the "real world." Soon, the mentees are the mentors, and the cycle repeats itself. The system perpetuates itself and maintains stability.

2. What can we do, as nurses, that would assist us in fostering a communal and compassionate approach in the provision of direct patient care?

If we are to foster a model of communal, compassionate provision of care, several things need to happen. I am sure there are other ways to approach this problem as well, but for the sake of brevity, I intend to address only a few. You will note that in all cases, I am talking about building a stronger power base for such a model of care. In some cases this can be done best by enhancing driving forces and in others, by addressing restraining forces. In the latter case, counter-forces are discussed that would offset or neutralize the restraining forces.

First, we (nurses) need to believe that we can achieve this goal. Such an attitude will be necessary if we are to be able to contend with restraining forces in the system and to mobilize the resources within ourselves, the system, and the environment that are needed to induce change. Coupled with this attitude, nurses need to sincerely believe that

Nursing is a unique, autonomous profession, and that nurses contribute significantly to the health care of society. We not only need to believe this, but also learn how to act as though we believe it. Thus, we need to learn how to believe in ourselves, to unfold, and to know that when we reach out and touch others, we are making connections that create driving forces. We need to act on this knowledge, become more politically involved and provide leadership for professional and consumer groups. But first, we must begin with ourselves, taking the time to know who we are; we cannot reach out, transcend restraining forces, and connect with others without an understanding of our own self.

If we are to transcend the current system, we must each clarify our own beliefs about humanity, our own philosophy of Nursing, and come to an internal understanding of how these two relate. Without this process, nurses have difficulty sorting through their feelings and thoughts. They experience discrepancies in the system and misunderstand the issues related to the driving and restraining forces [described above]. *Inherent in this discussion is the underlying issue of acceptance of the definition of our profession, i.e., ANA's definition of Nursing. It is essential that nurses not only clarify their own beliefs, but that they think about them within the context of ANA's definition of Nursing. Unless we do this, we will have difficulty building a cohesive group—a prerequisite for building a power base.*

We need to continue building a common language. We do this as we build our knowledge base, or our discipline. A common language is a prerequisite for building cohesion and power. It helps us define and explain what compassionate care is and predict what value it has for the total well-being of our clients. We need to learn how to label and articulate what we know intuitively, to find a way to explain and describe the essence of holism. As we build a common language, we will acquire additional power in the system. Power is necessary if we are to bring about change.

Collegial support is also essential. Cohesion can only be accomplished if, and when, we can learn how to support one another, and provide a safe environment for those who reach out, take risks, and try to achieve the desired goals. Such a state would mean that nurses would be reinforced for compassionate, professional, autonomous caring by other nurses. Without such support, nurses will tend to continue to seek reinforcement from members of other subsystems within the parameters of the larger suprasystem. When this happens, nurses are often reinforced by actions and thoughts that are related not to the profession of Nursing, but to the goals of another professional group.

Nurses will have to be willing to take risks, to be different, to aim toward goals that are different from those desired by members of Nursing, and to challenge the apparent goals of the suprasystem—goals which are usually set by the subsystem that holds the majority of the power base.

Unfortunately, nurses will never be able to be risk-takers unless they have the support from their colleagues. Such support includes reinforcement for diversity. Thus, nurses will need to use reward power, not coercive power, to reinforce the risk-takers. The risk-takers will need expert power, associative power, and legitimate power bases as they function within the suprasystem.

Up to this point, I've talked about strategies aimed specifically at nurses, for nurses. However, the nursing process is an interpersonal relationship between nurse and client. So, it is important to discuss the nursing process as it relates to what nurses need to do to foster change in the healthcare system with a purposeful movement toward compassionate care. Specifically, nurses need to learn how to address the needs of the client from the client's worldview. This means that nurses need to learn how to collect data, interpret it, analyze it, make diagnoses, plan and implement care—all based on the client's worldview. Stated in another way, the nursing process needs to be implemented with the client's worldview as the focus of care rather than what the nurse does as the focus of care. Such purposeful implementation of the nursing process requires that nurses use a theory base to guide their data collection and interpretation, and purposeful planning of care.

Modeling and Role-Modeling (MRM) is an example of such a theory (Erickson, Tomlin, Swain, 1983/2009). According to this theory, Modeling requires that the nurse enter the client's world in order to understand his/her needs, from his/her perspective. Simultaneously, the nurse must keep one foot in the theory of MRM in order to interpret these needs. Role-Modeling requires the planning of purposeful, health-directed, client-centered interventions that will facilitate holistic growth, health, and wellness. It must be noted that within this context, the primary source of information is the client; the secondary source is the family coupled with the nurse's observations. The tertiary source includes data collected from all other sources, including medical information. It should also be noted that health is a holistic state, not a physical state. That is, health is a state of physical, mental, and social well-being, not merely the absence of disease (WHO, 1947).

Nurses who use MRM discover that their referent power base has shifted. They are more interested in the view of the client and their families and less concerned with the views of members of other subsystems. I, personally, believe that nurses who make such a shift would soon discover that they have also acquired power, power attributed to them by the consumers and other members of the suprasystem interested in person-centered, humanizing care.

3. What would be the political impact of nurses' communal and compassionate response in administering direct patient care? In other words, what kind of changes might result for patients, family members, professional peers, and administration if nurses were to respond in this manner?

The last question I am to address has to do with the political impact such changes might produce. My final comments relate to this question. From my view, if nurses could overcome the restraining forces and build on the driving forces, we would see the desired changes in the healthcare system. First, we would see nurses who truly enjoy nursing. They would be spiritually and emotionally fulfilled. In addition, we would see care that is person-centered, holistic, health- and growth-directed as opposed to the fragmented, disease-oriented care currently provided by many health care personnel. This type of care would alter the power bases in the suprasystem; clients would become referent power bases for nurses, and nurses would take on new importance for consumers both within the system and within the environment. Rather than medicine being the most powerful subsystem, I believe that the consumer would achieve this status. I also believe that the consumer, currently kept outside the boundaries of the suprasystem, would penetrate the boundaries, providing even more reinforcement for system change.

We would see consumers and nurses taking more proactive roles in determining the structure of care, the type of care provided, the settings for care, and even the financing of care. There would be a greater emphasis on and investment in helping those who have been unable to demand care, such as the young, old, handicapped, and poor. More emphasis would be placed on providing primary and tertiary care to individuals, families, and groups. There would also be an increase in the care given outside agencies, but within the community. Nurses and social workers would become the primary contact for health care and would ultimately serve as triage consultants.

Compassionately administered care that is holistic, health- and growth-directed could result in individuals acquiring higher levels of development. If this happens, we could have a society constituted of more self-actualized people. Maslow has described these people as seeking love and well-being for their fellow man, promoting peace and justice for mankind, and therefore, increasing the quality of life for all. Conceptually, one could follow with an argument that as members of society grow and achieve higher levels of development and become more self-actualized, there would be a decrease in abuse within families.

Finally, I would like to propose that these changes might very well impact international affairs. If nurses could overcome barriers of the systems in the United States and provide more compassionate care, it is very possible that they would provide leadership for nurses in other countries. If this is possible, it is also possible that the potential effects described above would be seen internationally. It is clearly possible for nurses to assume such communal, proactive roles if they recognize and accept their own potential as change agents. If they do, they have the potential to initiate change that will produce a new international structure, promote peace, and enhance health and well-being for mankind in general. [Table 1.5 lists the potential impact of a communal, compassionate model of Nursing care.]

Table 1.5 Potential impact of a communal, compassionate model of Nursing care.

Person-centered, holistic nursing care;
Proactive nurses and consumers;
Shift in power bases in healthcare system, with client as the focus of care;
Changes in nature of health care delivery;
Increased health/well-being of society;
Potential for international influence.

Conclusions

Today, I've tried to describe selected factors in the healthcare suprasystem that impact the nature of its dynamics. I've talked about the interactions among the multiple systems embedded in the suprasystem, driving and restraining forces that influence the dynamics, and I've briefly discussed how some of these relate to the practice of Nursing. Now, I'd like to invite you to join me in my quest of impacting the type of care our clients can expect. Together, we can carve out tomorrow. We don't have to go to Africa or join the picket line, but we do need to learn how to both like and love our selves. When we do this, we will be better able to reach out to our fellowman, whether at home, the bedside, or even in an adverse environment. We have to take risks, practice and learn. If we can do that, we will soon discover the joy of communal, compassionate client care.

REVISITING THE PAST

What Goes Around, Comes Around

More From the Past

About the same time that I presented this paper I also wrote two other articles. The first I sent to Dimensions of Critical Care Nursing (Erickson, 1985). In that paper I proposed that the (then) new PPS model for health care would mandate that nurses be more efficient and more effective. I elaborated on the problems nurses faced that were related to the PPS model that cut back on hospital-stay, etc. And then I argued that nurses who practiced purposefully and systematically within the context of a holistic, health-oriented nursing theory base could prompt shorter hospital stay and decrease readmissions–two of the reasons for escalating health care costs. The editor of DCCN decided that the topic was important, but didn't want to publish the entire paper. As a result, what was printed was an overview of the paper, written as though the editor had interviewed me.[4]

The second article I mentioned above never made it off my desk. Although I thought it was important, the editors I contacted didn't. This paper addressed the importance of proactivity given the environmental climate of the 1980s. I focused on the influence nurses could have on the system if they took a holistic stance and discussed the difference between proactive and reactive nurses.[5] Today, we have a clear split in paradigms; nurses are divided between two worldviews. This issue will be discussed thoroughly in the next chapter.

I mention these unpublished papers from the past because the issues discussed in both are still relevant. Today, we are challenged more than ever to be efficient and proactive. To do this, I think we need to think about our beliefs, how we came to know what we know, and what is important for our practice. If we can ever find a way to be clear about our views, articulate them, and become proactive, we will be like the awakened sleeping bear.

Opportunities Today

Although a split in paradigms could have been predicted 25-30 years ago, little has been done to deal with the fallout. That is, Nursing hasn't discussed the

[4] For readers interested in this paper, it is reproduced in Appendix A.
[5] For readers interested in this paper, it can be found in Appendix B.

implications for the profession. Nevertheless, the American Nurses Association (ANA) recognized Holistic Nursing as a specialty in 2006 (AHNA, 2007). Recognition of a model or paradigm of care as a specialty implies that other models exist. If Nursing wishes to harness its potential power bases to effect change in the healthcare system at large, it is essential that we discuss our split in paradigms. We have to discuss how we wish to recognize diversity in the profession, the implications for the advancement of our discipline and practice models, and the impact on healthcare in general. Unless we discuss our status quo, our situation may seem so obvious that it will never be considered important. Instead, articulated power bases (such as medicine and funding agencies) will continue to impact the healthcare system, unfettered and unchecked.

I fully recognize that the discussion presented above is an over simplification of the situation, both then and now. If I were to be inclusive, there are many other factors that would need to be considered. Yet, I also know that we nurses have great potential; we can create a great power base if we simplify our orientation and focus on what we, as nurses, can do to bring about change. I am comfortable with this approach since I know that small changes in one system can affect changes in another—that a ripple-out effect can occur, and with time and consistency we can make a difference. Thus, this book focuses entirely on Nursing defined within the Holistic Paradigm with a focus on the use of Modeling and Role-Modeling as the theory base in many of the chapters.

As stated in the Introduction, this book was written to empower nurses in leadership roles with a focus on those who wish to practice from a holistic perspective, particularly those who use the Modeling and Role-Modeling theory to advance the discipline and profession of Nursing. Our goal is to offer you stimulation of thought, specific ideas, and a way of thinking that might help you as you take the lead in carving out the future of Nursing. As you can see from this 1984 presentation, the ideas raised in this book are not necessarily new ones. Yet, they are pertinent for today's reader. Healthcare is a greater, more powerful suprasystem than ever before. According to national statistics (Young & Olsen, 2009), about 6% of the national budget was dedicated to healthcare in the 1980s; today it is at least 17% of the national budget. However, we still don't have a healthcare model that is concerned with the health, growth, and well-being of all our citizens.

We can't take on the entire healthcare system, but we can explore ways to "walk the talk" and influence changes in our own system; and we can be proactive. Since Holistic Nurses talk about compassionate care, I started Section 1 with this challenge from the past, hoping to put the same questions that were put to me in 1984 out to you for your consideration. The interface between these questions from the past and those I proposed in the introduction of this book are shown in Table 1.6. As you consider them, you might note that there is little difference in the underlying issues in both sets of questions. What goes around comes around until it is addressed. Maybe the issues will be addressed a little differently each time, but still, the issues are the same. I wonder, are we ready for them this time around?

Table 1.6 Rhetorical questions from the past and today.

Questions from the Past	Questions Today
1. Nurses spend a great deal of time in direct contact with patients and witness patient's struggle to come to grips with their illness, suffering, and for some, their impending death. All these factors are highly charged with spiritual/religious meaning. Why is it that nurses are so reluctant or avoid involvements with patients, relative this dimension?	1. How do we advance the discipline of Nursing so that we can close the gap between knowledge and practice?
2. What can we do, as nurses that would assist us in fostering a communal and compassionate approach in the provision of direct patient care?	2. How do we best prepare novices of our profession so that they are not only competent, ethical practitioners, but also assertive, altruistic members of the profession, able to utilize Nursing's knowledge base?
3. What would be the political impact of nurses' communal and compassionate response in administering direct patient care? In other words, what kind of changes might result for patients, family members, professional peers, and administration if nurses were to respond in this manner?	3. What stands in our way of explicating the specific, unique role of Nurses?

SUMMARY

This chapter raised several questions about our healthcare system. A paper presented in 1984 served as a jump off point to discuss factors that influence our ability to move toward a more humanistic, person-centered model for Nursing. The indirectly stated argument was that nurses need to adopt a holistic paradigm of care if they wish to influence changes in a healthcare system that is focused on the health and well-being of the person rather than on disease, sickness and treatment. The arguments were based on our earlier discussion that there are two models of care, depending on whether one views the person as wholistic or holistic (Erickson, et al., 1983/2009, pp. 44-46)—two different paradigms, two different ways of viewing human nature.

Since our view of the world determines what we think about, how we interpret what we observe, what we call it, the value we place on it, and so forth, it is important for each one of us to assess our own view of the world before we proceed to discuss issues related to advancing the discipline of our profession. Chapter Two discusses factors that influenced Nursing's philosophical split and the two paradigms that resulted. My aim is to provide a brief overview of our professional history and to lay the background for you to explore the ontological nature of what you know to be true.

CHAPTER 2

PARADIGM CHOICES: IMPLICATIONS FOR NURSING KNOWLEDGE

Helen L. Erickson

The discipline of Nursing will advance as nurse scientists seek to understand the relations among the art of Nursing, relevant scientific findings, and observed outcomes of care. But first, it is important to consider how one's philosophy interfaces with the discipline. A nurse's philosophy influences how the art is practiced, concepts studied, methodologies used, data analyzed, and findings interpreted. In short, our philosophy motivates our behaviors. Therefore, it is imperative that nurses be able to articulate their own beliefs, so they can describe clearly who they are, why they act as they do, what outcomes they anticipate, and their potential power bases.

OVERVIEW

In the previous chapter I proposed that: healthcare is a dynamic suprasystem which creates a context or environment; interactions among the multiple systems within the suprasystem are continuous and ongoing; Nursing is one of the many systems which exists in that environment; changes in Nursing have the potential to bring about change in other systems in the environment, and, ultimately, change the suprasystem. I described the driving and restraining forces of the 1980s that had the potential to produce such changes, and finally, argued that we cannot hope to change the suprasystem, but we must understand that even as we take proactive positions in our own system, we have the potential to generate a ripple out effect, stimulating change in one system at a time and ultimately, affecting the larger suprasystem.

The ontological perspectives of nurses were identified as key factors throughout the discussion. While all nurses support the idea that the profession is focused on *person-centered care*, how individual nurses define person-centered care differs; it differs based on what they *believe* to be true, and therefore, how they carry out their role(s) in health care.

Since the 1950s, nurses have struggled to articulate Nursing's unique role in society. Recently, the American Nurses Association (ANA) revised the Scope of Nursing and said, "Nursing is a learned profession built upon *a core body of knowledge* reflective of its dual components of *science and art*" (ANA, 2004, p.10). An earlier document by ANA (2003) indicated that the *science of nursing* is based on "a critical thinking framework, known as the nursing process, composed of assessment, diagnosis, outcomes, identification, planning, implementation and evaluation" (pp.11-12), while the *art of nursing* is "based on a framework of caring and respect for human dignity" (p.12). ANA also stated that Nurses integrate "objective data with knowledge gained from an appreciation of the patient's subjective experience" (ANA, 2003, cited in ANA, 2004).

These statements indicate that nursing actions are based on a body of knowledge systematically applied with the nursing process and enhanced with the art of nursing. They also imply that the art of nursing is either a *set of beliefs that guide the caring-healing processes,* or it is the *artistic application of the nursing process*.

In either case, it seems clear that the nursing process, a scientific process for problem-solving, is based in a unique body of knowledge *that includes the art of nursing.* Nevertheless, confusion regarding what nurses do that differentiates them from other professionals persists, creating problems as nurses try to articulate and validate Nursing's unique role in society.

We think this situation exists because nurses are split in what they believe to be the core of Nursing. That is, nurses are split in their philosophical views about the essence of Nursing, what nurses do, nursing outcomes, and even, what nurses should study. As a result, although Nursing has struggled to link research and practice to create a sound discipline for the profession, the gap between research and practice only widens with time. Part of the problem is that some think that research is all there is to Nursing's knowledge base.

This chapter picks up on this issue of *ontology*. I start with a brief background to the problem and conclude with the premise that nurses are divided along two views or paradigms. Since this book is written for those interested in the holistic paradigm, I admit bias toward that perspective. It discusses how social changes have influenced our evolution as a profession—*an evolution that created a dichotomy in belief systems* among nurses. It also proposes that since this dichotomy is not often addressed, it has caused confusion about Nursing's role in society.

BACKGROUND

The Knowledge-Practice Link

Comforting, the Core of Nursing

As recently as the 1950s, nursing practice was considered an art. The focus of nursing practice was the *unique application* of skills and techniques, *artistically* designed to comfort patients, help them recover from sickness, heal and get well, and stay well. Information acquired from basic and behavioral sciences[1] helped nurses to make clinical decisions, but it was not considered the *core of nursing*. Instead, a *philosophy of person-centered caring* was taught as the *essence of nursing*. The sciences were taught as one way of knowing about the persons whom nurses served. Skills and techniques were also considered knowledge important to acquire, but most important was Nursing's philosophy *about the person and about the unique role of the nurse.* The *expertise* of nurses was evaluated by their artistic ability to *use* acquired knowledge to help their patients be comfortable, attain the best possible condition to heal and get well, and stay well. They were expected to do this within the philosophical beliefs of Nursing as described by nurse leaders starting with Nightingale (1915), and including Henderson (1960) and others.

Case studies, published in The *American Journal of Nursing*, described essential information about patients and their support systems, their life situations, and how the nurse cared for them. Skills and techniques were not usually mentioned; instead, the nurse's *artistic approach to individualized care of the person* was emphasized. These case studies served as exemplars of excellent nursing and were used to clarify the differences between Nursing and other professional groups. There was no gap between what was taught as Nursing and what was practiced. Nurses were clear about their roles and their service to society.

> At one time, the art of nursing, embedded in a philosophy of caring for the person, was the essence of Nursing. Expert nurses knew how to comfort patients and facilitate healing. This *knowing* set them apart from other professionals. *Nursing's role in society was clear.*

The Knowledge-Practice Gap

Emergence of A Disease-Orientation

The first issue of *Nursing Research* was published in 1952 (ANA, 2004, p. 7). Concurrently, the focus of nursing began to shift from care *for the person* to care *for the person's problems.* During the 1960s and early 1970s—the era of "information explosion"—modern technology and changes in society ushered in a wave of new science. Nurse leaders (Abdellah, 1957; Fry, 1953; McCain, 1965; Orlando, 1961) argued that we must become more systematic in our approach and

[1] For example, I (H. Erickson) studied chemistry, biochemistry, anatomy, physiology, microbiology, psychology, sociology, and other sciences in 1954-55; yet, it was clear to me that these courses provided information to help me better understand the holistic person, not just to understand how a physiological or psychological subsystem worked.

develop a *science* base unique to Nursing—a *science* that would guide the practice of Nursing.

Nurses refocused their care from the *person* to the *person's problems.* A medical model clinical assessment was adopted with emphasis placed on the pathology, systems, diseases and conditions. The patient's perceptions were considered subjective, unreliable data. Objective data were primarily those acquired by understanding diseases and disease processes learned by studying the basic sciences. The *art of nursing*, now considered unscientific, was relegated to the past. Most of the skills and techniques previously taught (such as PM care to help the client be comfortable, get sleep) were no longer considered important. They were traded for the *nursing process*, which became the *way of doing nursing*. Initially, the nursing process was considered to be the scientific[2] process. Later, however, it was recognized as a systematic, problem-solving approach that helped us *use science* (Rogers, 1983).

Nursing was no longer described as the caring of human beings, but refocused onto the medical problems presented by patients, the geographical setting of practice, or the population served. Medical-surgical nurses, community health nurses, pediatric nurses, diabetic nurses, cardiac nurses and other disease- or population-related types of nurses emerged. While many of these nurses continued to practice person-centered care, it was no longer recognized as the focus of nursing. The emphasis was on the *science of nursing,* not on the person who received the care.

Since the art of nursing was put aside, and no longer considered important, the philosophy of Nursing, too, slipped into the background. Sciences that explained disease processes took the forefront. When this happened, philosophy, skills and techniques previously taught as comfort measures were also abandoned. *Case studies* evolved into *care studies*[3]*;* the focus of professional practice shifted from *caring for the person* to *nursing interventions* designed to resolve problems.

An Academic Shift

A gap between Nursing education and Nursing practice emerged. Educators taught the basic and behavioral sciences as the core of Nursing's knowledge, and then taught students how to apply the science to the care of the person's problems. The art of nursing (and often the history of Nursing) that focused on the comfort of the person was no longer taught in schools. Simple

---

[2] It should be noted that the ANA definition of science still includes the nursing process (2008).

[3] Today we use the words "care and caring" to imply a focus on the person, rather than the interventions. We owe our thanks to J. Watson (1979) for this change. Nevertheless, when the language changed from case studies to care studies, the emphasis switched from the person to what was been done "for" the person, i.e. the nursing interventions.

comfort measures such as back rubs, a.m., p.m. and H.S care, soft touch, gentle voices, management of external stimuli, etc., were lost in many of the new curricula. The *nursing process,* considered a scientific approach that mandated critical thinking, was implemented across nursing settings. Nevertheless, many nurses continued to practice what they believed to be *true nursing; they continued to focus on the person, addressed comfort needs and aimed to facilitate healing.* However, they rarely discussed what they practiced and almost never charted these *actions which were usually based on their philosophy. Instead, they charted their observations as they monitored the identified medical problems.*

Many nurse leaders recognized that Nursing's unique role in society was no longer obvious, and that there was a growing gap between what was taught and what was practiced. They argued that nurses needed a conceptual framework to guide their practice, so they could clearly articulate what they were thinking, explain their decisions and actions, and predict outcomes. Yura and Torres (1975), working with the National League of Nursing, compiled curricula offered by Schools of Nursing to find common threads across the programs. They identified four major constructs that seemed to provide a base of reference for all Nursing programs. They included: Person, Health, Nurse and Environment. These constructs, linked together, became known as Nursing's Metaparadigm.

The Nursing Metaparadigm emerged as the conceptual framework for Nursing and was followed by Nursing theories. The theorists intended to clarify and articulate the major constructs embedded in the Metaparadigm. Soon it became clear, however, that Nursing theories seemed to create more confusion. As nurse theorists clarified their view of Nursing, the solution became part of the problem. As the focus of Nursing became clearer, the philosophical division among nurses grew. There seemed to be a split in how nurse theorists viewed the nature of Nursing, nursing actions, and Nursing science. This split was reflected in the clinical setting, research arena, and wherever Nursing existed.

> Nursing theories emerged as a way to articulate the uniqueness of Nursing and to specify the nature of Nursing knowledge. This was followed by a proliferation of research and knowledge dissemination through journals and educational programs. But Nursing theories seemed to split along two lines.

Science as a Solution

Nurse leaders recognized the need to rectify this debate in philosophy. In 1980, ANA published the first Social Policy Statement in an effort to clarify the role of Nursing. This document stated that nurses focus on the *human responses* to actual or potential health problems, *not the problems* themselves. While the attempt was to refocus Nursing onto the person, this description fell short as it failed to state that the *person, including his human responses to actual or potential health problems, was the focus of Nursing. Instead, it was left open to interpretation, depending on the nurse's personal philosophy.*

The schism among nurses continued to grow and with it a gap between education and practice surfaced. To solve the problem, academic nurses called for more research—research that would focus on nursing actions and, thereby, resolve questions about the nature of Nursing and provide the knowledge needed to practice nursing.

Research *is* Science

The National Center for Nursing Research (NCNR[4]) was established in 1986 to help nurses achieve this goal. Since then, millions of dollars have been spent on Nursing research; numerous Nursing journals reporting research findings have emerged; and thousands of students have graduated from research-oriented institutions. Yet, a recent IOM study (2001) indicated that the gap between Nursing knowledge and practice continues to grow. The science derived from extensive research has not produced the body of knowledge needed for the systematic practice of Nursing.

To compound the problem, although *science* is a *systematically organized body of knowledge about a specific subject,* the words *science* and *research* became synonymous. By the late 1980s, the only accepted way to *build* science was through the *research process*. This meant that other types of knowledge were less important. Knowledge acquired from practice was considered subjective until systematically researched.

Received or Perceived View: Which One?

Since most of the funded research was aimed at studying disease, disease processes and pathology, the accepted view of science was the *received view*. Nursing, still not clear about its focus of care or its role(s) in society, adopted this *positivistic view* of science, *which soon became* the mainstream model for knowledge-building in Nursing.

While most nurse leaders agreed that we needed to build a unique knowledge base, many disagreed with the *focus on disease* and the *received view of science* as the best way to do it. Some argued that nursing is contextual and that Nursing research needed alternative approaches to building knowledge; they argued for the *perceived view of science* or the post-modernistic orientation.

Supporters of the *received* view of science believe that research should be objective and detached from the process and findings, use deductive thinking processes, make predictions and control variables. They believe in results that can

---

[4] NCNR became NINR in 1993. That is, the center was advanced to a full-fledged institute of NIH in 1993.

be generalized. Supporters of the *perceived* view of science believe that research is both subjective and objective and that the researcher contributes to the process and findings. They use retroductive thinking processes, look for trends and patterns, believe in the holistic model of mankind, and seek understandings of the human experience.

Recently, Nursing adopted "evidence-based-nursing" (EBN) as the optimal solution for linking knowledge and practice. Evidence-Based-Nursing is the process by which nurses make clinical decisions using the best available research evidence, their clinical expertise and patient preferences (McKibbon, 1998). Today, nurse leaders offer conferences designed around EBN, with many arguing that this is the future of Nursing.

The Schism Grows

One would think that a movement toward evidence-based practice would strengthen the link between Nursing science and practice; instead, the gap continues to grow. Despite extensive efforts to improve research utilization and promote evidence-based practice, the gap has widened (IOM, 2001). One reason for this state of affairs is that research findings often fail to provide clear directives for nursing care (Leeman, Jackson & Sandelowski, 2006; McCaughan, Thompson, Cullum, Sheldon, & Thompson, 2002; McClearly & Brown, 2003). As a result, they have little meaning for clinical nurses who need to make expedient and proficient decisions. Consequently, they are more likely to act from knowledge drawn from experience or from their personal knowing.

To compound the situation, nurses who focus on the well-being of the patient (rather than the efficacy of their interventions), often create conflicts with colleagues—conflicts difficult for them to resolve. They believe that nursing is the comforting and caring of people, that the art of nursing is important, and that facilitating growth and healing are the goals of nursing care. Yet, often they are neither supported for these views nor rewarded for actions based on them. Instead, they are strongly urged (and sometimes told) to focus on the efficacy of interventions that address disease-oriented problems.

The schism among nurses continues to grow and with it debates have flourished. Nurse researchers debated the merits of the *received versus perceived views of science*, and nurse clinicians debated the merits of *task-focused nursing versus person-centered nursing.* While at first glance, it seemed that the debates varied by Nursing role (i.e. clinicians versus researchers), upon closer assessment it is clear that their differences are philosophical. Both, the clinician debates and the researcher debates are based on basic beliefs about the nature of Nursing and the kind of knowledge needed to practice Nursing. Nursing still has not resolved the basic questions: What *is* Nursing? What do nurses focus on? Until we understand that the answers to these questions depend on our philosophical view, we will have difficulty linking research findings and clinical practice.

> No matter how much research we do, and no matter how many times we revise our approach, we still seem to have trouble establishing and defining clear linkages among theory, research and practice—linkages that all nurses accept. It seems that the real issue is a disagreement about the focus of Nursing. Is it the person or the problem?

DELIMITING NURSING

The Metaparadigm

Today, we have a Metaparadigm accepted by most nurses that clarifies what Nursing is about. According to Fawcett, a metaparadigm is "the most global perspective of a discipline acting as an encapsulating unit or framework within which the more restricted structures develop" (1984/1995, p. 64). While there is general agreement that Nursing's Metaparadigm consists of four major constructs: *Nursing*, *Health*, *Person* and *Environment* (Fawcett, /19841995; McKenna, 1997; Yura & Torres, 1975), there are some who disagree. For example, some think that the inclusion of *Nursing* in Nursing's Metaparadigm is redundant, and that it can be exchanged for *Caring* (Leininger (1978), cited in Huch, 1995). We might argue, however, that such an exchange eliminates differentiation among professional groups. That is, other professional groups also embrace Caring as a major construct which defines their actions. Therefore, we conclude that Nursing (as a construct) is needed in the metaparadigm in order to differentiate the concept of *caring in Nursing* from caring in other disciplines.

Social Justice

Others (Schim, Benkert, Bell, Walker, & Danford, 2007) argue that a fifth construct, *Social Justice*, should be added. ANA supports this view (2003) by stating that "Nursing addresses the organizational, social, economic, legal and political factors within the healthcare system and society" (p.6). Therefore, we contend that the Nursing Metaparadigm contains five key constructs: *Nursing*, *Health*, *Person*, *Environment* and *Social Justice* (see Figure 2.1).

> The primary constructs in Nursing's Metaparadigm are Nursing, Health, Person, and Environment. Social Justice is an optional fifth construct.

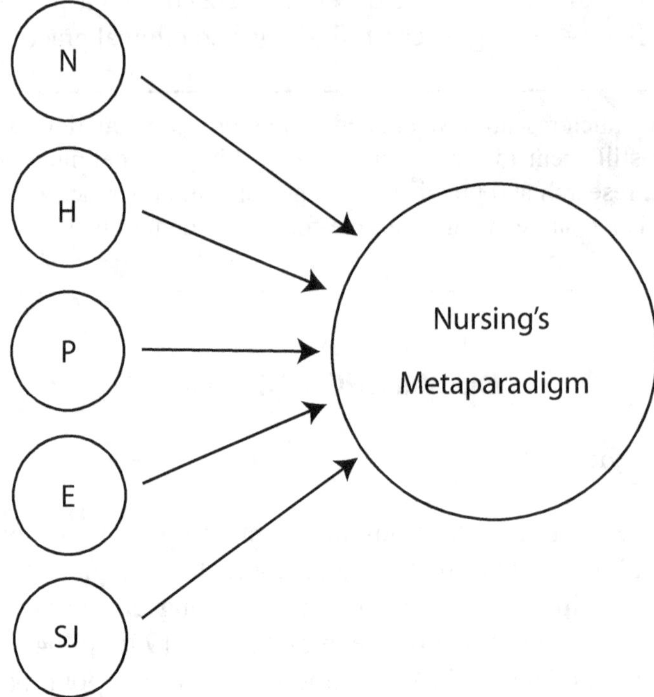

Figure 2.1 Relations among constructs of Nursing and Nursing's Metaparadigm.

These constructs set parameters or delimit the boundaries for the discipline of the profession of Nursing. They provide a structure for understanding the type of knowledge needed to guide the profession. That is, as large complex ideas, these constructs frame the discipline of Nursing. They serve to organize concepts in some meaningful way which provides a direction for our thinking processes.

But constructs do not distinguish Nursing from other disciplines. We have to *identify the concepts that create the constructs* before we can distinguish differences among professional groups. Furthermore, we have to understand the phenomena of the concepts before we can clearly articulate the essence of Nursing. That is, constructs are abstract, grand ideas while concepts are more specific parts or aspects of the idea. The phenomena delineate the specific dimensions of the concept. Concepts create constructs and the constructs create the Metaparadigm. Figure 2.2 provides an example of how these relate to create one of the constructs in the Metaparadigm, Nursing. The phenomena are important because they specify the essence of Nursing—that is, the phenomena *explicate the content of Nursing knowledge.*

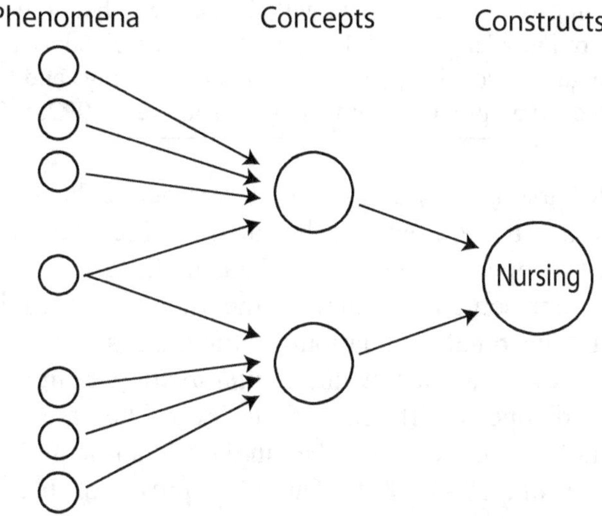

Figure 2.2 Relations among phenomena, concepts and constructs of Nursing. Reprinted with permission from Erickson, H. (1985), *Synthesizing Clinical Experiences.* Ann Arbor, MI: The University of Michigan Medical Center, Biomedical Communications.

> While our Metaparadigm helps us understand *what Nursing is,* it doesn't help us understand *what it is not.* Nevertheless, we can use the metaparadigm to identify and explore the knowledge needed to more explicitly articulate what Nursing is and what it is not.

Two Paradigms Emerge

The services of any profession are guided by a set of beliefs (i.e. a philosophy) that influence what is deemed important "knowledge and actions" for the members. Since nurses agree that our Metaparadigm explicates the constructs important for our profession, we might think that all nurses share common beliefs, act similarly, and carry out professional activities in comparable ways. Yet, we know this is not true. We know that thoughts and actions are influenced by the individual person's beliefs. As a result, although Nursing is a legitimate profession, sanctioned by society, mandated by law or practice acts consistent with the beliefs, guidelines, and framework of the Nursing profession, the actions and thought processes of individual nurses are greatly influenced by what that nurse perceives important, how he/she views the world and articulates nursing care.

Silva (1999) says a philosophy is concerned with the nature of being, the nature of reality and the limits of knowledge. A philosophy is also perceived as a "statement of beliefs and values about the world, a perspective on human beings and their world and an approach to the development of knowledge". (Fawcett, 1992, p.68)

According to Parse (1987) and Cody (1995) nurses have split along two points of view. That is, although Nursing has a single Metaparadigm that guides all of Nursing, how we operationalize our Metaparadigm varies. We have two paradigms[5] that are represented in Nursing theories, practiced in the clinical arena, and used as a conceptual foundation in Nursing research. These disparate paradigms were labeled as the *Totality* and *Simultaneity* paradigms by Parse and Cody. They represent distinctly different world-views. They are very comparable to the wholistic and holistic models described in the Modeling and Role-Modeling paradigm (Erickson, et al., 1983/2009). Table 2.1 provides an overview of the differences between these two models.

The Totality paradigm views the person as a wholistic being, composed of multiple systems that work together to create a whole. Within this paradigm, nursing can occur in an acontextual environment. On the other hand, the Simultaneity paradigm sees the person as a holistic being, composed of multiple interacting subsystems that have dynamic feedback loops. Nursing always occurs within a context, one that includes the immediate and more distant environment.

Wholistic nurses often define their role in terms of *what* they nurse, e.g. cardiac nurse, telemetry nurse, diabetic nurse, etc., while holistic nurses define their role in terms of *who* they nurse, e.g., Mr. Smith, Ms. Jane, Sally, etc.

These divergent life-views result in different practice foci, practice actions, and practice outcomes. Failure to be clear about our own philosophy results in ambiguous practice decisions, research designs, data interpretations, and clinical practice. This is because our view of the world, what we believe what we hold to be "true" about human life, impacts the meaning we give to phenomena, events, and life experiences. These beliefs impact how we practice Nursing and what type of knowledge we deem important for our practice.

Parse's paradigm model is similar to the MRM (Erickson, et al., 1983/2009, pp. 40-46) argument that nurses hold two world-views of mankind. The first view is that people are wholistic beings with multiple parts; nurses attend to the appropriate parts. The second view is that people are holistic beings, composed of multiple interacting subsystems that create a unit greater than the parts; holistic nurses facilitate growth and healing in the human as an indivisible entity.

[5] A paradigm is a pattern, model or organizing framework.

Table 2.1 Overview of the Wholistic and Holistic models.

	Wholistic (Totality)	**Holistic (Simultaneity)**
Metaparadigm		
Nursing	Can be contextual; evidence-based practice with consideration of patient preference; patients are often passive recipients of care; focus is on objective data; efficacy of interventions is important; personal knowing is unimportant; role defined by condition or system; nurse aims to maintain separateness of patient and nurse.	Is always contextual; reflective practice with emphasis on client perceptions; clients are always active participants in care; client's self-knowledge is primary; individualized, quality care is emphasized; personal knowing is essential; role defined in terms of relationship with client; nurse aims to build energetic field of interconnectedness between nurse and client.
Health	Clinical definition including absence or control of disease; ability to perform ADL.	Adaptive and eudemonistic definition; health is a degree of well-being and self-actualization.
Environment	Can be delineated, controlled, separated from human being.	Man and environment are in continuous, dynamic, interaction.
Person	The person is wholistic, composed of multiple dimensions that can be reduced to the parts; the whole is the sum of the parts.	The person is holistic, composed of multiple interactive dimensions so interconnected they cannot be separated out; the whole is greater than the sum of the parts.
Scientific process	Positivistic, received view; critical thinking; controlled, randomized studies with focus on efficacy.	Post-modernistic and/or neo-modernistic, perceived view; interpretive thinking with meta-narrative; qualitative studies; sometimes triangulation; subjective understanding of interaction between beliefs and scientific process.

Professional Implications

Although Nursing has a Metaparadigm that sets the parameters or boundaries of professional Nursing, an individual nurse's personal world-view will determine how phenomena are interpreted and translated within the

Metaparadigm (see Figure 2.3 below). This, in turn, affects how researchers and clinicians determine what is "true," what warrants attention and what does not. For example, J. Smith's (1981) content analysis of the literature showed that there are four different meanings attached to the word *health.* Accordingly, *health* can be: a lack of a disease; one's ability to perform daily-life activities; the process of adapting to stress; or a high-level of well-being. The meaning given to a concept will determine how it is operationalized and applied in research and practice. For instance, researchers who view *health* as a lack of disease will most likely find ways to study *health* from a disease orientation. They might look for instruments which assess compliance to a medical regime, changes in biochemistry parameters, symptoms of the disease, and so forth.

Parse and Cody described the Totality paradigm as a *received view* of knowledge building. As stated above, the person is seen as an organism whose nature is a composite of biophysical, psychological, social, emotional, and spiritual dimensions. In comparison, the *perceived view* of the Simultaneity paradigm holds that the person is a holistic human being with multiple inextricably interactive dimensions that cannot be broken down into parts.

While two separate researchers might study the same concept, how they might define it, operationalize it, and even measure it differs based on their world-view. Take, for instance, the concept *quality of care*. The Institute of Medicine (IOM) defines quality of care as "the degree to which health services for individuals and populations increase the likelihood of desired health outcomes and are consistent with current professional knowledge" (Gebbie, Rosenstock, & Hernandez, (Eds.) 2003, p. 23). From this definition you might think that the options for studying this construct are minimal, but in reality the differences are significant.

From the *received* (Wholistic or Totality) perspective, *quality of care* usually refers to outcomes of the nursing process, often evaluated in terms of the healthcare system's expected outcomes, like increased compliance, decreased hospital days, number of nosocomial infections, etc. While the context of the care provided might be considered when evaluating quality of care from a received perspective, it isn't always; nor is it deemed important. Usually, the outcomes are evaluated objectively—the whole can be reduced to its parts. What is important is the *efficacy* of the interventions designed to affect quality of care. From this view, the nursing process is based on science, is objective, and often acontextual.

In comparison, concepts viewed from the *perceived* (Holistic or Simultaneity) perspective are evaluated within the *context* of the individual's perception of an experience. From this view, the nursing process is a dynamic, ongoing, interpersonal and interactive relationship between nurse and client,[6] so

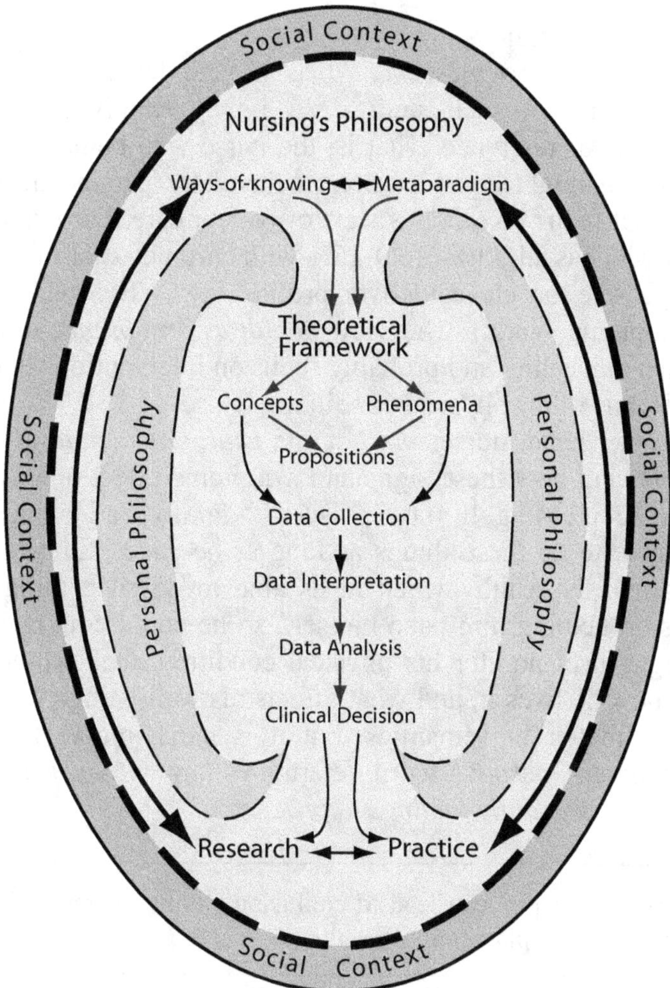

Figure 2.3 Relations among Nursing's philosophy, metaparadigm, ways-of-knowing, the nurses' philosophy and practice/research choices.

that *quality of care* incorporates the client's satisfaction with the process, the nurse's perception of her/his role in the process, as well as the role of other healthcare providers. From this philosophical view (i.e. the Simultaneity Paradigm), quality of care might better be thought of as *quality care, caring,* or even *facilitating healing*. Each of these exists within a context and is measured

[6] The nurse-client relationship is often independent of a doctor-patient relationship (Erickson, et al., 1983/2009, pp. 18-22, pp.103-115). Furthermore, the nursing process is built upon a trusting, functional relationship (Erickson, et al., 1983/2009 pp. 169-171).

accordingly. That is, outcome variables might be need satisfaction, loss resolution, perceived control, sense of well-being, and so forth.

Data Interpretation

Research-users who view *health* as a high level of well-being might disregard the findings of such studies since they simply don't apply to the practitioner's frame of reference. That is, the nurse who believes that *health* is a sense of well-being might consider the biochemistry parameters as part of the overall picture, but focus on other aspects of patient care. For example, we know an elderly man who has a LVEF of 20-25% with chronic atrial fibrillation, a pace-maker to compensate, an elevated liver profile, low WBC, and other abnormal biophysical symptoms. Nurses who view *health as an absence of disease* would consider this man unhealthy and probably focus on interventions that would slow-down further decline of his physical condition.

On the other hand, nurses who define *health as a state of well-being* are interested in knowing how these signs and symptoms affect quality of life. They might learn that he likes to golf, travel, visit with family, and be physically active, and that he is able to do these things as long as he paces himself. These nurses might say this man is healthy when he is able to do such things; they would probably focus on helping him pace himself, so he could continue to enjoy life. While they might also monitor his physical condition, they would focus on his quality of life, how he lives it, and what affects his well-being. We could say that this is merely a matter of semantics, but it is much more. The meaning we attribute to any given *operative* word determines how we *operationalize it, how we study it, and how we apply findings to practice.*

> An inarticulate philosophy can lead to confusion among operational definitions, research designs, and explanation of results.

The work by Ryan and Lauver (2002) further helps clarify this issue. They argued that tailored interventions (TIs) should produce better outcomes than standardized treatments (STs). To test this hypothesis, they undertook a secondary analysis of 20 studies to test the *efficacy*[7] of nursing interventions customized to match specific characteristics of the subjects. Their findings showed that TIs *were more effective* than STs, but in only half of the studies.

I think that Ryan and Lauver's interest in testing the *efficacy* of an intervention indicates that they held the *received or positivist* philosophy of science. At the same time, their interest in nursing interventions *customized to*

[7] Testing the efficacy of a nursing intervention indicates a *received view* and the *Totality Paradigm.*

match characteristics of subjects indicates that their view of the human being is more consistent with the *perceived* view of science.

Nevertheless, they did not distinguish the studies based on the received and perceived views of science, the way TIs were operationalized, or discuss their findings from these two different scientific philosophies. While they reported that TIs "were more effective than were STs in promoting health behavior outcomes in 50% of studies reviewed" (p. 335*), they did not attempt to explain why only 50% of the studies showed these relationships*. Instead, unable to speculate or explain why the findings did not hold up across the studies, they proposed that more studies needed to be done to determine whether "TIs *are or are not* efficacious" (p. 337), a positivist's view.

Had these researchers been more aware of the philosophical underpinnings of their research methods and the way the concepts were operationalized, they might have been able to think about their own design differently, and they might have been able to explain their findings more thoroughly. For example, they might have looked more carefully at the concept of Tailored Interventions to determine if there were differences in the outcomes when TI's were operationalized to mean patient *preference among limited choices* or patient *perceptions of the choices.* In the first situation (i.e. limited choices), it is possible that clients who are offered *limited choices* among a group of options *might perceive* that they are offered a choice among a set of interventions with *no good option; that they have to choose among several undesired interventions. If they had explored this more thoroughly, they would have had data to determine their subjects perceptions of the choices.*

It is possible that many researchers would interpret their data quite differently if they had been more aware of their own philosophy of science, beliefs about human beings and the nature of Nursing. They might also make different recommendations for future research and/or practice.

An example is provided in the discussion of a report written by Sidani, Doran, and Mitchell (2004). According to them, "a comprehensive and realistic evaluation of the quality of nursing care is critical for depicting nursing contributions to desired patient outcomes" (p. 64). These authors go on to describe factors that need to be considered when evaluating studies. They are:

•Attend to factors that affect the delivery of care and the outcomes expected;

•Identify aspects or processes of care believed to produce the expected outcomes;

•Select outcomes that are sensitive to nursing care;

•Measure the outcomes upon entry into and at exit from a care episode; and

•Delineate the relationships among the factors, processes, and outcomes to explain what contributes to the achievement of favorable outcomes (p. 64).

Although these authors write primarily from a *received view* and suggest that there are *cause* and *effect* relationships, they also demonstrate awareness that not everything is so simple—not everything important in Nursing can be broken down into its parts. For example, their conclusion that nurses need to *identify aspects or processes of care believed to produce the expected outcomes*, suggests that they recognize that nurses need to find ways to purposefully study both *processes* and *outcomes* although processes might best be studied using the perceived view of science and outcomes the received view. Furthermore, until the processes are understood, there is no way to comprehend the outcomes since one precedes the other! The implications for the advancement of Nursing knowledge are significant (Dickoff, James, & Widenback, 1968)[8].

Maybe the problem is that we are looking in the wrong direction. We tend to focus on the *application of science,* so we can provide more *efficient care.* Maybe we should refocus and explore *the science of the art of nursing so we can learn what facilitates healing and growth.*

> We need to explore the nature of the art of nursing. When we do that, we will discover what facilitates healing and growth.

IMPLICATIONS FOR THE ADVANCEMENT OF THE DISCIPLINE

Today, most nurses accept the notion that the health of the profession depends on the advancement of knowledge needed to guide the profession. This means that research is needed to better understand what nurses do, why they do it, and the significance of these actions. Research studies are usually designed within the context of the received or perceived view of science. However, not all researchers think through their own beliefs before conceptualizing their studies. Since the received view is more dominant in society (and Nursing) and the perceived view is often considered as "soft science" or "unscientific", some who believe in the Simultaneity paradigm of Nursing and mankind, use positivistic

[8] Readers might enjoy revisiting the work of Dickoff and James who argued that knowledge building requires four stages of research activities: identifying the phenomena, relating the phenomena, predicting outcomes and prescribing (interventions that will affect outcomes). Each stage requires unique methods aimed at answering the question.

methods (i.e. methods consistent with the received view of science) rather than methods that are more appropriate for their questions and belief systems.

This problem can't be resolved by using a Nursing theory unless the philosophical underpinnings of the theory are consistent with the nurse's belief system and the selected research methods. Researchers often borrow theories that are inconsistent with their own beliefs, their research question, and/or the methods used rather than exploring their own beliefs and seeking a theory consistent with their life-views and then designing a study philosophically consistent with their beliefs. The obvious outcome of this state of affairs is that they have difficulty interpreting their findings, and correspondingly, difficulty in linking research findings to theory and practice.

> Currently there are two views of science. Each is built on a specific philosophy of knowledge building. In our attempt to build knowledge, we have often overlooked basic philosophical questions such as: *What do we believe to be true about mankind and nursing? How does this impact our view of the essence of Nursing? How do our beliefs affect our practice, scientific processes, teaching, evaluations, and other roles we assume as professional nurses?*

Evidence-Based Nursing will not solve this problem until researchers and clinicians learn to articulate their beliefs upfront and explain how these influence their decisions. Until the philosophical beliefs of the researchers are consistent with those of the clinicians, it is unlikely that clinicians will attend to the research reports. Instead, they will continue to practice based on their own belief systems rather than steeping their clinical decisions in science.

For example, one nurse who worked in the Cardiac ICU said that she always kept track of her clients' oxygen saturation levels, but often chose to let a client rest rather than reposition (as indicated by research) even when the levels were down a "bit, sometimes even below 90%". She stated that she believed that rest was important in recovery and healing, and that sometimes the way the person "looked" was a more important indicator of his overall well-being than the monitor reading.[9]

> Sometimes we overlook the long-range effects of caring (designed to promote healing in the holistic person) for the immediate effects of interventions designed to deal with a part of the human being.

---

[9] This same nurse said she always tried to ask clients or their families if there was a favorite position, something that was comfortable, etc. before surgery, so she could model their world as much as possible.

Simply stated, the "evidence" (or knowledge) that clinicians use must be consistent with what they believe to be true before they will use it to *direct* their practice. The same is true for Nursing theories. If the philosophical underpinnings are not consistent with the clinicians' way of thinking about nursing and mankind, they are unlikely to adopt the theory as a guide for their practice.

This is also true for researchers. Unless they have considered how their own philosophical beliefs relate to a particular view of science and paradigm of Nursing, they will have trouble with designing studies, data analysis and data interpretations. While there *can be* inconsistencies in philosophical views of science and research methods, unless these inconsistencies are *articulated and critiqued*, researchers will often experience conflicts in designing research programs and pursuing knowledge important to Nursing. Clinicians have the same problem. Without a clear understanding of the linkages among personal philosophy, research and practice, and the importance of articulating and critiquing these beliefs, they will have trouble defining the uniqueness of Nursing, nursing practice activities, and nursing goals.

> Nurses need to learn to be comfortable with their beliefs and to articulate them clearly. They also need to recognize that there are two equally acceptable ways to view Nursing, and that each has implications for choice of theory to drive nursing decisions both in the clinical and academic arenas.

SUMMARY

Nurses recognize the importance of developing knowledge that articulates the nature of Nursing. Unfortunately, in our efforts to be more *scientific,* we have lost a clear understanding of what constitutes our uniqueness. Currently, nurses are split in their beliefs. Two paradigms of Nursing have emerged, and with it, two ways of thinking about research and two ways of thinking about practice. While it is possible that the two paradigms might be able to coexist, it is imperative that nurses learn to articulate their own beliefs and analyze how they interface with Nursing's axioms, their own practice and research activities. Until this happens, we will continue to have difficulty describing the nature of Nursing, nursing actions, and articulating the knowledge needed to advance the profession.

This is particularly important for nurse leaders who have the responsibility of preparing and guiding the next generation of nurses. Unless faculty are clear about their own beliefs and how they interface with the curriculum they develop and teach, they will have difficulty explaining how their personal philosophy guides their thought processes, evaluation of peers and students, their research, and so forth. Simply stated, our philosophy affects our thoughts and actions, our behaviors, and our outcomes.

The next chapter addresses Nursing's discipline, how it has evolved, and the roots of our epistemology. A matrix model links the Metaparadigm of Nursing with our patterns of knowing. Carper's Ways-of-Knowing serve as a starting point.

CHAPTER 3

WAYS-OF-KNOWING AND THE METAPARADIGM

Helen L. Erickson and Margaret E. Erickson

A discipline is a field of knowledge unique to a professional group.
(Loscin & Purnell, 2009, p. 9)

OVERVIEW

Nurses have confused the relationship between ontology and epistemology for ages. Educators rarely articulate their personal beliefs. Instead, they adopt the broad Metaparadigm as a framework, develop curricula around Carper's ways-of-knowing, and then independent of one another, develop course work that lacks internal consistency. Unless Nursing students are encouraged to articulate their own views to determine how they relate to their own practice, they will be confused about the relationship between philosophy and knowledge. As a result, they often abandon what they have learned and adopt alternative models of care, frequently losing sight of what makes Nursing a unique profession.

In this chapter we propose that nurses need to clarify the linkages between their philosophy and choice of knowledge and discuss linkages between knowing and knowledge. We think that the interface between philosophy and Nursing's ways-of-knowing help clarify these linkages. After a discussion of the various ways-of-knowing currently described in the literature, we propose a matrix model which links Nursing's Metaparadigm to its ways-of-knowing. It also provides a model for educators, so they can think about the type of knowledge needed to prepare professional nurses. Finally, two additional versions of the Metaparadigm and Ways-of-Knowing (MWK) Matrix Model are offered as illustrations of the variance that exists when alternative paradigms are purposefully selected.

BACKGROUND

The Context-Discipline Connection

Nursing, a person-centered, practice profession, is defined by its *Metaparadigm,* and differentiated from other professional groups by its *discipline* or *knowledge base*. Our Metaparadigm creates a context for our practice, and our discipline serves as a structure for purposeful practice. Our philosophy guides us in defining and delimiting both. The combination of philosophy, Metaparadigm, and discipline offers us a *way to think about who we are and what we do* as members of an autonomous profession. Together, their interaction defines the essence of the profession.

Since both our philosophy and our discipline have been part of our vernacular for years, one would think that philosophy, knowledge and practice would be seamless. Faculty could teach Nursing students how to think about Nursing and its context, and how to purposefully apply its knowledge base. Students would be able to transfer what they had learned to their clinical practice post-graduation. Yet, what nurses learn in their academic programs is not always what they practice in clinical settings.

Dissonance, An Ontological Issue

There are many reasons for this disconnect between what nurses learn and what they do. In the previous chapter we discussed the split in paradigms. Because faculty don't usually clarify their own beliefs, they aren't always clear about how they should operationalize their school's mission. That is, they don't always agree on what knowledge is needed, what outcomes should be expected, or what actions are uniquely Nursing.

This situation occurs even though the Metaparadigm serves as the context for educational programs, and Carper's Ways-of-Knowing have been accepted as patterns of knowing important to Nursing. In other words, most Nursing faculty agree that the practice of Nursing is person-centered and is defined by the Metaparadigm constructs: nursing, health, person, and environment. Most also agree that the knowledge upon which practice is based includes the empirics, esthetics, ethics, and personal patterns of knowing (Carper, 1978). Yet, there is disagreement about specific concepts and the content that is necessary to prepare nurses, so they are able to practice professionally. We think this is due to the educators' lack of clarity about their own philosophy which results in confusion when faculty select concepts and content that comprise the discipline of Nursing.

Most educators would agree that nurses need basic and behavioral sciences as a foundation, yet there is disagreement about the application of this information. Some argue that the practice of Nursing is concerned with the health and *well-being* of clients, while others argue that it is concerned with their clients' *health care problems*. The first emphasizes an understanding of what is normal, what interferes with normal processes, and, when interference occurs, what will help people restore health and well-being. The latter emphasizes pathology, what causes it, and what can be done to remediate pathological processes. While both views have merit, how nurses perceive the unique role of Nursing in society will determine what needs to be taught to students, and how students will be socialized to perform as professionals.

This problem is amplified when students discover that what they are learning is inconsistent with what they believe to be true about human nature, science, and their role in society. To compound the problem, since most programs don't encourage students to inductively articulate their own beliefs, they often confuse knowledge with belief systems. Such dissonance results in a disconnect between what is learned and what is valued. Rather than a seamless transfer of philosophy, knowledge and practice, they often adopt a patchwork model of knowledge, and practice without articulating the relationship between their choices and their belief systems.

> How nurses articulate their beliefs about the essence of Nursing determines what concepts, content and skills they think are important in the practice of the profession. If faculty members are not clear about their own beliefs, they have difficulty articulating the paradigm they adhere to and the implications for educational programs they design. As a result, students often experience educational programs that are inarticulate, leaving them to pick and choose what fits their beliefs and their views of what Nursing is and what nurses do.

Earlier we stated that the essence of Nursing is defined by *its Metaparadigm* and differentiated from other professional groups by its *discipline*. The previous chapter was dedicated to the philosophy of Nursing, its Metaparadigm, and two differing views of Nursing's philosophy. This chapter is dedicated to a discussion of Nursing's discipline with consideration of the interaction among Nursing's Metaparadigm and Ways-of-Knowing. We start with a brief, historical background, aiming to identify a few factors that have changed how we think about our profession.

An Evolution

What Nurses Do

Although society has always needed someone to care for those who are sick, ill or unable to care for themselves, *Nursing* was not identified as a unique profession until Nightingale's seminal work, *Notes on Nursing* (1859). Her work specified *what Nursing is* and *what it is not.* She stipulated that Nursing has a unique role, includes specific actions, and is based in knowledge. Accordingly, Nursing is based on the laws of health and healing, and its role is to "put the patient in the best condition for nature to act upon him" (p. 28) through actions that facilitate the health and well-being of the individual.

> Nightingale's book, *Notes on Nursing* (1859) served four purposes: it transformed Nursing from a job to a profession, clarified what Nursing is, specified what nurses do, and identified the knowledge base necessary for practice.

Later, Henderson (1961) built on Nightingale's description of Nursing when she stated that the nurse's responsibility is to assist "the individual, sick or well, in the performance of those activities contributing to health or its recovery (or a peaceful death) that he would perform unaided if he had the necessary strength, will or knowledge" (p. 6).

Both nurse leaders are clear that Nursing, a practice profession, is based in a relationship between nurse and client, and that the role of the nurse is to promote a sense of human dignity and well-being with the aim of facilitating healing, in life and death. Implicitly, both argue that nurses enact these roles, directed by a discipline which includes a *set of behaviors, skills, and ethics*. Also implicit is the understanding that Nursing's philosophy sets the parameters for these activities. It dictates how the "laws of health and healing" should be interpreted and applied—laws that contain the knowledge nurses need to practice professionally.

If we were to extrapolate from this, it would seem that educators, expert in Nursing's discipline, would be able to teach their students how to understand and use such *laws.* The discipline of health and healing would pass on and be built upon from generation to generation. But we know that it isn't that simple. Instead, by 1981 Smith had identified four models of health (shown in Table 3.1), each with unique implications for the type of knowledge needed to practice. Clearly, there isn't a single set of laws of health and healing that guide what nurses do.

Table 3.1 Smith's models of health (Smith, 1981)

Orientation	**Implications**
Clinical	Health is defined by the absence or control of an illness, sickness, or disease.
Functional	Health is defined by the individual's ability to carry out roles deemed important to society
Adaptive	Health is defined by the individual's ability to cope with stress.
Eudemonistic	Health is defined by the individual's quality of life and sense of well-being in spite of an illness, sickness, or disease.

Perhaps this is partially due to the shift in thinking. While Nightingale, Henderson and other nurse leaders of the past emphasized the art of Nursing and thinking about *what we do*, more recent leaders have emphasized the science of Nursing and thinking about *what we think* and about what we know.

> Both Nightingale and Henderson emphasized the person as the focus of care and described the role of the nurse as a facilitator of the human's natural ability to heal itself. While today's nurses might accept that our practice is person-centered, and that the laws of health and healing serve as a determinate for the knowledge needed to provide such care, our individual definition of health determines the knowledge we attend to, the value we place on it, the outcomes we expect, the research projects we design, etc.

What Nurses Think

Our shift from the *skills inherent in the art of Nursing* to the data derived from the scientific process swung the focus of Nursing *from what nurses do* to help people mobilize the natural resources needed to recover and heal, *to how nurses think about* what they are doing. That is, whereas Nightingale and Henderson emphasized that the focus of practice was to facilitate well-being of the client, today, the emphasis is placed on the nurse's thought processes, often identified as "critical thinking." For example, the 2003 American Nurses Association's Social Policy Statement defines Nursing as:

> *...the protection, promotion, and optimization of health and abilities, prevention of illness and injury, alleviation of suffering through the diagnosis and treatment of human response, and advocacy in the care of individuals, families, communities, and populations.* (ANA, p. 6)

This definition emphasizes the nurse's thought processes, not the acts of nursing; it also emphasizes the nurse as the dominant member of the nurse-patient relationship. The inference is that the patient is a passive recipient of what the nurse thinks about and what the nurse does. While earlier nurse leaders emphasized thinking about how to empower the patient, this model emphasizes empowerment of the nurse's thoughts and related actions.

Discrepant Views on Nursing's Role

Role Ambiguity

Through the years, nurse leaders have been clear that Nursing is concerned with the *person*, not the disease. This focus on *care of the person* distinguishes Nursing from other disciplines, no matter whether the care is provided to an individual, a family, community, or even to populations of people. Yet, there still seems to be confusion about the *unique role of Nursing*. Hamric and Hanson (2003) discussed the future of advanced practice Nursing, arguing that the service provided by advanced practice nurses doesn't clearly delineate nurses from other health care professionals. They stated that we have two alternatives to remedy the situation. Either

> *advanced practice nursing fades as a definable level of practice and merges into 'mid-level provider' status along with physician assistants and others…*[or they] *become preferred providers of care based on the important holistic and family-centered focus that they bring to patient and/or family interactions.* (p.209)

While Hamric and Hanson addressed role ambiguity in advanced practice Nursing, a lack of clarity exists across Nursing. Nurses seem to know that Nursing focuses on the person, not the disease, and that nurses provide care for the person, but they have difficulty articulating the specific role of nurses in society. Is it to empower the person or the nurse?

Is it Nursing—Or Not?

We think this situation exists because nurses are not clear about what nurses *do* that is uniquely Nursing. More specifically, while nurses can usually articulate what Nursing *is,* they often have difficulty distinguishing which *actions* distinguish a professional nurse from other persons who provide health care. Most nurses know that critical thinking is essential for professional groups, but they have difficulty determining what knowledge should be used. For example, many nurses have told us that giving a bed bath is no longer the action of a professional nurse; it is the work of a nurse assistant. These nurses often offer alternatives to nursing actions stating that administration of medications is a more appropriate example since it requires *critical thinking*—a requirement of a professional person.

Our response to this view is to ask why this action isn't more appropriately that of a pharmacist. After all, they are more knowledgeable in the actions and interactions of medications than nurses. Usually, when nurses are asked this question, they respond in two ways. Some respond stating that this is a good point, and that maybe we should relinquish this activity to the pharmacists. Other nurses disagree with those who think that Nursing might relinquish the administration of medications to pharmacists. This second group of nurses argues that medications are often necessary to help the whole person heal and grow. Frequently, they add that only nurses think about the multiple dimensions of the human being, take into consideration how the multiple parts interact with one another, monitor these interactions, and observe their effects on the well-being of the person. This latter group believes that *nursing occurs in a context and that the context determines whether the nurse's actions are uniquely Nursing or not. The the actions are defined, delineated, and operationalized by their world-view; the context is created by what nurses think and believe as they initiate and carry out their work.*

The key point in this discussion is that healthcare providers from various disciplines often carry out similar actions. What distinguishes an action as *a Nursing activity* is the thought process behind the action, not the action itself. For example, a nurse may administer an IV drug and call it a Nursing activity; it must be remembered, however, that many people can do the same thing—even seasoned drug addicts! From the perspective of the holistic paradigm, administration of drugs is a Nursing activity only if it is initiated *for the purpose of facilitating eudemonistic health in the holistic person.*

> Since the actions of professionals are preceded by purposeful thought, we need to be more explicit about what nurses think about. That is, the actions of professionals are based in critical thinking about explicit knowledge. What we think about will determine the knowledge deemed important for practice.

What Nurses Think About

What nurses think about is the best determinate of what nurses will advocate, what they will do, why they will do it, *and what they will use to plan and implement care*. Without coherent thought, actions are erratic, unpredictable, and arbitrary. Without purposeful, coherent thought, the only context for Nursing actions is a philosophical one. With purposeful, coherent thought actions are based on an understanding of succinct patterns of knowledge and the related outcomes. Interventions can be designed that affect and/or effect actions. Key questions are: What *do* nurses think about? What thoughts create a nursing context? Do they think about knowledge or do they think about how they acquired their knowledge? And do they sacrifice the latter for the benefit of claiming a unique base of knowledge?

Laws of Healing

According to Calabria and McCrae (1994), Nightingale provided some direction when she stated that nurses make careful observations to *discover the laws of healing,* so they can determine how much sleep, nourishment, quiet, ventilation, and cleanliness patients need in order to be able to participate in the healing process (p. xvi). Our interpretation of Nightingale's work is that there are ways to observe, to think about what we observe, and to label and articulate what we observe, and that these *ways of thinking* will guide us to understand or obtain knowledge. The implication is that Nursing Knowledge is needed before we can *do nursing.*

Since then, many have indicated what nurses should think about. However, they have shifted the focus from the thinking to the doing. For example, Watson (1979) shifted the emphasis from healing the client to the work of the nurse when she established that *it is the caring actions of the nurse that facilitate healing to occur in the client.* While her work often implies that it is how we think that will determine what we do, the emphasis has focused on the caring aspects of nursing.

Wendy Leebov (2008) provided an example of how this relationship between the nurse's caring actions and the client's healing is important to Nursing. In her article, *Beyond Customer Service*, she states that nurses need to "create truly healing environments for patients, families and caregiver teams" (p. 21) and offers actions that will communicate their intent. They are:

1) Provide care with compassion,
2) Make sure caring comes across (to the clients),
3) Pay quality attention,
4) Reduce patient anxiety, and
5) Indicate that Nursing is a personal calling (not just a job).

The implications are that these *caring actions will create a healing environment* necessary for client-recovery and well-being. They do not state that there needs to be a seamless connection between what we do, what we think, and client outcomes, or that there needs to be a connection between what we know, our thinking processes, and client outcomes.

Today, nurses are concerned with the relationship between nurse and client, often called caring-healing processes. We need to be concerned with how to operationalize this construct, so that our practice is both efficient and effective. We have often sacrificed understanding our ways of thinking (or knowing) to be able to claim that we have a scientific knowledge base for practice. We need to study both, what nurses know (or the knowledge they use), and how they acquire what they know (the thinking process). Without an understanding of how nurses think, we can lose sight of who we are as a professional group, what makes us different from other professionals, and what makes our discipline unique.

DEFINING THE PARAMETERS OF NURSING'S DISCIPLINE

Knowing, Knowledge or Both?

For years nurses have argued that Nursing is an autonomous profession, yet we've had difficulty defining our discipline. We know that a discipline includes knowledge, skills and attitudes and together, they create a knowledge base for Nursing practice. Nonetheless, we still discuss the nature of our discipline. Carper (1978) advanced our discussion when she proposed that Nursing has four ways-of-knowing, labeling them *empirical*, *esthetic*, *ethical*, and *personal knowing*. While nurses often think of these ways-of-knowing as interchangeable with the types of knowledge embedded in Nursing's discipline, there is a difference between knowing and knowledge and both are important to Nursing.

Silva, J. M. Sorrell, and C. D. Sorrell (1995) addressed this problem, stating that Carper's work is shown as end products, while her language, *ways-of-knowing,* suggests a process. Earlier Benoliel (1987) had also addressed this issue with the following:

> *Knowledge consists of concepts, theories, and ideas about an identified area of information, often presented in organized form in textbooks and monographs. Knowing can be viewed as an individual's perceptual awareness of the complexities of a particular situation and draws upon inner knowledge resources that have been garnered through experience in living.* (p. 151)

The problem has not been resolved although many have contributed to the discussion, sometimes expanding the question. For example, in the work edited by Locsin and Purnell (2009) Boykin proposed that our use of the "nursing process" is part of the problem. She argues that the Nursing Process is usually seen as an objective, scientific process used to solve problems. As such, it naturally distances the nurse from the nursed. In the Prologue of their work, Boykin stated,

> *At the heart of a thoughtful practice process of nursing is coming to know persons....Much has been written about knowing in nursing, initially stimulated by Carper's germinal study on fundamental patterns of knowing....Models of care which understand and appreciate that to nurse, the nurse must be fully engaged in the human situation...to nurse, the person(s) nursed must be known.* (pp. xv-xvi)

Boykin went on to say,

> *In this compendium Locsin and Purnell invite the reader to let go of the traditional nursing process as having served and outgrown its purpose, and to embrace a contemporary, substantive process of nursing grounded in knowing persons as participants in their care instead of being objects of our care.* (p. xvi)

The objective of the Locsin and Purnell book is to introduce the reader to philosophical, theoretical and historical perspectives of *knowing*. At the heart of this work is the view that Nursing's discipline should focus on the *persons nursed*, rather than what the nurses do, that nursing care should be aimed at facilitating their well-being, and that *how nurses think about* what they consider to be "knowledge" will impact their outcomes.

Modeling and Role-Modeling and Knowing

This view is consistent with the basic premises of Modeling and Role-Modeling that the primacy of nursing is an interactive, interpersonal, ongoing, cyclic process which starts when the nurse steps into the client's world with the intent of gaining an understanding of the client's world-view. The overarching aim of this interactive process is to nurture and facilitate the client's growth and development; the purpose is to foster eudemonistic health in life and death (Erickson, et al., 1983/2009, pp. 103-222).

Throughout this work, we argued for an alternative to knowing and knowledge, stating that what nurses need to know depends on how they think about human nature, i.e., their view of the nature of mankind. Specifically, we (Erickson, et al., 1983/2009) argued that there are two paradigms nurses use to think about people—that nurses either view humans as holistic or wholistic and these views determine what knowledge is important for the practice of Nursing. (pp. 44-45). We proposed that nurses with a holistic perspective needed knowledge about several concepts including (eudemonistic) health; stress and adaptation; affiliated-individuation; self-care knowledge, resources and actions; unconditional acceptance; nurturance and facilitation. We believed that these concepts interfaced with the larger constructs commonly accepted in the Nursing Metaparadigm. We didn't think that Nursing's problem arose from the Metaparadigm, nor did we argue with Carper's ways-of-knowing. Instead, we argued that the split in paradigms (holism versus wholism) determined what knowledge would be used to operationalize each of the constructs in the Metaparadigm. We, wholeheartedly, believed that basic and behavioral sciences are important since they inform nurses about normal biopsychosocial processes of the human, but how one uses that information varies. That is, *the patterns of knowing vary by paradigm choice* and so does the knowledge derived from knowing and thinking.

> There is a "subtle distinction between *what it means to know, as opposed to what knowing means"*. (Purnell, 2009, p. 7)

Today, we (the authors of this chapter), do not intend to return to the question of what knowledge best serves as core courses for nurses. We agree that basic and behavioral sciences are important core knowledge for Nursing; they teach us about the normal processes of humankind. And since Nursing is based in relationships, the multiple ways-of-knowing are also necessary. That is, relationships are complex, and in order to best understand them so we can be purposeful in our nursing processes, it is important to incorporate many ways-of-knowing. Beyond that, the knowledge needed depends on one's paradigm.

We also think that Carper's Ways-of-Knowing have served Nursing well as a starting point. Her work provides some structure needed to delineate the kind of knowing and knowledge needed to advance our discipline. Without some structure, our thinking can be erratic, unsystematic, and inconclusive. At the same time, we believe that it is time for us to expand, to consider how to incorporate alternative ways-of-knowing proposed by others. Therefore, we support models which help us think about what we know, realizing that models change as we acquire new insights and with the natural evolution brought about by changes in society. But, for the time being, we start where we are, with our ways-of-knowing.

Ways-of-knowing

Since Carper's identification of empirical, esthetic, ethical and personal knowing, additional *patterns* have been proposed: Patricia Munhall's *Unknowing* (1993), Jill White's *Sociopolitical knowing* (1995), and Christopher Johns' *Reflective knowing* (1995; 2004). Also, Richard Cowling (2007) has offered *Consciousness* as yet another way of knowing. This latter suggestion raised a question about the original work of Carper. Since there appears to be confusion between knowing and knowledge, we wondered about the basis of Carper's work. A review indicated that Phenix (1964) served as the foundation for Carper's work, and that Phenix had identified two additional types of knowing: symbolic and synoptic. According to Phenix, the symbolic realm of knowing is used to give meaning to all the other types (e.g. empirical, ethical, esthetic, etc.) of knowing while synoptic knowing integrates all types of knowing. According to Phenix, they serve to bring all types of knowing together, to create a "single, meaningful pattern" (p. 9). According to Purnell:

> *Patterns of symbolic knowing and synoptic knowing in nursing . . . are merely two different expressions of the same knowing, rather like a double helix, between which patterns of knowing such as personal, empiric, aesthetic, ethical, social political and unknowing come into view and reveal their unique characteristics. The fusion of all the patterns of knowing into a single pattern, with meaning grounded in the disciplinary knowledge of nursing is the pattern which we will now call synoptic or integrative knowing in nursing practice.* (2009, pp. 13-14)

This suggests two things: First, integrative knowing is essential for nurses, and second, that Cowling (2007), and Cowling and Repede's work (2008) offer a way to discuss *integrative knowing* within the context of Rogers' (1970) theory of Nursing rather than to offer a new category. This is not to discount this elegant piece of work. Perhaps at a later date, personal insight will enable us to more fully understand this work and recognize that which is not immediately obvious to us at this time.

For the time being, we will continue with our discussion as it relates to holistic nursing, and particularly, to the Modeling and Role-Modeling theory. As such, we will focus on seven ways-of-knowing. Four of these, Empirical, Esthetic, Ethical, and Personal were originally identified by Carper; Sociopolitical was identified by White, Unknowing by Munhall, and Reflective Knowing by Johns. We will also use the language, integrative thinking as a way of incorporating and integrating knowledge derived from the seven Ways-of-Knowing. Each of these seven is discussed briefly below.

Empirical knowing is based on an assumption that what is known is obtainable through the physical senses, i.e., seeing, touching, hearing, tasting, or feeling. It is grounded in scientific theories and expressed as competence in the "scientific process." *Empirical knowledge* consists of information obtained either by direct or indirect observation or measurement. It is verifiable and usually thought of as *the science of Nursing.* Empirical knowing involves the critical thinking required to obtain the knowledge.

Esthetic knowing involves being able to understand a situation, so that the individual is able to creatively draw from personal experience to transform a situation into reality. *Knowledge derived from Esthetic knowing* is subjective, individual, and usually unverifiable. It is often discussed as knowledge related to the *art of Nursing*. It is the *unique application* of skills and techniques *artistically designed* to comfort patients, help them recover from sickness, heal and get well and stay well.

Ethical knowing guides and directs how we do our work and live our lives, moment-to-moment and decision-to-decision. It is based on what we value as important and where we place our priorities. *Ethical knowledge* relates to our moral obligation to society, and tells us what is acceptable behavior in Nursing. Generally speaking, Nursing's Ethical knowledge is articulated in *Nursing's Code of Ethics.*

Personal knowing involves tapping into one's "inner self." It requires opening up to one's self and becoming aware of how our relationships affect us.

> While Carper proposed that Nursing has four *ways-of-knowing*, according to her description, they might be more appropriately called types of knowledge. Yet, we will call them ways-of-knowing because, according to us, how nurses think is as important as what they think about.

Personal knowledge evolves as one becomes increasingly authentic; it is what nurses *know* about themselves. It relates to their inner self, and is individualized. No two people have the same personal knowledge. Personal knowledge may sometimes be known by others, but, in general, it is what we know about ourselves, consciously and subconsciously that no other person knows. Personal knowledge includes likes, dislikes, beliefs, behavioral motivations, and everything that facilitates us to understand who we are as human beings.

Sociopolitical knowing (White, 1995) is closely aligned with ethical knowing, but differs because it is partially based in ethical knowledge. It is the "knowing" that comes from maturity of the profession and society's mandate that nurses become more proactive advocates for the well-being of mankind. ***Sociopolitical knowledge,*** closely aligned with ethical knowledge, tells nurses how and when to act politically.

Unknowing (Munhall, 1993) involves suspension of all that we think or believe to be true about another human being, so we can discover the essence of that person. It involves being open to another, stepping into the "intersubjective space of two people . . . it is the space for human interaction and human understanding to unfold" (Munhall, 2008, p. 156). Unknowing is based in the belief that as human beings it is impossible to know everything about another human—that we can only learn as we step into the intersubjective space of the unknown. Without conscious awareness of *what is not known,* we may overlook important information.

Reflective knowing (Johns, 2004) involves being open to an alternative type of knowing, both subjective and objective. The process of actively using reflective knowing to acquire Reflective Knowledge is called *Reflexivity* (Johns, 1995), and will be discussed in detail in Chapter 14. Building on Huxley's belief that "there is a mind at large that few of us rarely tap into that opens up possibilities for human growth" (Johns, 2007, p. 2) and Shön's work, *The Reflective Practitioner* (1983), Johns proposes that nurses need to pause, reflect on their past experiences, and revisit those times when they seem to be totally connected to another human being. In these moments, we can uncover a new knowing about self in relationship with the client. Johns (2007) states that reflective knowing emphasizes the impact of past experience on the present turning-back on itself, to reflect on the way it has evolved, from past experience. *Reflective knowledge* is the "fusion of sensing, perceiving, intuiting, thinking related to a specific experience" (p. 3). Such knowledge "reflects the contextual…" (p. 4).

We think that nurses discover the essence of their *spiritual being* during moments of reflection; they connect with their Selfs (Erickson, H., 2006, pp. 6-11) at these times. What they learn in these moments of illumination provides the resources needed later as they center themselves and focus their intent (Erickson, H., 2006, pp. 310-312)—prerequisites to creating a healing environment.

> Carper's four Ways-of-Knowing, commonly accepted in Nursing as the basic patterns of knowing, can be enriched with three others: Sociopolitical, Unknowing, and Reflective knowing. Whether or not nurses use alternative patterns of knowledge depends on what information they value. Integrative knowing is the bringing together of multiple ways-of-knowing, integrating and creating new knowledge.

THE METAPARADIGM AND WAYS-OF-KNOWING MATRIX MODEL

Philosophy, Metaparadigm, Knowing and Knowledge

We started this chapter with the following statement:

> *Nursing, a person-centered, practice profession, is defined by its Metaparadigm, and differentiated from other professional groups by its discipline or knowledge base. Our Metaparadigm creates a context for our practice, and our discipline serves as a structure for purposeful practice. Our philosophy guides us in defining and delimiting both. The combination of philosophy, Metaparadigm, and discipline offers us a way to think about who we are and what we do as members of an autonomous profession. Together, their interaction defines the essence of the profession.*

This statement indicates that interactions exist among our philosophy, our Metaparadigm, ways-of-knowing, the knowledge we have acquired, and what we do as nurses. The implications for nurse educators are daunting. We struggle with our responsibilities, not only seeking ways to help students *learn how to understand* these complex aspects of our profession, but also teaching them how to integrate their knowledge.

Through the years, we have accrued considerable experience having merged practice, teaching, and research with our personal lives. We have learned that students learn best when we make complex issues as simple as possible by showing them how the parts interrelate. With that in mind, we developed the Metaparadigm-Ways-of-Knowing Matrix Model, hoping to help readers visualize relations between the ontology and epistemology of Nursing. Initially, we created a model that included the original constructs of the Metaparadigm and Carper's four ways-of-knowing (see Table 3.2), indicating the type of *knowledge nurses use as they study their profession.* It did not delineate specific information, but provided guidelines for conceptual discussions regarding Nursing's Metaparadigm and Nursing's knowledge, and what nurses think about.

Table 3.2 The Metaparadigm and Ways-of-Knowing Matrix Model (MWK Matrix) Reprinted with permission. (Erickson, H., & Erickson, M., 1995).

	Nursing	**Health**	**Environment**	**Person**
Empirical (Science)	Science connects theory, interventions, and outcomes.	Science specifies outcomes within the context of health.	Science addresses the environment as having an impact on Nursing.	Science addresses nursing that is client-directed.
Esthetics (Art)	Nursing philosophy.	Strategies that complement health of the client.	Creating a healing environment with caring strategies.	Client as a member of the nurse-client relationship.
Ethical (Morals)	Self-evaluation of own role in respect to focus and scope of Nursing.	Self-evaluation of role of own practice in health promotion.	Self-evaluation of own role in management of environment.	Self-evaluation of own role in terms of person-centered caring.
Personal	Knowing of self, self-awareness in practice.	Personal philosophy of health.	Self awareness, stress management, ability to use self to manage environment.	Awareness of self as member of nurse-client relationship.

Expanding the MWK Matrix Model

Since we first started using the MWK Matrix Model in 1995, alternative ways-of-knowing have been added to the literature. Table 3.3 provides an example of knowledge that might be deemed important for those who wish to add these *ways-of-knowing* to their framework. Neither Table 3.2 nor Table 3.3 considers the importance of paradigm choice discussed in the previous chapter.

Table 3.3 The Expanded Ways-of-Knowing Matrix Model.

	NURSING	HEALTH	ENVIRONMENT	PERSON	SOCIAL JUSTICE
Empirical knowing					
Esthetical knowing					
Ethical knowing					
Personal knowing					
Sociopolitical knowing					
Reflexivity					
Unknowing					

Table 3.4 An alternative expanded ways-of-knowing matrix model based on philosophical orientation.

	NURSING	HEALTH	ENVIRONMENT	PERSON	SOCIAL JUSTICE
Personal Knowing					
Unknowing					
Esthetical Knowing					
Sociopolitical knowing					
Ethical knowing					
Reflexivity					
Empirical Knowing					

When paradigm choice is taken into consideration, the order in which the ways-of-knowing are presented and the knowledge included in the cells might vary, such as shown in Table 3.4. Table 3.5 (Appendix C) offers a detailed use of the MWK Matrix Model within the context of the Holistic (Simultaneity) paradigm. Table 3.6 (Appendix C) offers an alternative use with MRM added as a theory base. Table 3.7 (Appendix C) offers an example of the MWK Matrix Model used with the Wholistic (Totality) paradigm as a comparison.

INTEGRATIVE KNOWING

Most people would agree that there are constructs common to Nursing and that they comprise Nursing's Metaparadigm. Most would also agree that there are patterns of knowing which link these constructs; patterns that are associated with specific knowledge necessary for professional practice. We have proposed a matrix model that illustrates these linkages. We have included five constructs in the Metaparadigm and seven ways-of-knowing. Assuming that there are specific constructs and ways-of-knowing common to all of Nursing, others using this matrix model might add or subtract from either of these. Some will use knowledge as it is identified in each of the cells; others will combine knowing and knowledge, sometimes confusing the two. Still others will add their own version. And, there will be those who wish to use a Nursing theory. This requires that they go to another level of thinking, i.e. integrative knowing.

Nurse theorists have integrated Nursing's Metaparadigm and Ways-of-Knowing to create new models. Some are based on the Holistic Paradigm and some on the Wholistic Paradigm (Erickson, et al., 1983/2009 pp. 44-6). Of course, when ideas are integrated, new concepts are created. This holds true for Nursing theories. Yet, they are only true to Nursing if they have, as a base, the philosophy and ways-of-knowing common to Nursing at large. Some think that Nursing theories help them to clarify and explicate the type of knowledge included in each of the matrix cells. We agree; specific knowledge helps *specify the phenomena* of caring and healing. Because the matrix model is a product of threading Nursing's Metaparadigm with Ways-of-Knowing, specification by theory can also help explain how these phenomena relate with one another, what might be predicted as outcomes, and even what prescriptions are needed to facilitate outcomes.

There are many extant Nursing theories used today. This chapter is not intended to review them, or to propose that one is better than another· Instead we wish to remind the reader that professionals base their work on an explicit knowledge base acquired through formal and informal means. Integration of our ways-of-knowing creates new understandings. Theories are derived from integrative knowing. But before we think about Nursing theories, we have to think about Nursing. We have to understand the relations between Nursing's philosophy and ways-of-knowing, and only then we can move on to knowledge acquired by integrative thinking.

Some nurses choose to use Nursing theories to focus their work. Nursing theories do not replace Nursing's Metaparadigm or Ways-of-Knowing. Instead, they help nurses to be more purposeful in their observations and actions, and to evaluate their outcomes.

SUMMARY

This chapter addressed issues related to the discipline of Nursing. We stated that the discipline is the knowledge upon which Nursing is based, and that it includes information (i.e. cognitive knowledge), skills and attitudes We also stated that Nursing's philosophy and Nursing's knowledge interface, creating a model that can be used to understand relations among our philosophy (metaparadigm) and our ways-of-knowing. We proposed the Metaparadigm and Ways-of-Knowing Matrix Model (MWK Matrix Model) as a way to structure Nursing's discipline. The cells created in this model can be used to specify the type of knowledge needed to practice professional Nursing.

We suggested that the paradigm choice, as described in the previous chapter, will affect which ways-of-knowing are included in the model and the order in which they are presented. We also stated that the paradigm choice will *affect* the knowledge deemed essential for the professional nurse. Examples are provided for the reader. Finally, we stated that integrative knowing is the assimilation of various Ways-of-Knowing and that integrative knowing has led to Nursing theories.

Since this book is written for nurse leaders and educators interested in the Holistic (i.e. Simultaneity) Paradigm, the following chapter was written to help those responsible for curriculum development and implementation. The first part describes how educators can develop a seamless curriculum for their educational programs. The second part offers an example of the MWK matrix model based on the MRM nursing model. A discussion related to each of the ways-of-knowing is included.

CHAPTER 4

LOOKING TO THE FUTURE: CURRICULUM IMPLICATIONS

Helen L. Erickson

Limited only by the parameters set by the mission and philosophy of the parent institution, faculty members determine the mission and philosophy of their educational programs, the structure of the curriculum, the courses offered, their description, course objectives, content, and placement in the program, but not necessarily how their plans will be implemented. Instead, faculty members who teach the course will determine how they do this and how they socialize their students. Their personal beliefs will have a major effect on what is taught and how it is reinforced.

OVERVIEW

Our Code of Ethics, a "succinct statement of the ethical obligations and duties of every individual who enters the nursing profession [is a] nonnegotiable...expression of nursing's own understanding of its commitment to society" (ANA, 2001, p.5). This code confirms that we are ethically bound to "practice with compassion and respect for the inherent dignity, worth, and uniqueness of every individual" and that "the nurse's primary commitment is to the patient, whether an individual, family, group or community" (p. 4). These are core obligations of all nurses. The responsibilities of faculty go beyond these ethical mandates.

Faculty are also responsible for preparing novices to understand the scope of Nursing, conceptualize key components of the Metaparadigm, articulate the discipline, and practice their profession based on Nursing's Code of Ethics and the Standards of Nursing. Simply stated, they are responsible for preparing novices to *link philosophy, Metaparadigm, and knowledge with practice.*

Stated in another way, educators, responsible for the learning experiences of their students, must prepare their students to jump the gap from learning to thinking (Bruner, 1966). It is not enough for students to acquire knowledge; they must also learn how to *think about* what they know, so they can purposefully and proactively make decisions and provide effective, compassionate and respectful care. When students can close this gap from learning to thinking, they are able to *make the observations needed to discover and test the "laws of healing"* (1915, p. xvi) *as described by Nightingale.* This chapter addresses issues for faculty responsible for developing programs and related curricula that provide learning experiences for their students. The first section describes a number of factors for consideration for those aiming to develop or revise their curricula. It is not intended to provide specific details, but instead, general guidelines for discussion. Table 4.1 can be used to facilitate the reader. The second section of this chapter provides a detailed discussion of the Ways-of-Knowing for those who use Modeling and Role-Modeling as a base for their programs.

Table 4.1 Phases of curriculum development.

PROCESS	**PURPOSE**	**CONSIDERATIONS**
1) Review Nursing documents.	Review Nursing's current literature.	Update faculty orientation to Nursing's philosophy, Scope and Standards of Practice, Code of Ethics, and Social Policy Statement.
2) Review belief system	Identify dominant faculty paradigm.	Determine general orientation of faculty; clarify faculty values.
3) Review institutional Mission and Philosophy.	Clarify the culture of the "parent institution."	The purpose for the existence of the institution; implications for Nursing programs; resolve contradictions.
4) Review and revise Nursing mission and philosophical statements.	Specify the purpose of Nursing programs and their philosophical bases.	Faculty clarification of: •language used in the mission and philosophy statements of the Nursing programs; •latest versions of Nursing's Social Policy Statement and other documents delineating Nursing's role(s) in Society; •paradigm selection by faculty (wholistic versus holistic); •implications; •Necessary and sufficient ways-of-knowing to fulfill program expectations.
5) Write program goals.	Specify the purpose of individual programs included in the curricula.	Clarify and specify: •similarities and differences among programs. •relations of program objectives with Nursing's guidelines.
6) Organize presentation of ways-of-knowing.	Determine order for introducing the ways-of-knowing and related concepts.	•Review relations between ways-of-knowing, Metaparadigm, and paradigm choice. •Determine which way-of-knowing (and related knowledge) serves as a base for other ways-of-knowing.
7) Concept selection.	Identify concepts to be included in each program.	•Clarify how concepts relate to ways-of-knowing; •Use Bloom's Taxonomy (1956) to help "level" presentation of concepts.

> Nurses in authority positions influence others through their actions in the classroom, clinical and research arenas, as well as how they, as individuals and as a group, develop and implement programs. They are ethically responsible for mentoring and socializing novices in the ways of Nursing. This means that they are responsible for mentoring students, helping them acquire the philosophy of Nursing, develop patterns of thinking which incorporate our ways-of-knowing, and identify and learn specific knowledge. Moreover, they have to help them apply all that they have learned.

EDUCATIONAL CONSIDERATIONS

Defining the Context

All Nursing programs exist in a context. Most are part of a larger system or parent institution, established for specific purposes delineated in the Mission statement and clarified with a philosophical statement. The smaller units of the system are expected to help the parent institution carry out its mission in a manner consistent with its philosophy. As a result, faculty members are limited, to some extent, by the mission and philosophy of the parent institution.

Still, educators have considerable freedom to determine what they teach in the classroom and clinical setting. While the parent institution's mission and philosophy *set the parameters* in which faculty members are able to create curriculum, they do not determine what is *designed within those parameters*. Faculty members make those decisions. While they have to be consistent with the parent institution, they are responsible for conceptualizing and articulating a mission and philosophy for their own programs that is consistent with Nursing's philosophy and standards. That is, they have a responsibility to society to produce nurses who "practice with compassion and respect for the inherent dignity, worth, and uniqueness of every individual . . . and know that they are committed to the patient, whether an individual, family, group or community" (ANA, 2004, p.4). Additionally, they have a responsibility to the parent institution to develop programs consistent with its mission and philosophy.

It would seem simple at face value. Faculty should be able to create a program of study consistent with the mission of the parent institution—a program that will help students learn what Nursing is, how to think about Nursing, and how to purposefully, proactively apply what they have learned. Yet, students often have difficulty jumping the gap from learning to thinking and from thinking to doing because inconsistencies exist in many programs. Sometimes it is because faculty members haven't attended to the relationship among the institutional,

Nursing, and school philosophies and missions (see Table 4.1 above). But usually, the problem exists at a more personal level.

> Relations between the mission and philosophy of Nursing and the parent institution create a context for Nursing programs.

Faculty Beliefs

One reason why inconsistencies exist in a program of study is that faculty members do not always clarify their own beliefs before they develop a curriculum. Unfortunately, an individual faculty member's personal beliefs often have a greater impact on what is taught and how it is taught than the mission and philosophy of either the parent institution or the Nursing program. For example, school philosophies often include words such as *holistic persons, person-centered caring,* and other jargon-type words, but the specific course content and learning experiences fail to demonstrate how these ideas are carried out. This state of affairs exists even though the course objectives, descriptions and titles suggest consistency with the philosophy. Even though these include language such as holism, person-centered caring, etc., concepts consistent with a Holistic paradigm, what is taught is that patient care is acontextual, nurses are concerned with conditions, and the important nursing skills are those which address problems related to disease processes.

Students learn how to perform tasks, use the nursing process as a problem-solving approach, and how to work in complex systems. Yet, they often fail to learn the importance of clients' perceptions, their values, beliefs, and how these relate to the context of their lives. Furthermore, these students often fail to learn about themselves as an important member of the nurse-client relationship. They learn about *doing* not *being* (Erickson, H., (2006a), pp. 6-20; Erickson, H., (2006b), pp. 309-316; Erickson, M., Erickson, H., & Jensen, B., (2006), pp. 205-207).

> Unless there are consistencies among the mission of the larger institution, the mission of the School of Nursing and Nursing's philosophy, faculty members will have difficulty staying true to their beliefs. However, they still have considerable freedom in carrying out their responsibilities. This is why personal philosophies are so important. Personal philosophies affect what faculty members believe students should be taught and how they should be taught. Personal philosophies are often the unspoken, unwritten underpinnings of curricula.

Semantics. Another reason for this *disconnect* between faculty intent and student learning might be called a matter of semantics. Faculty don't always agree on the language that should be used in a philosophy, so they compromise, sometimes stating that their differences are really only a matter of *semantics.* They fail to understand that semantics or *meaning* of a word will determine how it is operationalized and applied. And sometimes, they haven't thought about it enough to be able to articulate the difference between a holistic human-being and a wholistic person.[1] Instead, they focus on language such as *critical thinking, evidence-based nursing,* and *research*—language that addresses what the nurse does, not what the nurse aims to facilitate.

Is a Nurse a Nurse? Other times, individuals become members of a faculty without first examining the school's philosophy or considering how it relates to their own beliefs. They don't understand the importance of underlying belief systems, and how a philosophy statement should be the foundation for *what* is taught and *how* it is taught. Sometimes, they decide to *go along with* what is written, but are unprepared to implement the course objectives or provide learning experiences for their students. While they may have good intent, they are in the wrong place to carry out what they believe to be *good nursing* and *good teaching.* While there are many examples of this situation, one stands out in my mind. This example occurred in an institution where the Nursing program philosophy was current with Nursing, consistent with that of the institution, and included such language as "whole-person" and "caring." The faculty member in this example had several years of clinical experience, more than five years as a clinical faculty and was well-respected in the school for her "expertise."[2]

> *A number of years ago a senior student made an appointment to see me because she had decided that "Nursing was not her calling after all." When she arrived at my door, she explained that her faculty member and she had decided that she needed to leave Nursing and find another vocation. The problem had started the day before. Her faculty had*

---

[1] A common way to think about this is that holism is greater than the sum of the parts while wholism is equal to the sum of the parts. Another consideration is in the language human-being and person. While they might be interchangeable, the concept, *human-being*, often goes beyond the concept *person.* The *person* is usually considered to consist of biophysical, psychological, social, emotional and sometimes spiritual dimensions that interact. On the other hand, the *human-being* consists of multiple dimensions continuously interacting in such a way that they cannot be separated. Furthermore, these "human" aspects of the individual are interconnected with the "Being" aspect, i.e., the Soul.

[2] This is just one of many examples I have encountered through the years where a well-respected faculty member and a good student come together with potentially disastrous results. I am not aiming to fault the faculty or the student, but to point out what happens when persons in power fail to understand how their beliefs affect what they do, how they think, and what they value. Nursing cannot afford to lose good nurses simply because they happen to have a perfectly acceptable belief system that is inconsistent with that of another nurse who has power over them.

assigned her to the care of an elderly lady, so she could get experience with a "total care patient."

When the student reported on the unit, she said she noted that her patient had an NG tube, catheter, IV, and cardiac monitor, and appeared to be comatose. Her faculty asked her what she planned to do that day for this lady. She responded appropriately, including all of the technical care, but also talked about the lady's personal needs, talking with her family, and other options that might help comfort the patient and family. Her faculty agreed.

The student said that she immediately returned to this lady's room to find that she was near death. She called the charge nurse who advised her that there was little that could be done other than to comfort her. She proceeded to do this. She talked soothingly to her, held her hand, calmed her family, encouraged them to tell their mother they loved her, to thank her for a good life, and to tell her that it was okay to pass when she was ready. The lady passed within a few minutes.

About the same time, the instructor walked into the room, saw what was happening, took the student from the room and immediately reassigned her to another patient, so she could learn "total patient care." She was reassigned another patient with numerous tubes and equipment and told to leave the first patient for the charge nurse.

The student said that she was so upset that she cried. She felt that she had left the lady and her family precipitously; her care was unfinished. She concluded that she hadn't provided good nursing care. She went on to say that she had thought that Nursing was not about the tubes and equipment, although she admitted that was important, that Nursing was about caring for the holistic person. She stated that she didn't think the family was ready for her to leave, and that she hadn't had time to say goodbye to them or to the patient. Her faculty told her it was unprofessional to cry, to buck up and go get her work done. She concluded saying that she was so sad, she couldn't stop crying, and that she had decided to leave Nursing.

Because this faculty member adhered to the wholistic paradigm, she emphasized the knowledge and skills consistent with treating the patient's conditions, rather than caring for the person who needed complex nursing care. On the contrary, the student who appeared to adhere to a holistic paradigm had missed the mentoring necessary to learn how to deal with a normal part of the human experience. As a result, she had decided that she wasn't qualified to be a nurse.

Since I could understand the difference between the student's beliefs about Nursing and those of the faculty who supervised her, I was able to help both of them learn from the experience. This young woman, now 20 some years later, is a wonderful nurse who is clear about her beliefs, practices within the context of the holistic paradigm, and says so.

The faculty continues to practice from the wholistic paradigm, but now she knows how to recognize students who adhere to a holistic paradigm and how to facilitate their learning experiences. She is a wonderful team member to work with; she knows how to *do* and is one who knows when to seek guidance from those who know how to *be.*

Clearly defined personal and professional philosophies serve to link theory, practice and research. When faculty members are clear about their own beliefs and can articulate them to colleagues, they will be better able to articulate a school philosophy consistent with their own views, identify and define major concepts in the philosophy, prioritize the importance of these concepts, and develop curricula accordingly. They will also be able to implement curricula, guide students, and be clear about their clinical decisions.

The Mission and Program Philosophy

Before faculty can define the specifics of their curriculum, they need to articulate their school's mission and program philosophy. The mission articulates the school's purpose, and the philosophy provides a general description of their beliefs about each program. *The philosophy will determine what type of knowledge* will be selected to guide practice.

The MWK Matrix Model, as shown in Table 4.2, can be used to facilitate the discussions necessary to articulate a philosophy. Start with the constructs in the Metaparadigm; decide whether all five shown in the matrix model should be included and then determine if others should be. Next, review the ways-of-knowing and decide which should be included in your program. Fill in the cells of the matrix as you proceed. Although there is no specific starting point, i.e., no "right" cell to start with, it is important to discuss the topics in every cell of the MWK Matrix Model. As the discussion proceeds, faculty may add topics, clarify their beliefs about topics, and articulate clear understandings with one another about relations among their own beliefs and those of Nursing. Notes should be taken throughout the process listing key discussions and highlighting decisions. These can be used to write common belief statements. Together, these statements create a philosophy.

Table 4.2 A working form of the MWK Matrix Model.

WAYS-OF-KNOWING	NURSING	HEALTH	ENVIRONMENT	PERSON	SOCIAL JUSTICE
Empirical knowing					
Esthetical knowing					
Ethical knowing					
Personal knowing					
Sociopolitical knowing					
Unknowing					
Reflective knowing					

Side Trips

Sometimes, faculty discuss topics that seem to be outside the cells in the matrix model. This might be because the discussion springs from the paradigm alternative to the one selected. For example, nurses from a wholistic perspective might be concerned with pain management while nurses from a holistic perspective might argue that pain management is not as important as facilitating comfort. Although both faculty members might use a person immediately post-mastectomy as an example, the first would argue that the nurse is responsible for controlling the pain while the second might argue that the nurse is responsible for facilitating comfort in as many ways as possible. The first might focus care on patient-controlled-anesthesia (PCA) pumps, while the second might *include a PCA,* but would also be concerned with other needs as perceived by the individual.

Another reason why faculty members seem to take these "side trips" in their discussions is because the proposed topic is *inconsistent* with the Scope of Nursing, outside of Nursing Standards, or unsupported by Nursing's Code of Ethics. When this happens, faculty must revisit the essence of Nursing to determine if they are being true to their profession or if they are being swayed by the views of other professional groups.

The goal is to articulate a program philosophy. Decisions made throughout this process should be cross-referenced with Nursing's Scope of Practice, Standards for Practice and Code of Ethics to ensure that they are consistent with the Nursing profession and contribute to distinguishing Nursing from other professions.

A Circular Process

The above process of defining a school mission and program philosophies is not a neat and tidy linear occurrence. Instead, it is an ongoing, spiral process, with ever deepening faculty understandings. Throughout discussion it is important to remember that the goal is to articulate program philosophies that are consistent with the parent institution, Nursing, *and* the faculty's paradigm choice. At each step, individuals have the opportunity to learn and discover, to evolve and grow. As a result, faculty will discover that they will want to revisit their own beliefs, revise the program philosophy, and tighten their linkages as they work.

It is important to embrace growth and evolution, to provide time for both process and task work, and to expect that even as you move forward, it is sometimes necessary to revisit and rework "finished work." However, it is equally important to recognize disagreement when it occurs. Sometimes individuals who seem to agree at one point disagree at another. This can be because continued work results in new insights.

But, more often, it is because they are in disagreement with the selected paradigm. While the ideal situation would be that all faculty members would adopt a single paradigm, this is not usually the case. More typically, faculty members are split between the two paradigms. (Table 4.3 provides an example of a working form that can be used to identify faculty paradigm choice.)

Table 4.3 Working form for faculty paradigm clarification.

FACULTY NAME	HOLISTIC PARADIGM	WHOLISTIC PARADGIM

When the faculty, as a group, conclude that there is a split in paradigm perspectives, it is important to agree that diversity can strengthen a faculty *if and when* faculty agree that there are two paradigms in Nursing, that each has its merit and each mandates specific course content and clinical expectations, the faculty are matched paradigm to course, *and* students are informed of the differences. Otherwise, within a short period of time, individuals tend to sabotage the intent of the program; they revise course objectives and alter course content.[3]

> A philosophy statement, derived from faculty discussion, consistent with the school's mission (and that of the larger organization), provides a sound base for the next step in curriculum development, writing program objectives.

[3] Emphasis is placed on the Holistic Paradigm within the MWK Matrix Model.

Program Goals and Level Objectives

Now that the school's mission statement is clear, and the philosophy has been articulated, it is time to write specific program goals and level objectives. Goals written for each of the programs specify expected student outcomes at the completion of each program, i.e., ADN, BSN, MS, PhD, DNP, etc. That is, Program Goals operationalize the mission statement and are written *within the context of the philosophy* of Nursing. For example, a mission statement might declare that the institution aims to *prepare professional nurses at the baccalaureate and graduate level; a* related program goal might state that the program will produce nurses *who are able to provide leadership in the professional practice setting and the profession* (ANA, 2004, p. 44).

Program Goals identify faculty expectations at the completion of each program (for e.g., the completion of the baccalaureate program). Program Goals provide the structure for delineating Level Goals and related Level Objectives. The number of Program Goals identified by a faculty can be as minimal as one and as many as the faculty determines appropriate (See Table 4.4).

Table 4.4 Working form to set *Level Goals.*

	PROGRAM GOAL 1	PROGRAM GOAL 2	PROGRAM GOAL 3	PROGRAM GOAL 4
Level goals				
Level 1.				
Level 2.				
Level 3.				
Level 4.				

Level Goals specify the faculty's expectations at *the completion of each level* in a specific program, while ***Level Objectives*** identify the specific parameters needed to accomplish Level Goals.

Table 4.4 provides a working form for identifying Level Goals that will meet Program Goals. This table indicates that faculty members have identified four program goals and are working on a curriculum for a four year (or four level) program, as one would expect to see in the generic baccalaureate program. Table 4.5 provides a working form faculty can use to specify Level Objectives designed to meet the Level Goals.

Simply stated, faculty members move from a Program Philosophy to Program Goals, to Level Goals, and to Level Objectives with each becoming more specific.

Table 4.5 Working form to set multiple *objectives for each level.*

	LEVEL 1 GOAL	LEVEL 2 GOAL	LEVEL 3 GOAL	LEVEL 4 GOAL
Level 1 objectives				
Level 1.1.				
Level 1.2.				
Level 1.3.				
Level 1.4.				

Educational Considerations

Since Nursing is a practice profession, Nursing programs are designed to produce a *competent, professional person.* Therefore, Level Goals are designed to assess the practitioner's knowledge, skills *and* attitudes. There is an assumption that learning builds on previous learning, that knowledge becomes increasingly sophisticated, and the knowledge base becomes increasingly interactive and integrated. What might seem very complex at an earlier level might become simple at a higher level.

Nurse leaders have talked about the importance of *integrative knowing* (Locsin & Purnell, 2009), a process whereby multiple ways-of-knowing are integrated, resulting in knowledge that is unique to the situation. The notion that integrative knowing is possible suggests that not only are there ways-of-knowing, there are also *levels of learning* that occur.

While a number of authors have written about levels of learning and domains where learning occurs, the most commonly recognized is the work of Benjamin Bloom (1956), revisited and revised by Anderson & Kratwohl (2001) as shown in Table 4.6. Bloom argued that there are three domains or *areas of educational activity* that are important when considering how people learn. These include cognitive knowledge or mental skills; psychomotor behaviors or skills; and affective learning or attitudes.

Bloom also identified *levels of learning,* arguing that higher-level learning can only be achieved after learning has occurred at the lower levels. For example, he argued that students can not *apply* knowledge until they have first mastered *comprehension* of the said knowledge, and that *comprehension* precedes the ability to *recall* this knowledge. So, before students can evaluate or synthesize knowledge, they must comprehend it, know how to apply it, and so forth.

But according to Bloom, cognitive learning is not enough in a practice profession. The learner must also have the psychomotor abilities needed in the practice arena. More specifically, for practice professions, application of knowledge depends on one's ability to *act or behave* in ways necessary to demonstrate that such knowledge has been acquired.

Table 4.6 Bloom's taxonomy of cognitive, psychomotor, and affective domains of learning. Extrapolated from the work of Anderson, & Kratwohl, (2001); Bloom (1956, 1972); Kratwohl, Bloom, & Masia (1973).

BLOOM'S LEVELS OF LEARNING		
(Cognitive)	**(Psychomotor)**	**(Affective)**
Cognitive Acquisition (Remembering): Recalls information (defines, identifies, lists, recalls).	Perception (Perceiving): uses sensory cues to guide motor activities (chooses, detects, isolates, selects).	Receiving phenomena: intake of stimuli, identification of parts (asks, chooses, identifies).
Cognitive Comprehension (Understanding): Understands the meaning, translation, and interpretation (distinguishes, explains, interprets).	Set (Connecting): knows and acts on a series of connected activities (explains, reacts).	Responding to phenomena: labels, recites, discusses parts (tells, discusses, writes).
Cognitive Application (Applying): uses concept in new situations (applies, demonstrates, solves, uses).	Guided Response (Practicing): imitation, trial and error; expertise acquired by practice (copies, traces, reproduces).	Valuing: demonstrates belief in and acceptance of phenomena/behaviors (initiates, shares, proposes).
Cognitive Analysis (Analyzing): deconstructs concept or construct into parts to understand organizational structure (analyzes, compares, discriminates).	Mechanism (Performing): habitual responses to a set of activities; movements can be competently performed (assembles, manipulates).	Organizing: prioritizes values, resolves conflicts (integrates, explains).
Cognitive Evaluation (Evaluating): judge the merit of the "new whole" (appraises, contrasts, critiques).	Complex Overt Response (Creating): proficiency is demonstrated by quick, accurate performance (builds, calibrates, measures).	Internalizing: takes on a value system which guides behaviors that are pervasive, predictable, and characteristic of the learner (i.e. professional person); influences, qualifies, questions, revises, verifies.
Cognitive Synthesis (Creating): Combines or compiles parts into new whole with new meaning (combines, creates, reconstructs).	Adaptation: performer can alter patterns to accommodate the situation (adapts, alters, rearranges).	
	Organization: creation of new patterns of behavior (constructs, creates, designs).	

Finally, the *attitudes* of the learners affect their ability to proceed from lower level cognitive learning to the higher levels; what they perceive important will determine what they attend to, value, prioritize and act on.
Nurse educators, usually, address most of the cognitive and psychomotor domains of learning, but overlook affective learning. Yet, we have argued in this chapter and in earlier ones that it is important to proactively address affective learning. Now, we state that is also important to reflect these values in the Program Goals, Level Goals, and Level Objectives. Table 4.7 provides an example of a working form which can be used to identify Bloom's learning domains as they interrelate with Level Objectives. This model is not limited to Level Objectives; additional work forms can be developed for Program and/or Level Goals as needed. Table 4.8 provides a working form that can be used simultaneously while faculty consider which of Bloom's levels of learning are required to prepare students to meet Level Objectives.

Table 4.7 Working table to determine which domains of learning are required to meet level objectives.

	LEVEL OBJECTIVE 1.1	LEVEL OBJECTIVE 1.2	LEVEL OBJECTIVE 1.3	LEVEL OBJECTIVE 1.4
Cognitive				
Psychomotor				
Affective				

Table 4.8 Working form to specify relations among learning domains and ways-of-knowing.

COGNITIVE: PSYCHOMOTOR: AFFECTIVE:	Remember Perceive Receive	Understand Connect Respond	Apply Practice Value	Analyze Organize	Evaluate Perform Internalize	Create Create
Empirical knowing						
Esthetical knowing						
Ethical knowing						
Personal knowing						
Sociopolitical knowing						
Unknowing						
Reflective knowing						

Curricular Specifics

Once Program Objectives have been clarified, it is time to identify where and how students will be introduced to the concepts and content specified in the matrix model. Tables 4.8 and 4.9 will be particularly helpful with this process. First, working in Table 4.8 above, concepts and content that require a specific way of thinking (knowing) can be identified according to Bloom's Levels of Learning, and then they can be "plugged into" Table 4.9 to indicate which concepts and related content address each of the Level Objectives.

Table 4.9 Working table to determine types of knowledge (concepts, content, & skills) required to meet specific level objectives.

	Level objective 1.1	**Level objective 1.2**	**Level objective 1.3**
Empirical knowledge			
Ethical knowledge			
Esthetical knowledge			
Personal knowledge			
Sociopolitical knowledge			
Reflective knowledge			
Unknowing			

Grouping concepts by Level Objectives enables faculty to visualize the concepts and content that need to be addressed at each level of the program. It will also help them think about the type of knowing they want to encourage in their students and their expected outcome for students, by level. Finally, concepts can be grouped, course descriptions written and course objectives specified to complete the process. Previously completed work forms, including the MWK Matrix Model can be used to help faculty members clarify and refine their thinking and concept grouping, course descriptions, and course objectives. Finally, course objectives should be matched with Level Objectives. Table 4.10 provides a working form for this activity.

Table 4.10 Working table to determine types of knowledge (concepts, content, and skills) required to meet specific course objectives.

	Level Obj. 1	Level Obj. 2	Level Obj. 3	Level Obj. 4	Level Obj. 5
Course 1 objectives					
Course 2 objectives					

USING MODELING AND ROLE-MODELING

Some faculty use Modeling and Role-Modeling as the base for their curriculum. While Table 4.2 (p.77) can be used to guide their thinking, I offer an alternative that includes some basic considerations when using MRM. In Table 4.2, the ways-of-knowing are presented in the order in which they are often discussed in Nursing; the cells include some concepts/knowledge common to Nursing. On the contrary, the listing in Table 4.11 suggests an alternative order for presenting the ways-of-knowing. When using this table, the cells can include concepts and some content important for those teaching MRM, and they are discussed below.

Table 4.11 An alternative order for presenting Nursing knowledge.

	NURSING	HEALTH	ENVIRONMENT	PERSON	SOCIAL JUSTICE
Personal Knowing					
Ethical Knowing					
Unknowing					
Reflexivity					
Esthetical knowing					
Sociopolitical knowing					
Empirical knowing					

Personal Knowing

Personal Knowing or knowing of the Self is expressed as a "state of being, a personal experience reflecting inner and outer harmony" (Clements & Averill, 2006, p. 270). It involves tapping into one's inner knowing. Personal Knowledge involves discovering Self-knowledge, responsibility, and engagement with life. It is acquired as we open ourselves to explore our belief systems and clarify our philosophy.

Since Nursing is based in a relationship that starts with the nurse as an authentic person, Personal Knowing and Personal Knowledge are important to nurses and Nursing. To be open to developing personal knowing skills, nurses need to be aware of their own beliefs and how they impact their thinking processes—values important to clarify before they engage others in a caring or healing process.

Recently, Silva, J. M. Sorrell and C. D. Sorrel (1995), critiquing Carper's model, discussed the philosophical shift that is occurring in Nursing. They stated that Nursing is shifting from an epistemological focus to ontological reflections on ways-of-being. We believe that our "ways-of-being" are strongly influenced by our own Self-knowledge or Personal Knowing.

Implications of Personal Knowing

According to the Holistic paradigm, people live in a context—a context that is continuously evolving. A part of this context is the relationship between nurses and clients. When nurses interact with clients, they affect the relationship and alter the context either positively or negatively; all behaviors, words, actions and attitudes serve as communication cues to this end. As stated by Watzlawick (1967) (as cited in Erickson, H., (2006b), pp. 307-309) *we cannot not communicate*. We communicate even when we don't intend to do so. The more we are aware of our own *Self* (Erickson, H. (2006a), pp. 5-32), the more *proactive and purposeful* we can be in our communications.[4] And the more we are able to create a positive, healthy, healing context for ourselves and our clients.

Nurses need to be aware of their inner knowing, their beliefs and attitudes, so they can understand how these affect the context, and thus, the nurse-client relationship.

Personal Knowledge and Reason for Being

While our Self-knowledge always exists, it is often suppressed or overshadowed by the demands of everyday life. We learn to focus on material issues and physical problems of living, rather than the larger issue of *the meaning of the relationship in which we are engaged.* Self-knowledge connects us to our Soul and helps us understand our Life Purpose and Reason for Being (Erickson, H., (2006a), pp. 5-32). It helps us seek greater understanding of how we affect others, and they us, and a deeper purpose for our interactions. While we know in our Souls why we have chosen to be nurses *and* the importance of the moment-to-moment interactions in our relationships with others, we often lose sight of this "knowing" because of the immediacy of daily living. Fortunately, when we are encouraged to embrace Personal Knowing (Erickson, H., (2006a), p. 8) as essential information, we can become more fully integrated—mind, body and soul—an integration needed to help us achieve our goals as *professional nurses*,

[4] In an earlier publication (Erickson, H., 2006b), we discussed the reasons nurses have difficulty connecting with their clients, suggested a few strategies that facilitate connecting, (pp. 300-323) and offered a few suggestions for Self growth and Self-actualization (Erickson, H., (2006c), pp. 433-444).

purposeful in our practice, clear about our focus, and dedicated to serve clients and society.

> Bottom line: the more we learn to understand ourselves, the more purposefully we can facilitate the growth or healing of another human being, design research studies that will answer our practice questions, provide leadership in the community to improve health care delivery, and contribute to the well-being of society at large.

Ethical Knowing

Ethical Knowing is closely aligned to Personal Knowing, except it is a way of *thinking about* our attitudes and beliefs and how they impact our clients rather than about how they affect ourselves. Our ethical knowledge is stipulated in our Code of Ethics which sets the standards for our moment-to-moment actions and decisions.

As professional practitioners, it is imperative that we remember to keep the ethics of our profession in our thoughts, to use them as parameters for our practice. Ethical knowledge helps us to understand the unique roles of a professional nurse and to distinguish Nursing from other professions. Without ethical knowledge, nurses might apply acquired knowledge (especially empirical knowledge) within the context of the Metaparadigm of another professional group. And without ethical knowing, nurses might lose sight of the reasons for their decision to be a nurse.

Ethics and Morality

While the concepts 'ethical' and 'moral' are often used interchangeably, they are different. According to ANA, "'Ethical' is used to refer to reasons for decisions about how one ought to act [while] 'moral'…is more aligned with personal belief and cultural values" (2001, p.5). Nurses must be clear about the parameters of the Nursing profession and the similarities and differences among the professional groups before they can be clear about the parameters of our practice and research. For example, while some might argue that a guideline for ethical knowing is "do more good than harm," this holds true for any human being. Furthermore, it does not distinguish among the professional groups. On the other hand, when we refer to our Code of Ethics, the parameters of health problems of importance to nurses are clear:

> *The measures nurses take to care for the patient enable the patient to live with as much physical, emotional, social and spiritual well-being as possible. Nursing care aims to maximize the values that the patient has*

treasured in life and extends supportive care to the family and significant others. (ANA, Code of Ethics, 2001, p.7)

This statement indicates that nurses are concerned with the person's well-being and not a condition or disease. Each nurse has to decide the importance of this *ethical knowledge* and how it will impact their own behaviors.

Ethical knowledge is important if nurses are to focus on and delineate their actions and decisions. Ethical knowing helps nurses keep their focus.

Unknowing

Unknowing, also important for holistic nurses, relates to Ethical Knowing. Munhall (1993) argued that no matter how expert the nurse, no human completely fits into our preexisting model; there are always some things about the client and self that are unknown. She called this *Unknowing* and said that if nurses are to be open to discovery, they need to be open to these *unknown* factors. Heath (1998) described this pattern of Unknowing as follows:

> *This unknowing is an awareness that the nurse does not and cannot know or understand the client when they first meet, and by recognizing this unknowing, the nurse remains alert to the client's perspective of the situation.* (p. 1055)

Unknowing is consistent with the MRM belief that nurses have a responsibility to facilitate clients in *telling their story* (Erickson, H., 2006b, pp. 315-17). MRM stipulates that people have Self-care Knowledge (SCK) and that SCK is the primary source of information (Erickson et al., 1983/2009, pp.48, Hertz, & Baas, 2006, p. 118). While some might say that Unknowing is incorporated in esthetic knowledge, we think it warrants exclusive discussion. Unknowing is an attitude—an attitude that determines whether or not nurses perceive their clients as the primary and most important source of information. Recognition of Unknowing helps nurses to focus on, seek and value Self-care Knowledge (Brekke & Schultz, 2006, pp. 61-62; Erickson, H., 2006b, pp. 315-317; Erickson, et al., 1983/2009, p. 48; Erickson, M., Erickson, H., & Jensen, B., 2006, p.193; Hertz & Baas, 2006, pp. 97-122).

Unless the nurse is aware of the clients' ability to provide information about their well-being that no other individual can provide, they often fail to seek it, or when it is offered by the client, to value it. Instead, it is considered subjective or irrelevant.

Chinn and Kramer (1995) described *knowing* as the individual human process of experiencing and comprehending the self and world in ways that can be brought to some level of conscious awareness. This suggests that knowing, which is a conscious process, is linked to unknowing. And unknowing can be both about the self and others. This description illustrates that is necessary for nurses to value MRM's concept of Self-care Knowledge. SCK is defined as "[Our] personal understanding of what is needed to help us grow, develop, or heal. It includes awareness of personal needs and goals, as well as strengths, capabilities, characteristics, values, and liabilities. It also includes recognition of what is not needed" (Hertz, & Baas, 2006, p. 98).

> Frequently, nurses talk about the differences between subjective and objective data. Self-care Knowledge is subjective; it is perceived. It is also the basis of an individual's health and well-being and, therefore, must be the basis of a nursing care plan. We think that recognition of our own Unknowing helps us be more aware and respectful of another person's Self-care Knowledge.

In previous work, Kinney, in discussing Heart-to-Heart Relationships (2006, pp. 278-299), refers to Watson's *Caring Field,* and then goes on to discuss connecting, spirit-to-spirit. She states:

> *Our intention influences the nature of the relationship we build with others. Relationships can be built at the spirit level when it is our intent to do so! When we build such relationships, we can help people connect with their Soul and initiate understanding of their Soul-work. We can do this by having the intent to create heart-to-heart relationships with our clients and connect spirit-to-spirit with them. When we incorporate into our Way-of- Being an intent to make heart-to-heart connections and build a relationship within the context of the client's worldview, we create a Caring Field.* (Kinney, 2006, p. 291)

Intention, then, is the aim to discover what is unknown. The Recognition of Unknowing as a Way-of-Knowing encourages nurses to be mindful of their clients' Self-care Knowledge, the primary source of information. When we not only recognize, but *embrace* Unknowing as a Way-of-Knowing, nurses are able to help others *discover what they know, but don't know they know*, what they need in order to grow, and to discover the essence of who they are at a deeper level. Because nurses don't understand this concept, the next pattern of knowing is extremely important. As illustrated in Chapter 14 of this book, Reflexivity helps nurses get in touch with their own Self. That is, it helps them connect with their own spirituality and opens them to better understand the importance of Unknowing as a Way-of-Knowing.

Reflective knowing

Reflection, originally coined by Schön (1983/1991, 1987), is described as a process used to gain understanding, insight and new knowledge about practice. Johns has written extensively on Reflexivity and Reflective practice (1995, 2002, 2004a, 2004b, 2005/2007). Recently, he proposed that Reflective knowing is a unique way of experiencing our relationship with clients. He describes this concept as follows:

> *Reflection is being mindful of self, either within or after experience, as if a window through which the practitioner can view and focus self within the context of a particular experience, in order to confront, understand and move toward resolving contradiction between one's vision and actual practice.* (2004a, p.3)

Later, (2005/2007) Johns stated:

> *Reflection is both subjective and particular. It is the fusion of sensing, perceiving, intuiting and thinking related to a specific experience in order to develop insights into self and practice. It is vision-driven, concerned with taking action toward knowing and realizing desirable practice….In doing so it intends to resolve contradiction so that people can lead more meaningful lives. In other words, reflection is purposeful.* (p. 2-3)

Opening oneself to reflective knowing is also a way for nurses to learn about themselves both as individuals and as professionals. Schaefer (2006) stated that nurses often have difficulty facing the day-to-day challenges of nursing; they feel victimized, develop feelings of helplessness, and fail to take leadership roles. She stated that nurses need to call on their inner strength to help them face everyday challenges. She proposed that they learn to cultivate self-reflection and broaden their perspective so they can see where others are coming from, and learn to let go of the past, so they can move toward the future. I would add that reflective knowing is essential if we are to better understand ourselves, connect with our spiritual being, and gain insight into our reasons for choosing Nursing as a profession.

Helping students reflect on their practice is one way of facilitating them to link philosophy with theory, practice and research. It is a necessary part of learning how to use integrative knowing, learned through discovery learning methods. Chapter 5 and several chapters in Section II and III describe our position on a learning process we have developed through the years as we synthesize and integrate knowledge using discovery learning methods.

> *Reflective knowing is an open, dynamic process. It produces knowledge about ourselves in connection with others. It also helps us connect directly to our own Self, to better understand our Reason for Being and our Purpose in Life.* (Erickson, H., 2006a, pp. 5-32)

Esthetical Knowing

Esthetical knowing is the next pattern of knowing according to our model. Esthetics, the art of Nursing, "is experiential, often non-verbal, and shared by the nurse and the client" (Clements & Averill, 2006). From the MRM perspective, the art of Nursing is the provision of professional nursing care based on the client's view of the world. It includes artistically designed interventions planned to meet the client's needs.

According to Carper (1978), empathy is a basic tenet of esthetic knowing. We agree with this perspective. Without empathy, it would be impossible to understand the meaning of a client's world-view. Empathy helps us have the ability to step into the world of another, to create a mirror image of that world, and to comprehend what might be helpful to that person.

MRM argues that there are specific Aims of Interventions, each related to a specific Principle of Nursing. The Principles of Nursing help set parameters for our practice while the Aims help direct or focus it within those parameters. Three strategies, proposed previously (Erickson, H., 2006b, p. 309-317), provide some guidelines for application of esthetic knowing (see Table 4.12).

Intuition, also known as tacit knowledge, (Polanyi, 1962, pp. 69-243) is often used by expert nurses in clinical decision-making (McCaffrey, 2009, pp. 346-349; Smith, 2009, p. 143). We, the authors of this chapter, believe that *Intuition* is a type of Esthetic Knowledge. We gain intuition by integrating various types of knowledge, (such as personal, ethical, reflective, and empirical knowledge), recycling knowledge acquired from the various ways-of-knowing, each time gaining a deeper understanding of the essence of Nursing. As with other growth experiences, it is not a "once-and-for-all" experience, but a continuous deepening of understanding and knowing—knowing about Self and others.

Table 4.12 Strategies common to Nursing. Adapted with permission, *Modeling and role-Modeling: A view from the client's world*, 2006b, p. 310. Unicorns Unlimited: Cedar Park, TX.

Establishing a Mind Set:		
	Self-care Preliminaries	•Explore own philosophy. •Identify beliefs. •Identify ways to enhance own Self-knowing.
	Moving Forward	•Develop centering skills. •Learn to focus on client, not skills. •Open self to energetic intra-connection with client.
Creating a Nurturing Space:		
	Sources of stimuli	•Decrease negative stimuli. •Enhance positive stimuli.
	Respecting space of others	•Recognize environment is client's context. •Ask before manipulating environment.
	Spirit-to-spirit contact	
Facilitating the Story:		
	Tapping Self-care Knowledge	•Address the stimuli. •Attend to client's Self-care Knowledge.

Glaser and Strauss (1967) maintained that insight is the source of all significant theorizing. We think that nurses who are comfortable with their own intuition often seek insight; they try to understand why they make their decisions. This search is a natural stimulant for theorizing. The intermediate step between intuition and theory has been labeled Reflection.

Sociopolitical Knowing

Sociopolitical knowing, proposed by White (1995), is our next way of knowing. Nurses work in a context that includes society, culture, economics and politics and as such, need to understand how this context impacts them and the well-being of their clients. Previously, we stated that there are strategies which can be used to facilitate connecting and building a trusting, functional relationship. Knowledge about the system one works in is important. Without such knowledge, nurses, with the best intentions, are overwhelmed and unable to do what they know is ethical and moral.

> Nurses have a responsibility to society. To fulfill our responsibilities, we need to understand the sociopolitical environment in which we work and live.

Empirical Knowing

Empirical knowing is our last way of knowing. Empirical knowing, a logical, problem-solving way of thinking is often thought to incorporate only objective thinking. Some actually identify empirical thinking with the scientific process. And although it does include an objective problem-solving approach, it is much more than that.

During the 1960s nurse leaders argued that we needed to nurse by *process not by intuition.* Some, such as McCain (1965) argued that nurses needed a problem solving approach to care-giving, suggesting that we needed a *nursing process.* Most nurses agreed. But we failed to be clear that being objective does not exclude other types of knowing. For some, being objective means that we can only use knowledge acquired by objective means. Since we have not carefully studied the *art of nursing*, this version of empirical knowledge excludes a large portion of what nurses know that is important to creating, maintaining, and expanding human relations and client well-being. Simply stated, nurses need to use *all types of knowing, integrate all types of knowledge and use it in an objective, problem-solving way.* According to us, this is the value of using a Nursing theory; it helps nurses use multiple ways-of-knowing, draw on multiple types of knowledge and be purposeful in their thoughts and actions. This view of empirical knowing and empirical knowledge is not the same as that held by those who believe that empirical knowing is the same as science.

Trouble with Empirical Knowledge

Since the word *science* is used to mean both the research process and the resultant findings, (depending on how it is used), then empirical knowing can be either knowledge *about* the scientific process and/or knowledge acquired *from* it. To further complicate the issue, there are also two types of empirical (or scientific) knowledge used by nurses: shared knowledge and unique-to-Nursing knowledge. Shared knowledge is knowledge common to all professional groups that provide care to the human being—knowledge about the scientific process and knowledge acquired from the scientific process (i.e., research results). Unique-to-Nursing knowledge is knowledge derived by studying Nursing phenomena and concepts as defined by the discipline of Nursing.

When we talk about the *scientific process*, there are research designs used by various disciplines. As indicated before, there are basic assumptions that underlie various research designs. For example, the positivist view indicates that randomized, controlled studies should be used to study the efficacy of the phenomenon of concern. Therefore, it is important for nurse researchers to explore their own belief systems before adopting specific research designs.

There are also *scientific findings* which are shared across disciplines. For example, information obtained about the "normal" parameters of human nature (from the basic and behavioral sciences, for example) is used by many healthcare providers. While such knowledge might be studied primarily by a group of scientists interested in the phenomenon, it is a shared knowledge base.

Shared scientific findings (i.e., a type of knowledge) are important to Nursing because they help us understand the parameters of the average human being under usual circumstances. They also help us understand when there are deviations in the norm—important information when attending to the holistic being. This common, shared knowledge is important to Nursing, but is *not* Nursing science. Nursing science is based on an assumption that what is known can be accessed through the human (Chinn & Kramer, 2004). It is knowledge about the health and well-being of dynamic, interactive, bio-psycho-social-spiritual human beings; the environment in which they live; their interactions with the environment; their relationships with their caregivers (including their nurses); and the processes that influence these relationships.

Until recently, Nursing's empirical knowledge was heavily influenced by the positivist view of science. At its best, this state of affairs caused confusion in the profession. While not all nurses supported the positivist view, they didn't always consider the philosophical orientation of science when selecting a design, or when accepting research findings. At its worst, it stymied the advancement of Nursing knowledge. More specifically, it created problems for nurses who held an alternative view of Nursing as a discipline. For example, nurses who believed in the Holistic paradigm.

When the mainstream sociopolitical environment adopts a particular way of thinking about knowledge building, novice researchers are often discounted and sometimes even jeopardized if they don't follow the "norm." When the positivist view is believed to be the premier scientific orientation, others are often considered second-rate or inferior. This was the case in Nursing during our early years of research advancement. Studies designed to test for factor-relating and factor- predicting were more easily approved and funded than studies designed to test the first two levels of knowledge building. And knowledge acquired through alternative methods (e.g., case studies) was considered anecdotal, unimportant, and unscientific. Nurses who believed in the Holistic paradigm of Nursing often felt disenfranchised, had difficulties obtaining funding, and claimed that the findings from such research studies did not reflect their view of Nursing.

A number of nurses who believed in the Holistic (Simultaneity) Paradigm of Nursing felt disenfranchised from mainstream Nursing, where the majority of nurses viewed humans from the Wholistic (Totality) Paradigm. Early in the 1980s, they convened to establish the American Holistic Nurses Association (AHNA). In 2006, Holistic Nursing was recognized by the American Nurses' Association (ANA) as a specialty, indicating recognition by nurse leaders that the Holistic Paradigm is an acceptable way to view the nature of mankind, Nursing science and Nursing practice (AHNA, 2007).

> Predominant acceptance of the positivist view of science created a problem for Nursing since we had not yet had time to clarify and name the phenomenon of *Nursing*. Instead, we accepted the science of other disciplines as a way of "knowing" about the phenomena of concern to Nursing rather than seeking our own understandings and ways of science.

Nursing Today

Today, Nursing is moving toward a neo-modernistic view of science, one that values both paradigms of Nursing: the Wholistic (or Totality) and the Holistic (or Simultaneity). Still, nurses often fail to state their philosophical beliefs upfront and discuss their findings in respect to what they believe to be true about nursing, science, and society.

We think it is important for nurses to base their research in a Nursing theory that has a philosophical base consistent with the researcher's. We also think it is important for nurses to be clear about these beliefs when they report their findings. Without clear definition of who we are, what we are studying and why, our scientific knowledge is not unique to Nursing.

> The science of Nursing must be based in a sound theoretical framework and grounded in an explicit philosophy. Only then will the clinical implications be clear and only then can we design and teach a well-articulated program.

SUMMARY

This chapter served two purposes. First, it proposed numerous factors that needed to be considered when developing a curriculum. It started with the mission and philosophy of the parent institution and progressed through the logical steps needed to develop a consistent curriculum based on faculty beliefs and designed to prepare students who could link knowledge with practice. The second purpose of the chapter was to provide more specific information for those who wish to use the Modeling and Role-Modeling theory and paradigm. This section described, in detail, the ways–of-knowing as they relate to MRM. The following chapter, building on the ideas presented in this chapter, presents Bruner's Discovery-Learning theory as a way to facilitate students' learning of content, attitudes, skills, and behaviors consistent with their personal belief system, yet within the context of Nursing's framework.

CHAPTER 5

DISCOVERY-LEARNING METHODS: LEARNING TO THINK

Helen L. Erickson

And, may I say a thing from my own experience? No training is of any use, unless one can learn to feel, and to think things out for oneself.
(Nightingale, 1915, p. 27)

Our job, as teachers, is to facilitate the learners to discover what we want them to know [and] *to jump the gap from learning to thinking.*
(Bruner, 1966, p. 68)

OVERVIEW

Educators have many responsibilities: to recognize their students as active learners with predispositions; to structure and sequence the course content so it can be easily learned; and to pace and reinforce learning experiences so students can learn how to think and act like professional nurses.

Bruner stated this more eloquently with the following comments:

> *There is nothing more central to a discipline than its way of thinking. There is nothing more important in its teaching than to provide* [the learner] *the earliest opportunity to learn the way of thinking—the form of connection, the attitude, hopes, jokes, and frustrations that go with it. In a word, the best introduction to a subject is the subject itself. At the very first breath, the young learner should...be given the chance to solve problems, to conjecture, to quarrel as done at the heart of the discipline. But, you will ask, how can this be arranged?* (Bruner, 1965, p. 29)

Since this book is designed primarily for those who have accepted formal educational responsibilities, this chapter will address structured teaching-learning considerations. It is based on and extrapolated from Bruner's Discovery-Learning Model, as well as the work of Carl Rogers and Milton Erickson. There is no intent to misrepresent the exemplary work of these scholars, but to extrapolate from it. The bottom line: I believe that people want to learn, and that they seek opportunities to learn, but they enter such learning experiences with a frame of reference derived from past experiences. That is, they have ways-of-knowing and knowledge that precede interactions with formal educators. These affect how and what they attend to in new learning situations, what they identify as important, and even how they interpret what is taught. This chapter provides an overview of Bruner's Discovery-Learning Methods with adaptations made by incorporating techniques and strategies I have learned through the years.

BACKGROUND

Teaching and Learning

Many people think that the educational process is two-sided—that the teacher's responsibility is to teach and evaluate, and the learner's responsibility is to learn and demonstrate what they have learned. I agree that the educational process involves both teaching and learning, but question the division between teacher and learner. Instead, I choose to think about teaching-learning as a unitary, dynamic process that is spiral in nature; one that produces an ever-increasing depth of *knowing.* And I believe that the teacher and learner is often one and the same person. That is, teaching and learning are best facilitated when they are interconnected to create a singular process. Learning is ongoing, builds on previous knowledge, creates ways-of-knowing, and often occurs in an individual in the absence of another person. At the same time, I know that learning can be facilitated and expedited by a teacher, and that learning does not always bring about positive growth, but it does always effect change.

I have concluded that teaching is not about preparing notes and slides, giving lectures, planning seminars or clinical experiences. It is about facilitating growth in the learner—growth related to acquisition of new knowledge and discovery of new ways of thinking. I didn't learn this overnight; nor did I learn it in a class. I learned it because a few of my teachers (some formal and some informal) had the wisdom to build on what I already knew, (but sometimes didn't know I knew), to stimulate my curiosity, and to open the door so my imagination could take flight. I have written about some of these *teachers;* others I just hold dear in my heart. Yet, they are all part of who I am, a part of what I *know* to be true, a part of what I wish to share with you today.

My perspective comes from years of experience and exposure to many great teachers. Some in formal settings, others in informal; some in person, others in writings. I remember, for example, an interaction I once had with Carl Rogers. We were exiting a lecture hall, talking superficially about the conference we were attending. I turned to him and said something about how much I appreciated his work, elaborating on how much I valued his attitudes and teachings. He stopped, looked me in the eye, humbly thanked me for my "kind words," and then went on to say that he was just doing what he was meant to do. That he did not intend to tell people how to live their lives or how to teach or practice; he was just sharing with us some of what he had learned. And then he added that he was happy if I benefited from his work, but that he was the one who had learned the most.

I learned more about teaching and learning in that 2-3 minute interaction than I had in the previous three days at the conference, and it didn't stop there; the importance of what he said has deepened with time. As humans, we are inherently prone to growth; it occurs throughout life when, by serendipity, we make new discoveries or develop insights about what we know. It also occurs when we purposefully seek knowledge, sometimes in formal settings, sometimes not. I have concluded that great teachers never intend to teach, but instead, aim to facilitate others in their own quest. This holds true for those who are formal educators and those who teach by the way they live.

> I know, now, that *to be a teacher* I must focus on *facilitating the student to learn.* Although we talk about teaching content which addresses specific course objectives, I think this is ineffective if we don't first consider the readiness of the learner. When we focus on the learning process (rather than the teaching activities), we encourage our audience to be active participants in the process, not passive recipients of our lecture.

Accommodation and Assimilation

Years ago, I attended a conference advertised to teach beginners *all there is to know about stress.* The speakers were all considered experts on stress and adaptation. We attended one of the sessions advertised as "Scientific Explanations of Stress." One of my colleagues, a well-respected professor, who had a basic understanding of Selye's work on stress, attended the session with me. The speaker spent three hours describing some rather simple concepts on mind-body relations *using psychoneuroimmunology* (PNI) as the science for explaining his hypotheses. Although the session had been advertised as a discussion on stress and the effects of stress on the body, the lecturer never once used the word *stress* or any of the other words used by Selye to describe the Stress-Adaptation-Syndrome (Selye, 1976). Rather than starting with *pieces of information* consistent with Selye's work, he used words unknown to my colleague; he discussed bio-psychological interactions using current PNI literature and posed related rhetorical questions.

Since I was well versed in the psychoneuroimmunology literature and had been thinking along the same lines, I was able to follow his lecture and the rhetorical questions he posed; I was excited about what I had heard. My colleague, interested but unread on PNI literature, turned to me as we left the lecture hall, saying, "I heard everything he said. I don't have the foggiest idea what any of it meant, so it went in one ear and out the other. I've just wasted my time and my money. I should have gone to a different lecture."

Others around us agreed with her; it seemed that many were disappointed that they hadn't had the learning experience they had anticipated. When I restated what I'd learned in the lecture, using what I thought my colleague knew about Selye's work, she looked astounded, and said, "That's what he said? *I didn't hear him say that at all!* You should have given the lecture!"

This raises two problems commonly seen in formal teaching-learning situations: First, the lecturer failed to start with language common to the audience. As a result, participants were unable to *recall, comprehend, integrate or use what they had heard.* That is, the teacher presented content without an understanding of the potential learner's readiness to learn. Add to this the second issue, previous learning of the audience. While most of the audience had a cursory understanding of the concept of stress, they lacked the information for a related concept, psychoneuroimmunology. As a result, they were unable to accommodate their cognitive schema to assimilate the new information. While the learners may have *learned* about the lecturer and about themselves, what they learned was not cognitive information that would complement their understanding of their disciplines. Bruner argued that learning to *know* is best done by discovery methods—methods which focus on the learners' needs and their ability to accommodate and assimilate new information (1965, 1966, 1967, 1968, 1986, 1996).

> Just as the caring-healing process is without purpose unless the focus is on *facilitating healing*, the teaching-learning process is a waste unless the focus is on *facilitating learning.*

About Bruner's Discovery-Learning Methods

Bruner believed that the instructor must be interested in helping the student develop skills that provide a base for future learning, and should focus on the *process of learning, not just the presentation of content.* He argued that the intent of teaching is to involve the student in the learning process, and that active learning helps the learner make the transition from *learning* to *thinking*. He explained that this instructional model requires that educators *structure knowledge* in such a way that learners can understand what we want them to know, integrate the *pieces of information,* and create new understandings. He stated that the knowledge acquired should lead to interest in the learning process, and curiosity about what is *yet to be learned*. He stated that

> *a curriculum should involve the mastery of skills that in turn, lead to the mastery of more powerful ones, the establishment of self-reward sequences....The reward of deeper understanding is a more robust lure to effort than we have yet realized....If there is a way of adjusting to change, it must include the development of a meta-language and meta-skills for dealing with continuity in change....It has to do with the need for studying the possible rather than the achieved.* (1967, p. 35)

Later, Bruner said, "It matters not what we have learned, but what we can do with what we have learned (1966, p. 29). He argued that students learn best by "discovering" new knowledge. The idea is that faculty members should have a clear understanding of what they want their students to learn, should tell them what they are going to learn, and then guide them to *discover* what they wanted them to know. He proposed that the learning which occurs through discovery methods results not only in *new knowledge*, but also in *a way of knowing that can be used again and again.*[1] It also helps the student learn how to learn, and how to shift from extrinsic to intrinsic rewards. Moreover, it helps to conserve memory and facilitates retrieval.

Table 5.1 Principles for teachers interested in Bruner's model, extrapolated from his work.

1. Meet learning preconditions.
2. Decrease competition and facilitate cooperation.
3. Break content into small units and sequence learning experiences.
4. Facilitate "chunking" of information.
5. Personalize knowledge.
6. Encourage intuition.
7. Facilitate identification and labeling of intuitive knowledge.
8. Clarify differences between inductive and deductive thinking.
9. Encourage retroduction.
10. Resolve intrinsic and extrinsic conflicts
11. Pace positive reinforcements.
12. Minimize negative reinforcements.
13. Guide discovery.
14. Teach discovery as a means *and* end for learning.
15. Encourage curiosity, being aware of being aware.

Bruner's model of Discovery-Learning includes four major components and related sub-components. The first deals with factors that address the students' predisposition toward learning. Accordingly, faculty members need to consider

[1] Assuming that nurses need to learn how to use the *ways-of-knowing* discussed in previous chapters, Bruner's discovery-learning methods might be important to nurse educators.

Table 5.2 Components, subcomponents, characteristics and potential strategies based on Bruner's discovery-learning model.

	Sub-components	Characteristics	Strategies
PREDISPOSITION	1. Act of Learning	a)Acquisition of knowledge	Pace; break into small units; chunk information.
		b)Transformation of knowledge	Personalize; present knowledge in several ways (Piaget)
		c) Evaluation of new knowledge	Follow Bloom's Taxonomy for formative evaluation.
	2. Motivation	a) Intrinsic	Reinforce past learning; encourage intuition and curiosity.
		b) Extrinsic	Focus on learning, not teaching; reinforce discovery; reframe "failures."
	3. Cognitive facilitators	a) Activation	Stimulate curiosity; provide security for exploratory behaviors.
		b) Maintenance	Critique, don't criticize; support, don't ridicule; maximize strengths.
		c) Pacing	Consider students' worldview; expect that students want to learn.
		d) Direction	Challenge, don't threaten. Specify nursing, not personal goals; use models to demonstrate concepts; decrease competition.
STRUCTURE OF LEARNING	1. Mode of representation	a) Enactive	Use concrete examples, e.g. anatomy, physiology, Selye, etc.
		b) Iconic	Use graphic presentations, show relationships among parts.
		c) Symbolic	Use alpha-numeric presentations and measurements.
	2. Economy		Use memory-learning theory; e.g., no more than 7 + or - 2 pieces of information at a time.
	3. Effective powers		Chunk, condense, and recode information.
SEQUENCING OF KNOWLEDGE			State/restate problem, expectations; organize knowledge so it can be built upon. Explain relation of course to curriculum; describe retroductive processes.
NATURE AND PACING OF REINFORCEMENT			Use positive reinforcement; reinforce for corrective purposes, not punitive; Link reinforcement with behavior ASAP; Reinforce when and where information can be used to learn.

their potential students as they plan their course content and presentations. The second component of Bruner's model deals with the way in which faculty structure the learning process. The third component deals with the sequencing of knowledge; and the last component addresses the nature and pacing of reinforcements. Each of these contains sub-components and specific characteristics important to the learning process. Table 5.1 above, provides general guidelines for discovery-learning methods. These will be addressed more fully as we discuss the four components of Bruner's model, shown in Table 5.2 above.

Predisposition Toward Learning

Bruner argued that educators who aim to help students learn *how to think* about their observations, to *jump the gap from learning to thinking*, must attend first to the students' predisposition to learning before structuring the learning process. In other words, before we start teaching content, we need to focus on our learners, consider their biases or inclinations toward learning, and consider cultural, motivational, and personal factors that influence the need to plan strategies to contend with these preconditions, including negative attitudes and fatigue.

My experience with undergraduate students supports these premises. I've learned that beginning students are often fearful that they don't know enough to interact with a patient and that seniors are "*tired of being taught*." Paradoxically, the beginning student doesn't understand that nursing is based in a relationship, and that the most important thing they will ever offer a patient is their own time and caring. On the other hand, seniors often think that they have learned what they need to know to practice, and now, they need to *just practice.* At the same time, faculty members often perceive that they have a great deal to teach their students. They think it is their responsibility to deepen their students' experience, increase their competency, and ensure that they are ready for "the real world."

According to Bruner, educators have a responsibility to respect what students *already* know, to activate their curiosity and interest in discovering new perspectives about what they already know, and to help them develop *thinking* skills necessary for continuous learning. He proposed three major factors which need to be considered when planning at this phase in course development. They include the act of learning, motivation and cognitive facilitators, all of which are discussed below.

The Act of Learning

Acquisition of knowledge. When thinking about *learning* and what it is, we have to think about the *acquisition of knowledge* or what helps students acquire new knowledge. From this perspective, Bruner says that the instructor's first responsibility is to ensure that students are clear about the expected outcome of the course. If students are not clear about what they are expected to learn, it is easy for them to get lost in the process! At the same time, it is important to reassure the students that they *already know what they need to be successful students*. They just need to add to their repertoire of knowledge, learn new ways to use it, and learn when to use it. And, they need to be reassured that they can learn what is necessary—that it will happen a bit at a time.

When we use these simple techniques, we remind students that they have already learned how to learn, that they have already acquired the knowledge needed for them to build on, and that they are competent learners. Sample statements about past learning experiences and current expectations that stimulate curiosity can be found in Table 5.3.

Table 5.3 Examples of statements used to facilitate the acquisition and transformation of knowledge.

Statements used to encourage curiosity.	•You have repeatedly demonstrated that you can learn; there is no reason to believe that it will be different this time. You many not remember, but there was a time when you didn't know the ABCs, and now you can read full sentences! •It will be fun for you to discover something new, perhaps about yourself, and certainly about your profession. •I don't know what you will discover as you journey through this class, but I do know that it can be fun for you; that you can do it without being distressed. All you have to do is let yourself learn!
Statements used to encourage transformation of knowledge.	•You already know what you need to know to be successful; now you need to learn how to reorganize what you already know. •You have a lot of knowledge that you haven't begun to think about. •Soon, you'll discover how what you already know can be used elsewhere.

Pacing. *Pacing* involves teaching content in a way and at a rate so that the student can learn it. It involves understanding the student's readiness and ability to learn new content. Pacing the student's learning experience seems obvious, but it isn't. While some faculty members are inherently focused on the student's world-view and ability to learn, others are more focused on teaching. Pacing requires that faculty know where they want the student to go, and simultaneously, fully understand where the student has been *and where the student is at the moment of teaching.* Simply stated, if educators want *to lead* students to a level and depth of understanding, then they have to *pace* the students first. Pacing always precedes leading.

There are two aspects to pacing. The first is to pace the students' rate of learning. This is done so that learners do not get overwhelmed with what they need to learn. It is like learning to drive a car; you can't drive fast until you have mastered the skills, knowledge and attitudes necessary to drive slowly! Moreover, you can't drive too fast if you want to avoid a crash. And, of course, our goal is to help students learn how to be *curious about the process* and interested in *how* to learn, not to have them crash and burn before they leave school! Therefore, faculty members are responsible for pacing the students' *rate of learning*.

The learner's world-view is the second consideration when pacing the learning experience. That is, pacing requires that the instructor understands the learning experience from the learner's perspective. There are two key reasons why learners might perceive an experience differently from the instructor. The first is because they have different life philosophies. We discussed this in Chapter 2. I only mention it here to remind the reader of its importance when trying to teach our students what we want them to know. When faculty and students have differing world-views, any single observation can be experienced differently. As discussed in previous chapters, it is important for faculty to clarify their own world-view, so they can understand their students' world-view. Otherwise, they will have difficulty communicating with one another—a prerequisite to pacing a student's learning experience.

It is also important for faculty to be able to recognize behaviors related to various ways-of-knowing, so they can understand a student's behavior. While most nurses practice using Carper's Ways-of-Knowing, there are times when a situation reminds us of an earlier experience. At such times, personal knowledge acquired from prior learning emerges; many students don't know what to do with it. *They need help transforming the knowledge—a prerequisite to reframing the experience.* If faculty members aren't alert to such teaching opportunities, they might not pace the student, and when this happens, the faculty loses the opportunity to facilitate important learning. Let me provide an example.

> *The non-responsive, elderly person lying in the hospital bed was approaching death. Her vitals were gradually slowing down as her body shut down; she was in renal shut-down and her potassium level was rising. The room was dimly lit by a nightlight, but bright enough so that all the monitors in the room could easily be seen. The oxygen saturations, vitals, etc., were obvious from the bright green lights. The monitor alarms had been turned off—no need to hear the constant beep-beep-beep of the alarm because either the oxygen was getting too low or the pulse was declining. Instead, the room was filled with songs loved by the patient playing quietly in the background. The family knew that it was only a matter of time. Her wishes had been discussed with the doctors and the evening nurses; now it was time to simply comfort her, be with her, and let nature take its course. The aim was to create a quiet, peaceful*

environment which would facilitate the patient's transition. Her daughter, an older, experienced nurse sat with her. We'll call her Doreen.

It was 12:30 at night—time for shift change. Ann, a young nurse who had graduated a few months before, entered the room for the first time. She looked around, then walked over and turned on a bright light and turned down the music, stating that she needed to be able to see. She then proceeded to examine all the machines, taking note of their recordings, charting them carefully. She turned back to the bed, straightened the sheets, failing to touch her patient. Then she bent down, squatting at the bedside, supposedly looking at the empty drainage bag; the patient had not produced any urine in over 12 hours.

Doreen sat in a chair on the opposite side of the bed, watching. No words were exchanged between the two nurses. Ann remained in a squatting position for several seconds, seconds that turned into minutes. The daughter, frustrated that Ann seemed to be focused on the things in the room, but seemed to show no interest in facilitating a peaceful transition, finally asked her what she was doing. The young nurse mumbled something about the catheter bag. Doreen stated that it was empty, that there had been no output for several hours, that the goal now was to comfort the patient, to facilitate her in her journey. She suggested that it was time for her (Ann) to finish up so that the lights could be turned down and the music restored. The young nurse didn't move, didn't respond. Irritated, Doreen walked around the bed, ready to confront Ann and demand that she finish up and leave. As she approached the young nurse, she noted that she was sitting on the floor! What nurse sits on a dirty floor and then goes and takes care of other patients! What was she thinking? And then she noticed that she had her face in her hands. WHAT WAS SHE DOING?

And then she noticed that Ann was wiping her eyes, wiping her nose, crying quietly. Doreen bent down and pulled Ann to her, asking if it was her first time. The young nurse responded that this was her first patient, but not the first time she'd seen someone dying. She stated that her grandmother had died two months before, and that this lady reminded her of her grandmother. She added that she, as the nurse in the family, had to be strong, not cry, and help the family get through their loss.

Doreen recognized the importance of the situation for Ann, and thought that she needed an opportunity to express her personal needs, so she could learn and become what she had the potential to be—a loving, compassionate nurse who could be in a relationship with patients, even as they were dying. Doreen said that it is important to know many things and things in many ways, and to build on past experiences. She went on to tell

Ann that she would soon learn how to facilitate others in their natural life journey, even when it was hard. Ann wept quietly for a few seconds, then embarrassed, pulled herself away, stating that she was sorry, that she just couldn't help herself. She said that she would try to behave herself and be a better nurse, but then started to cry again.

Doreen told Ann that her only problem was that she hadn't yet learned what it meant to be a good nurse, but that she <u>*would*</u> *learn. She suggested that she just needed to discover that we can't always change another person's journey—we can't change their journey, but we can join them; we can comfort them as they continue on their journey, and we can learn as we go. Doreen continued, stating that life is like a cherry pie; if you eat the pie, you are likely to find some pits. You just have to learn how to distinguish the pits from the rest of the pie, spit them out, and keep going. She then suggested that Ann might want to take the patient's hand and tell her how honored she was to be with her that night, that she'd do what she could to make her comfortable, and that she'd always remember her. Doreen reminded Ann that people* <u>*can*</u> *hear what is being said right up until they transcend.*

The young nurse was relieved. She stood up, dried her eyes, dimmed the light, restored the music, and then went to the patient. She spent several minutes gently providing comforting measures such as applying lip-chap, wiping her mouth with glycerin, turning her body, fluffing her pillows, etc. Finally, she took her hand and talked to her. When she was finished, she turned to the daughter, hugged her and asked if she could do anything for her. Doreen thanked Ann and then asked her if she had learned anything new by caring for her mother. The nurse immediately responded that she had learned that it was okay to have feelings, to care about what she is doing, and that she wouldn't be a very good nurse if she didn't let herself feel. And then she added that she knew that she would be a good nurse someday, because now she knew how to comfort people even when they were dying. She commented that she no longer felt helpless, but instead thought she could learn to be a good nurse. Doreen confirmed that indeed she had demonstrated that she could learn, and that she was already a good nurse. She told Ann that she would continue to learn about herself, about nursing, and about her relationship with her patients, and as she did, she would get better and better, and some day, she would be able to teach a young nurse something when she needed help learning.

Interestingly, Doreen received a card from Ann two years later, stating that she had not forgotten what had happened two years before. Ann added that she hoped Doreen was doing well, and thanked her for helping her "discover her calling." She ended by saying that she had become a hospice nurse and loved what she was doing.

Pacing requires that the instructor, mentor or teacher focuses on the learners' immediate experience, and builds on that, one piece at a time. If Doreen, in the above example, had reprimanded the younger nurse for her unprofessional behavior, told her to toughen-up, or simply ignored her, the young nurse *would have learned*, but not what she needed to learn in order to become what she had the potential to be. Rather than to learn that she had the potential to become a competent, compassionate, holistic nurse, she would have probably learned to isolate her feelings and detach herself from the needs of others. She may have missed her chance to learn how to be *in a relationship with a client*—the essence of Nursing.

Fortunately and unfortunately, people learn from every experience. Our responsibility, as educators, is to try to remember what we want them to learn, and then to pace the learning experience so they can learn it. This is fortunate because it offers us hope that people can become what they want, *if* they are facilitated. It is unfortunate, because without assistance people often learn to withdraw from relationships, to isolate and protect themselves.

Learning a piece at a time. The way we structure content is also an important consideration related to the *act of learning.* Content should be broken down into small units, so that the student can master the pieces of information before trying to link them or comprehend what they create when linked together. Bruner calls this *breaking content into units* and then *chunking* it once it has been learned. He stated that educators often try to teach complex concepts (and sometimes even constructs) without ever identifying the parts. When this happens, the student is left to make meaning out of the learning, without ever understanding the relationship.

People learn through both inductive and deductive processes. Small children learn initially by inductive processes. Let's use the example of a child observing a dog for the first time. The dog approaches the child; he has never seen a dog before. The dog sticks out its tongue and licks the child's hand. The child notices parts of the dog. He sees the tongue, the nose, and the eyes of the dog. The mother tells the child it is a *dog.* Now the child has a label for the "thing" he has seen; the tongue, nose, eyes is a *dog!* A few days later, when the mother and child are out for a walk, something new appears in the child's line of vision. It has a tail, four legs, and ears. Mom calls it a *dog*! The child combines all of the parts; now a *dog* includes a tongue, nose, eyes, tail, four legs, and ears. The child has taken the parts and chunked them together; he has learned a new concept. The next day they go out again and "Aha-ha!" He spies a dog. He knows it is a dog because it has a tongue, nose, eyes, tail, four legs, and ears, all arranged in about the same order! He points and says, "Dog." The mother laughs and says, "No. That is a cat." The child has learned inductively that the parts can be put together to create a new whole—that together, the parts create an idea which differs from the parts. Since he has also learned that the "whole" is called a dog, he knows how to recognize a dog. Until he learns that there are more parts (such as the sound they make) that distinguishes a dog from a cat, the child will continue to call other animals who have a tongue, nose, eyes, tail, four legs, and ears, a *dog*.

Breaking content into small units enables the instructor to guide the student to "discover" how the parts fit together to create new concepts. It also enables the instructor to help the student *learn how to think* about the parts—how, when linked together, they create something new. When educators are purposeful in their instruction, linking parts to create a whole, they also teach students *how to think about learning*!

Chunking. It is interesting to note that many educators understand the idea of breaking content into parts, but forget to help students chunk it back together or integrate it with new knowledge. That is, students are often required to learn information considered basic to the practice of Nursing, but they fail to know what to do with such knowledge. Instead, they think that the learning process is just a "hoop" to jump through, a step required to prove that they can learn, etc. For example, nearly all Nursing schools require that students take basic science courses such as chemistry, biochemistry, anatomy and physiology; yet, many upper level students say that they don't remember what they learned, and that they don't use it. The truth is that they probably do use what they have learned, but they aren't very purposeful or creative in their use of previously acquired knowledge. Furthermore, because they frequently fail to see the relations among the pieces of information, they aren't very efficient learners. They have trouble using higher level thinking processes described by Bloom and described in the previous chapter (Table 4.6, p. 81).

One way to help students to chunk information is to assign readings which provide concrete pieces of information about a concept discussed in class. When students are able to associate the pieces of information with the larger concept, they are able to recode the pieces. They are no longer seen as isolated pieces of information, but as part of a bigger concept. According to Bruner, students acquire *effective power* when selected readings help them recognize and recode past learning. Recoding is necessary, as it helps students to chunk information. That is, recoding helps students take *pieces* of information and chunk them together to create a new single piece of information. As a result of recoding, students have fewer pieces of information to juggle at any given time. It helps them be more effective problem-solvers.

An important teaching strategy is to break new knowledge (including skills and attitudes) into multiple parts, so that the student can easily learn them.

Once the parts are learned, the educator assists the student in chunking it together to create concepts and constructs.

Transformation of Knowledge

The second factor to consider is facilitating students to learn, so that they can *transform what they have learned and discriminate its appropriate use in other situations.* Specifically, the instructor's responsibility is to facilitate the students' ability to adapt what they have learned, so they can appropriately apply it to new situations. ***Personalizing knowledge*** is one strategy faculty can use to help students acquire the skills necessary to apply what they have learned, and to be able to distinguish *when* it is appropriate to apply it.

Personal knowing. While this may seem obvious, it is not. The story about Doreen and Ann, above, is a good example of personalizing knowledge. In this case, Ann needed help in recoding information and reframing past experiences. Since learning is a personal experience, it is important to help students build on past experiences to acquire new knowledge. Sometimes when we personalize knowledge, it surprises the learner, opening them to discover new information and deepening their ways-of-knowing. As stated by Wood, Bruner, and Ross, "*The triumph of effective surprise is that it takes one beyond common ways of experiencing the world....Creative products have this power of reordering experience and thought ...*" (1976, p. 22).

Personalizing knowledge can be done by encouraging students to build on what they already know at multiple levels, to use various ways-of-knowing, to make educated guesses, and to evaluate their understanding. Before students can take advantage of this strategy, they have to be in an environment where they feel safe to use their personal knowing and intuition, to be inductive and creative. They have to be assured that they have the freedom to learn, to make mistakes, and to adjust their thinking.

Piaget's cognition. A related faculty consideration is the language used to present new information. Piaget has described various levels of understanding, ranging from sensorimotor to abstract. Faculty members often present abstract ideas without breaking them into parts, discussing them from a perspective that the learner can understand, or even from their cognitive way of thinking. Students who are very concrete thinkers (Erickson, et al., 1983/2009, pp. 63-68) tend to see things as very discrete pieces of information; they are "black" or "white." There are no gray areas. For these nurses, information is right or wrong, good or bad. When instructors present new ideas, students can understand what is being taught if the instructors repeat the content using language consistent with Piaget's cognitive levels of understanding. This facilitates comprehension—a prerequisite to application, discrimination, and/or evaluation of knowledge.

Evaluation of Knowledge Acquired

Students need consistent feedback to help them determine whether they are learning, and educators need to have some means of evaluating whether they have learned. The problem is how to evaluate honestly and accurately without interfering with the students' natural drive to learn. Formative evaluation is one option that works. Content is broken down into small parts, designed to go from Bloom's lower level domains of learning to higher levels. Learning is then assessed or evaluated at each step. Both faculty and students must be clear about the criteria used for evaluation. That is, faculty must understand what they want their students to learn, and students must be clear about the criteria that will be used to evaluate them. Bruner states that formative evaluation helps students to assess their own mastery, to pace their learning, and to identify learning difficulties. It also helps faculty identify points of instruction where students need additional assistance.

Feedback. According to Bruner, evaluation isn't nearly as important as feedback. This is because feedback is what the student will learn from, and *that* should be the reason for evaluation. Some faculty members perceive that they carry the burden of ensuring that their students are adequate to progress, so they must be careful, and sometimes, harsh evaluators. The irony of this perception is that most students have been admitted to their institutions because their credentials indicate that they have already learned what they need in order to be successful in the institution. So in most cases, faculty can relax and enjoy their teaching, knowing that their job is to facilitate learning, and not be on the lookout for those who haven't learned properly.

Evaluation is often viewed as a test of effectiveness or ineffectiveness—of materials, teaching methods, or whatnot—but this is the least important aspect of it. The most important is to provide intelligence on how to improve these things (Bruner, 1965/1971, p. 166).

Just as Bruner said that content to be learned should be broken down into small units, he argued that evaluation should evaluate what has been learned, unit by unit. Furthermore, feedback should occur as close to the learning time as possible. It should be done with positive comments, remembering to critique, not criticize. It is important to point out which learning criteria have been met and which have not. It is also important to use evaluation comments which encourage learners to continue to try. Chapter 10 in the next section will provide examples of how to evaluate students without criticism.

Guiding Future Growth. I have one final comment about evaluation. Through the years, I have encountered a number of students who have not met end-goal criteria in the required period of time. Sometimes they had difficulty with a class, and sometimes it was with the program. Some would say that they failed either the class or out of the program.

I have learned that most people are receptive to an evaluation of their learning when it is done with respect for the person and stated in a way as to encourage future learning. While we have a responsibility to the community to ensure that nurses who graduate from our programs are competent nurses, we also have a responsibility to our students to help them explore alternatives, to encourage them to find ways to accomplish their life-goals, and to seek outside assistance if and when needed. A student I worked with years ago serves as an example.

> *This student graduated from her high school close to the top of the class and entered the School of Nursing the following fall. The first year was uneventful; she took basic and behavioral courses and did fine. Then, the second year she entered Nursing courses including pathophysiology, biochemistry, clinical nursing, and others. She floundered and failed courses the first semester. She was advised that she had to repeat two courses and increase her GPA. The alternative would be dismissal from the program. She again failed the courses specific to Nursing. Her GPA was unacceptable for continuation in the program.*
>
> *When I called her into my office to discuss the situation, she looked very nervous, upset, and ready to cry. My first interaction was to ask her if she knew why she had been asked to come see me. She responded that she had failed, and she was going to have to leave. I responded that I did want to see her about her future, and after we had talked about the courses she'd taken at the university we could discuss what we should do next. Then, I commented about the courses she'd successfully completed and commented that obviously, when we offered her something that interested her, she did very well. I waited for her response. She commented that she really liked the courses I'd mentioned. I then said that she hadn't been as successful in some of the other courses, and I wondered if she knew why. She immediately commented that she was a failure as a nurse. I responded by saying that she was not a failure; she just hadn't successfully completed the courses. I then pointed to a sign in my office that said, "There are no failures, only discoveries." I asked her what she thought about that. She commented that she didn't really know why she wanted to be a nurse—maybe it was because she didn't know what else to do with her life. And then she added that she'd discovered that she didn't like being a nurse and now she wasn't going to be one. I complemented her on making an important discovery, suggested that her learning had only begun, that now that she knew, she could be successful if she chose the right path, and that it would be fun for her to discover what she really did*

want to be. I added that most university students changed their majors at least one time, some as many as four or five, and that she was on her way to finding something that worked for her.

She smiled and thanked me, left my office looking quite different from when she arrived. My secretary came in and asked me if I had told her she could stay another semester. I said that I had just told her that discoveries are important, and that she was on her way to discovering what she would become. She has kept in touch through the years and is now a principal at an elementary school. From what I hear, she is loved and respected by those who work for her because she is smart and knows how to help her teachers and students do their best.

The example above is not unusual. As an administrator, it has been my responsibility to inform a number of students that they had not successfully achieved end-goal criteria of a Nursing program. I've also had a number that have failed my classes. It happens. Sometimes good people are in the wrong place at the right time. It is not my job to tell them that they are failures, but to help them learn about themselves, identify their strengths, and find alternative pathways. It is all a matter of remembering that all humans have a need for dignity, self-respect, and esteem from others. As persons in a powerful position, educators need to remind themselves, periodically, of their long-term goal, and act accordingly.

Motivation

Motivation is the second major consideration when planning for students. The first major component of Bruner's model was the students' *Predisposition Toward Learning*. According to Bruner, there are both intrinsic and extrinsic factors that affect students' motivation to learn. Supposedly, as students develop a sense of learning for its own intrinsic value, competition among group members decreases and cooperation increases.

Intrinsic Motivation. Our goal as educators is to encourage the learner to develop an internal desire to problem-solve and continue learning. When we do that, students enjoy learning; they jump the gap from learning to thinking. Although learning for the sake of learning is natural to us, many external factors can impede an individual's development of an intrinsic reward system. For example, when students spend time and energy trying to determine what they should learn, they focus on what they think the teacher wants them to know, rather than thinking about what they want to learn. As a result, they focus on external rewards for learning and fail to develop an internal desire to problem-solve. Paradoxically, the reward for learning is crossing the gap from learning to thinking. The faculty's responsibility is to help students resolve the conflict that exists between internal and external rewards. When people are paralyzed by fear of failure, they have few resources left for successful discovery. I have often reminded students that there are no dumb questions, only basic questions important for their learning, and that there are no failures when we aim to learn about learning—there can only be discoveries.

The example provided above, under *Guiding Future Growth*, is one where the intent was to increase the student's internal motivation for learning, even as she was being informed that she had to *change her major*. Guidelines or principles already listed in Table 5.1 and other strategies shown in Table 5.2 and 5.3 help faculty remember that their goal is to motivate their students to be active learners.

Extrinsic Motivation. Just like intrinsic motivation, external motivation can be based on both positive and negative reinforcement. Often students enter Nursing because they want to be like someone else who happens to be a nurse, or because someone in their family wants them to be a nurse. When an individual perceives that another has a power base, they tend to feel pressured by the "desires" of that other person. This might mean that they become nurses because of another, or that they want to do well in a class because of an instructor. Facilitating students to learn for the benefit of learning, and not to please another person, is essential for successful discovery learning. This means that educators need to consider their own attitudes toward learners, and to ask themselves whether there is more than one way to learn, more than one way to carry out a technique, or more than one way to practice professional Nursing?

If the answer is no, then discovery learning methods do not fit with that faculty member's view of the world. On the other hand, consider how many ways there are to touch your nose. Or say, "Hello." Is one way better than another? Why? Extrinsic motivation is very powerful. Educators who use discovery-learning methods will have no doubt that there are many ways to do any one thing. What is important is how a student thinks about what they are doing, and why.

I have one last example to illustrate this issue. I remember an incident that demonstrates how often students learn to apply knowledge, but don't learn how to adapt it to new situations. This happened many years ago.

> *A group of students had learned about "clean technique," and were taught that when transferring "dirty objects" from one room to another, they should cover a tray of instruments (to prevent contamination of the air/environment), back out through the swinging doors (to prevent touching the door), and go into the next room, i.e., the treatment room.*

One student, known by her classmates as an A+ student because she could memorize and recite everything, was asked to demonstrate "clean technique." She was told that the treatment room door was open. Nevertheless, after careful preparation of her dirty tray for transportation, she proceeded toward the treatment room door, turned and backed into the open door! We all gasped! The instructor asked her why she had done that. Didn't she realize that the door was open? She responded that she was following protocol; she had followed the steps precisely. The instructor asked her to think about it, and do it again. She tried two more times, each time repeating the exact steps she demonstrated the first time. Finally, the instructor told her to stop and asked one of her classmates what she had done wrong. The classmate explained that when the door was open, it was a waste of energy to back in and it might confuse anyone coming out, precipitating an accident. The student was mortified. She was always so intent on being perfect, doing what the instructor told her to do, that she had difficulty using what she knew in new and/or appropriate ways.

The student in this latter example had developed strong extrinsic motivation for her work. Although she was very intelligent and had the potential to think about what she was learning, she was unable to adapt to a simple piece of information, i.e. *the door being open.*

Motivation *to learn and think* is facilitated when students are encouraged to use their intuition, make educated guesses, and test and evaluate them. When this happens, students learn to think about their observations, uncover knowledge they are unaware of, and discover new knowledge.

Cognitive Facilitators

The third consideration important to understanding the students' Predisposition for Learning is described as "Cognitive Facilitators" by Bruner. Cognitive facilitators can be thought of as the strategies and techniques used to facilitate students to learn and to think about what they have learned. Accordingly, Bruner states that there are four dimensions of cognitive facilitators: *activation, maintenance, pacing* and *direction.*

Activation. To some degree, we've already discussed activation of learning. Most important here is that we stimulate curiosity about what will be discovered. Keep in mind that we want our students to be curious about knowledge related to all ways-of-knowing, not just empirical or esthetic knowing. For example, we want them to be curious about the sciences which provide a context for Nursing and about themselves as professional people! Activation requires that we create a safe environment, one conducive to exploratory behaviors.

Maintenance. Once students have started to learn, it is important that we maintain an environment conducive to continued discovery. Usually, students involved in discovery processes are a little anxious. They aren't used to learning without first having the instructor explicitly tell them what they are supposed to learn! This creates a little tension and sometimes anxiety. During this time, faculty using discovery-learning methods will want to be careful to *critique* student learning and to *avoid criticizing* what they have not learned. Students need to know what they are doing well; they need to be supported for what they have learned. They never need to be embarrassed, ridiculed or discounted.

Sometimes students seem to learn more slowly than others; this doesn't mean that they can't or won't learn. Just as with other things in life, growth has to occur before development. Learning is like that, too. Often, students have to learn a lot of things before they can demonstrate that they have learned. This is because there are many ways of knowing. Students have to deepen their understanding about each of these in order to be able to demonstrate that they have learned. Faculty simply have to continue to support them, critique clearly and specifically, and be clear about what it is they want the students to learn.

Pacing. We have already discussed pacing. We now identify two issues important to pacing as a cognitive facilitator. First, it is important for faculty to remember that students want to learn, but they should also understand that students have differing worldviews regarding the importance of the information we want them to learn. While they may want to learn, they may not value what is being taught, or they may think that they have already learned it! This is an interesting problem when teaching concepts that seem to be common sense. For example, I've had many students tell me that they think learning about communication is silly. After all, they've been communicating for years! Pacing is important if we are to help these students learn that they don't know everything there is to know, and to help others discover that they already know what they need, they just don't know that they know!

Direction. The fourth Cognitive Facilitator identified by Bruner that is important to Predisposition Toward Learning is *Direction.* This means providing guidance, so that learning moves in the planned direction. Faculty can facilitate students' movement in the right direction by clearly stating and restating desired end-goals, providing examples so that students can understand the end goals, and by decreasing competition among students. The latter issue is important so that students will internalize their learning rather than learn for extrinsic reasons.

Structure of Learning

The second major component of discovery-learning methods is the Structure of the Learning process. According to Bruner, learning is structured so that students can build from concrete thinking to more abstract thinking. There are three sub-components related to how we structure learning. These are, the *mode of representation*, the *economy* of what is taught, and its *effective powers.*

Mode of Representation

When we think about the mode of representation, we have to decide how we want to present the information we want the students to learn. We can choose among three modes, going from simple to complex or from concrete to symbolic representations. Bruner calls these *enactive, iconic,* and *symbolic* modes.

Enactive to Iconic. When we aim to be concrete, we start with the most basic pieces of information and put them together in such a way as to create something new, and then expect the students to be able to imitate us. For example, we might demonstrate a set of skills and provide practice opportunities. When we want to build on concrete data, we might use an iconic mode of representation. This type of presentation includes the use of graphics or images to represent the skills; it summaries information. When using this mode of representation, it is important to stimulate as many of the five senses as possible. That is, it is important to show students graphically what is being presented, to carefully discuss it, to help them personalize the information, and internalize it as much as possible. To use this mode to present information we might use graphs, diagrams, and/or illustrations that represent a concept. Information presented as a summary or in the iconic mode never fully includes all the information about the concept. This is because some information is lost or glossed over when it is chunked together with other pieces of information. Faculty need to decide which is more important: learning at a higher level of thinking or being able to identify all the pieces of information embedded in the concept. Consider for example, teaching students the Creb Cycle. This is often done through illustrations, demonstrating the interactions among the parts. Keep in mind that when students learn this if they don't understand the parts and how they function, they are unable to understand the elegance of the Creb Cycle.

Symbolic mode. The symbolic mode of representation of information is even more abstract. It is usually presented as a formula or equation which symbolizes the aggregation of information and follows a set of rules. When students don't understand the basic set of rules that serve as an underpinning, they are often unable to use symbolically presented information. Although they can memorize and recall the symbols, they are unable to transform the knowledge, or to build on it. The television show, *Numbers* provides a great example of this problem with the use of symbolic representation for problem-solving. Charlie and his colleagues clearly understand the rules underlying each of the formulas he uses to problem-solve; they know how and when to use them, and they know how to evaluate their accuracy. Interestingly, other members of the cast always seem confused, but respectful. They don't understand, and they can't evaluate the merit of the solutions offered. A more practical, realistic example is the statistics class many students are required to take so they will be able to do research or understand research findings. For many, the statistics class is something to "get through," not something to use. Not many really understand the *workings* of a regressional analysis, even though most researchers use it to test their hypotheses!

Faculty should never present information symbolically unless students have already acquired comparable information through the use of concrete and summary modes of representation of knowledge. Simply stated, while there is merit in all three modes of representation of information, and we may use all three at different times, if we want our students to be able to do more than recall, recite, or describe information, we have to be careful about how we structure it.

Probably, our best bet is to try to encourage students to keep learning by the use of positive reinforcement and encouraging the internalizing of information. For example, we can tell students that our goal is to help them learn to think systematically, to use multiple ways-of-knowing, to integrate knowing and knowledge, and to be able to apply it in their professional practice. When this is coupled with an example that motivates their learning, you are not only informing the student that knowledge builds on knowledge, but that it can be enjoyed and used, even as it evolves. You are also helping them internalize their learning, to own it, and to enjoy the learning process. A motivational statement might be something like this:

> *Learning is like the unfolding of a shrub in the spring time. First you see the branches, then the buds, then flowers, then leaves. As you watch each part come into view, you will notice that as one emerges, the other changes. While you may call this plant a shrub, it is really much more than that. It is a living, evolving thing, just as your thoughts are evolving, growing, changing; they are real and can be used.*

Economy and Effective Powers

These two concepts add to the understanding of how information should be structured. According to Bruner, it is essential for faculty to structure knowledge so that there aren't too many pieces of information to "juggle" at any single point in time. As the student is able to "juggle" more pieces of information by "chunking" them together in a way that has personal and professional meaning, it becomes easier to acquire new knowledge, and to go to higher levels of thinking. The instructor's responsibility is to help the students to chunk information, and to make it *economical* to use so that it takes less energy to learn and to use. The more efficient the chunking, the easier it is to use and the greater its *effective power.* Along this line, assigned readings should not only provide concrete information, but also provide ways to recode and chunk past learning with current information. Bottom line: assigned readings should never be busy work, but should help increase the students' effective power.

Sequencing of knowledge

Sequencing of Knowledge, the third major component of Bruner's model is closely related to how information is structured. Both these components deal with how faculty members plan to present their courses. Faculty members consider their students' *predisposition toward learning,* described above, as they plan for the structure and sequence of content presentation. That is, there are relations among the four components that must be thought about throughout the planning and implementation processes of courses designed to facilitate student learning.

To be efficient, knowledge must be sequenced so that the learner can grasp, transform and transfer what is to be learned. Movement from concrete to abstract concepts is important in this process. That is, educators need to sequence information so that the learner goes from learning the pieces, to chunking information, to creating new concepts, and so forth. It must also be organized in such a way that the student can incorporate past learning, restructure it as necessary, aggregate, synthesize and create new knowledge.

> The key value in sequencing knowledge is to simplify the learning process, to generate new propositions, and to increase the students' ability to manipulate knowledge. Since how knowledge is structured depends on the status and gifts of the learner, how knowledge is sequenced is, too. The two, structuring and sequencing of knowledge are interactive, ongoing processes.

Nature and pacing of reinforcements

Bruner identified four major themes in his Discovery-Learning Model. It should be obvious by now that these themes are interwoven in such a way as to create a way for faculty to think about their work as educators. We've talked about three of them above. You may remember that the first component was labeled *Predisposition Toward Learning.* Some of the strategies we discussed under the first subcomponent, Act of Learning, included the idea of the use of pacing students' learning and the use of reinforcements. Here we need to reiterate the importance of pacing reinforcements for learning. Simply stated, it is important to continuously reinforce curiosity and interest in learning since the faculty's goal is to move the student from learning *how to do things* to learning how *to think about things*. This includes learning how to think about what they are doing! If students can learn to value their own perceptions and to think about what they are doing and observing, they can be taught how to label and articulate their experiences, to practice purposefully.

According to Bruner, it is important to use positive reinforcement for corrective purposes as well as for setting direction. Explicit statements reminding students of *their past learning experiences* and encouraging them to remember that they can learn as well today as they could *then, serve as a reinforcement for chunking.*

Table 5.4 provides a few considerations for faculty to keep in mind as they use Bruner's Discovery-Learning methods. Faculty may wish to embellish these with their own reminders.

Table 5.4 Reminders for faculty using Bruner's Discovery-Learning Methods.

1.	Constantly encourage and reinforce:
	•retroductive thinking
	•divergence in conceptualization
	•having fun learning
	•trusting perceptions and ability to aggregate/integrate
2.	Expect:
	•expressions of anxiety
	•frustration
	•delight in achievement
3.	Use directive statements repeatedly,
	•repeat, repeat, repeat

SUMMARY

Through the years, I have concluded that teaching per se is ineffective. What we have to do instead, is to focus on facilitating the student to learn. Although we talk about the teaching-learning process, we need to focus on their learning, and style our teaching accordingly. This chapter presented the four components of Bruner's discovery-learning model with some detail about each component and related sub-components. Two of the components, Predisposition Toward Learning and Nature of Pacing and Reinforcement addressed the students' readiness to learn and considered how faculty could build on these factors. The other two components, Structuring and Sequencing of Knowledge discussed the planning and implementation of the teaching of content. Relations among the four components are ongoing and spiral in nature so that what and how the faculty teaches is in constant play with how the students learn, i.e., their predisposition and what reinforces their learning. Our job as teachers is to facilitate the learner to *discover* what we want them to know! Discovery learning encourages learners to be active participants in the process, not passive recipients of our teaching. The next section expands on this chapter, describing processes that can used to teach students to learn how to think and to continue to learn, to learn how to deepen their ways-of-knowing, and to link knowledge with practice.

SECTION 2

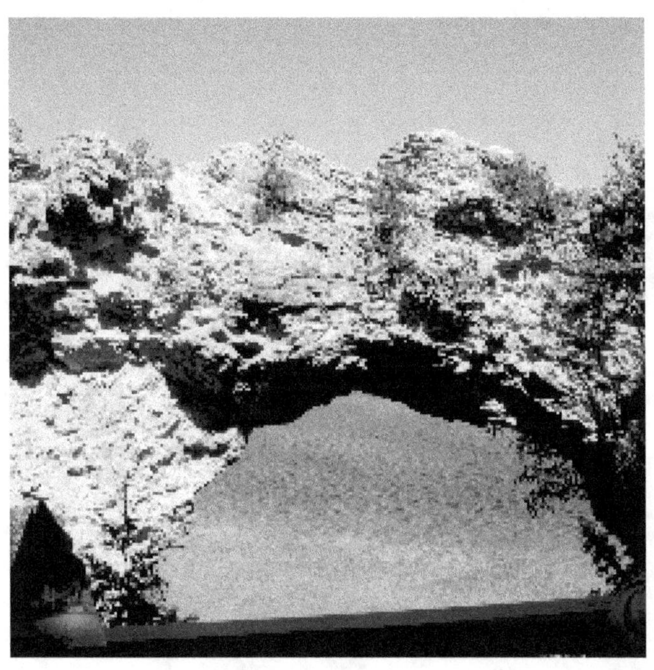

SECTION II

FACILITATING GROWTH

How can we prepare novices of our profession so they are not only competent, ethical practitioners, but also assertive, altruistic members of the profession, able to utilize Nursing's knowledge?

Nurse educators are challenged with the responsibility of teaching students how to think about and use Nursing's discipline. They also have the responsibility to assure the public that those who enter the profession are able to practice according to Nursing's values and ethics. These are daunting responsibilities. This section is designed to provide some help to those responsible for mentoring competent, ethical, altruistic holistic nurses. A special emphasis is placed on the use of Modeling and Role-Modeling (MRM), an extant holistic nursing theory (AHNA, 2007).

Chapter six discusses how to facilitate nurses to learn and integrate the MRM philosophy. Specific MRM concepts are addressed followed by a discussion of faculty considerations. Chapter seven discusses factors relevant to teaching undergraduate students how to implement MRM concepts. Although the text addresses teaching in an academic setting, the content is also relevant to those mentoring novices in the clinical setting. Chapter eight addresses factors important to graduate students' integration of knowledge.

Chapter 9 presents a discussion of a course taught using Bruner's Discovery Learning Methods. The aim of the faculty was to facilitate students' ability to synthesize and integrate what they had learned. The techniques and strategies described in this chapter have been used in numerous academic and clinical settings. Chapter 10 presents several factors that warrant consideration when evaluating the novice learner. This chapter, also written by an academic nurse leader, is relevant for those responsible for the evaluation of nurses in any setting.

Chapter 11 discusses factors related to teaching MRM in diverse cultural groups, in academic and clinical settings. Two of the authors spent several months in Taiwan, teaching MRM. All three have had experiences with diverse cultural groups. Chapter 12 discusses the importance of evidence-based practice, how it relates to the advanced practice holistic nurse, and offers suggestions on how to bring the two together.

CHAPTER 6

FACILITATING EXPLORATION OF THE MODELING AND ROLE-MODELING PHILOSOPHY

Helen L. Erickson

They must know that she cares for them even while she is checking them; or rather that she checks them because she cares for them... [The teacher] *may sometimes show a probationer the unspeakable importance of this year of her life, when she must sow the seeds of her future nursing in this world, and of her future life through eternity. For although future years are of importance to train the plant and make it come up, yet if there is no seed, nothing will come up.*
(Nightingale, 1915, p.14)

OVERVIEW

This chapter is designed to help those who wish to facilitate novices interested in learning about the philosophy of the Modeling and Role-Modeling (MRM) theory and paradigm. It addresses issues for educators to consider as they facilitate others in grasping the essence of the MRM philosophy.

The MRM philosophy and theory are not presented in this book, but in earlier publications (Erickson, H., 2006a; Erickson, et al., 1983/2009). This chapter addresses how faculty can help novices explore the MRM philosophy, compare it with their own, and decide if they wish to adopt it. First, a discussion on the essence of a philosophy is offered. This is followed by a discussion of three phases of the teaching-learning process which address how to stimulate interest and curiosity, initiate exploration, and facilitate growth in the learner.

THE ESSENCE OF A PHILOSOPHY: FRAMING OUR THOUGHTS

A philosophy is a very personal thing. *It is what we believe to be true;* sometimes others agree, sometimes they don't. A philosophy is not born in science, but comes from our life experiences. It isn't something we can teach, nor is it something we can force someone else to learn. We *can tell* people what they *have to* say, what they *have to* do, and even what they *have to* write, but we can't tell them what *to believe* no matter how hard we try. All we can do is to help others explore their own beliefs, and acquire insights about what they believe to be true.

Most of the time, we do not discuss our philosophy as a significant component of our learning. Nevertheless, it serves as an underpinning for what we think, a motivator for what we do, and an inspiration for what we want to learn. Educators interested in teaching the MRM theory and paradigm will need to consider some of the issues related to facilitating others to explore relationships among what they *know to be true* and the premises of MRM.

> The interesting thing about a personal philosophy is that most people don't talk about their own, but they act on it.

As educators, we are challenged with finding ways to stimulate interest and curiosity, initiate exploration, and facilitate growth in the learner. Each of these is discussed below. But first, it is important to revisit the concept of *power* raised in the first chapter. This is because the very nature of a teaching-learning experience creates a relationship. Faculty interested in teaching MRM need to remember that all humans have a need for affiliated-individuation (A-I). Therefore, the faculty-student relationship is designed to enhance the student's A-I with the faculty.

Remember the Context

While I discussed power bases from the systems perspective, the same concepts apply when we talk about a relationship between two people.[1] From this perspective, people who are viewed as having expertise, authority, or a legitimate status are also perceived as having a power base. This means that such people are *perceived* by others as having the potential or actual ability to affect their lives.

This issue of perceived power permeates everything else. When we are in formal educational settings, there are always legitimate and reward power bases; students know that we have the potential to determine what happens to them academically. Usually, students also perceive that we have expertise, and sometimes, they want to learn how to think like we do, adding referent power.

Our aim, from the MRM perspective, is to decrease students' external motivation for learning, while increasing their internal motivation. That is, we want to enhance their affiliation with us as their mentors or teachers, so they will

---

[1] The relationship between two people creates a system. This is the essence of what Watzlawick means when he says that communication between two people is an ongoing process, dynamic and evolving in nature (1967).

develop a strong sense of individuation as learners. This is the essence of the teacher-learner or faculty-student relationship.

This means that we need to use our power wisely. For example, expert power is appropriate when we are trying to facilitate the students' ability to learn, recite, and recall content. On the other hand, when we want them to explore their philosophies, our expertise is limited; we cannot be an expert on someone else's philosophy. You might ask, "How then, can faculty really grade a student's philosophy paper?" My response is that we cannot evaluate their beliefs *per se*, but we can evaluate how their beliefs compare to those held by Nursing, the school, and in our case, MRM.

Students have these possibilities in their minds when they interact with faculty. They are always concerned with the faculty's potential ability to affect them, reward them (or not), and impact their lives. This also holds true in other settings where the educator has some *perceived* relationship with the learner.

> We want to use our power bases wisely. Expert and referent powers are important, and with it, we can help people grow. Coercive power is counter-productive; it inhibits learning and impedes growth.

Educators who wish to stimulate interest and curiosity, initiate exploration and facilitate growth in the learner will want to be cognizant of how and when they use their power and which types they purposefully use. The type of power they use will determine the nature of the relationship they have with those they wish to teach or facilitate.

FACILITATING THE LEARNING PROCESS

Stimulate Curiosity and Interest

Being Aware

Unlocking Doors. All Nursing students come to Nursing with a set of beliefs about the nature of human beings although many have not consciously thought about them. Furthermore, most Nursing students and young nurses have never been challenged to think about how their beliefs relate to their practice, or Nursing's Standards and Code of Ethics. Many faculty members assume that people who choose to become nurses share a philosophy with Nursing. And, therefore, if they have chosen Nursing, their beliefs are consistent with those of MRM. But, this is not always the case.

I have learned that there are many who have always believed in and practice by a personal philosophy consistent with that of MRM. They rarely have any problems with either the philosophy or the theory. They are usually delighted to be able to put words to what they believe to be true, and usually embrace the MRM theory because it gives them a language that legitimizes their past nursing actions, and it helps them to be more proactive and purposeful in the future.

I have also learned that there are many who don't agree with the MRM philosophy. Most have not thought about it; nevertheless, they "just know" that they are uncomfortable with some of the practices we advocate in MRM. Some decide soon after our first interaction that MRM is not for them; others continue to stay connected and to ask questions. I believe that most of the time people ask questions (even defensive ones) or make comments because they are still interested in staying engaged in the discussion. They want to learn, but are not sure that they *really* want to accept what they have learned, or change what they believe, or how they practice.

> There is always a trade-off when we adopt new values and beliefs. In order to take on something new, we have to be ready to let go of competing values or beliefs. If we do not, we become ambivalent, and often retreat to what we know to *be true.*

As educators and mentors, our responsibility is to recognize the differences in individuals and to accept them as they are. We cannot change people, nor should we try. Instead, we should be aware of the differences among people and know that each person is on his or her own journey, learning and discovering what he or she needs to know to grow. Our responsibility is to recognize each person as worthy, offer ideas that might stimulate curiosity, and remember that curiosity will grow into something more in its own time. We cannot stop growth; it is inherent, and when nurtured, takes on a life of its own. Let me provide an example.

> *Years ago, I was sitting in a classroom with a group of doctoral students and faculty enrolled in an introductory course on Modeling and Role-Modeling (MRM). We had spent the previous few weeks discussing the philosophical underpinnings of MRM, and were now moving on to discuss the theoretical components of the model. On this particular day, I was talking about human needs, the various types of needs, and how need-status affects an individual's behaviors. I had just commented on linkages between a person's behaviors and their needs. I'd used, as an example, an individual who demonstrated behaviors which indicated feelings of anger, and then commented that anger is often secondary to loss. I'd asked the*

group what they could tell me about the concept of loss. One person said that loss made her feel sad. Another said that loss made her angry, which of course opened the door for a discussion about the relationships among feelings of sadness, anger, loss, grief and unmet needs. Everyone seemed to understand and accept the concepts and their relationships, except one member of the group. I could see the puzzled look on her face—her body language suggested that she was pulling back, closing herself off to what had just been discussed.

I turned to her and asked if there was anything that she wanted to add to the discussion, stating that as humans we each understand and experience ideas differently. I added that even though it might seem that there is only one way to think about any given idea, there are always many. She hesitated a little, and then, using a slightly aggressive tone, commented that she didn't understand how I could expect that she, as a nurse using MRM, could be confident that we knew how someone else felt. She went on to say that how we experienced any given situation was personal, that it would be presumptuous of us to think that we could label someone else's feelings.

My initial reaction was one of surprise, more by the tone of her voice than the content. Immediately, questions flooded my mind. "What did she just say?" "What does she mean?" "What is her world-view?" I responded by commenting that I was happy that she had spoken up, and I would love to hear more about what she was thinking and experiencing. I asked if she would be willing to say more about what she'd just said, so that I could answer her appropriately and as completely as possible. Her body language responded by opening up; her voice tone became less aggressive as she proceeded to tell me that as nurses we couldn't begin to know what someone was experiencing; that was personal. Our job was to use all that we knew and to do what we knew was best, to set good examples, and to try to be professional.

In response, I totally agreed that nurses used all the information they had and then did what was best, and that it was important to remember to be professional—after all, that is the nature of our relationship with clients—it is a professional relationship. I purposely ignored the issue of "setting good examples" for the time being. But I did go on and say that this was precisely why the client is the primary source of information and the nurse is a secondary source.

Using her words, I restated that we couldn't possibly know how someone else experienced a situation, and that each life experience is very personal about which we can't know unless we ask. And then I paused before I again stated that this was why we asked clients to describe their perceived situation in their own words. We don't ask the doctors, nor do we ask the family. First, we ask the clients. I then commented that the only way we really set examples is by demonstrating that we care about our clients' perspectives, that we value what they have to say, and that we think their perceptions are valid and important.

She looked puzzled and said that she thought that MRM was about modeling behaviors for others. I repeated that I thought it would be hard to model behaviors for people if we didn't know what they valued, what they thought was important, and the way they wanted to live their lives. I commented that we modeled or tried to create a mirror image of another person's world, but in truth, we can never fully understand how another person feels or thinks or experiences their life. That is why it is a mirror-image; it isn't exactly the same as the experience itself. She still looked puzzled. So, I commented once again, that from an MRM perspective, it is the client's model of the world—his self-care knowledge—that is the primary data upon which we make our nursing decisions, not the medical record.

She jumped from her seat, pulling back from the group as though I had touched her with a hot iron, exclaiming, "Oh my God, you're calling for a revolution in Nursing! You want nurses to ask the patients what they think is wrong with them!" I could not help but laugh with joy as I responded that yes that was what I wanted.

She responded by stating again that I was calling for a revolution and adding that she didn't know what to think about that. Nevertheless, she sat down, joined the discussion, and we started all over, talking about the philosophy of MRM. The only difference now was that we were at a deeper level of understanding, a different point in knowing. While some students had previously brought their esthetic knowing to the conversation, they now used multiple alternative types of knowing.

Several years later, this same person approached me at a conference. We greeted one another, spent several minutes talking about "the good old days," and then she suddenly commented that she'd noticed that MRM was still alive and well, that it was spreading, and that many were using it now. I just smiled and nodded; I knew there was more to come.

After a brief pause, she went on to say that she now used many of the ideas embedded in MRM, but she didn't call it MRM. She didn't know why, but even though she used many of the ideas, she thought her practice wasn't exactly MRM.

I commented that I was glad that she'd found some concepts in the model that were useful to her, and then asked her what she used the most.

She hesitated and then said that she thought about her patients' needs, and she was fairly good at recognizing their adaptive potential, but she never did "get the hang of asking them what they thought was important."

I smiled and then said that maybe that was because she really didn't believe that the client's view was primary in nursing. She nodded and commented that she'd just had too many years in research; she thought that science was more important than "soft, subjective stuff."

Again, I nodded and said that she was in good company. Many people agreed with her—that there was a need for many views in Nursing. Then I added that maybe someday she'd discover that there was a relationship between science and understanding another person's world-view—or maybe not—it really didn't matter.

What matters is that each one of us be aware of what we believe, and that each one of us learns how to be true to ourselves so we can be purposeful. When we are, we don't have trouble being consistent, setting priorities in our lives and in our practice, and linking knowledge to practice.

About then we both realized that we were behind schedule and late for a meeting, so we parted ways, hugging and remembering.

I received a message from her about a month after that meeting. There was no return address. She thanked me for understanding her and being willing to let her grow in her own time; she ended the note with a statement that she hoped that she could be like me when "she grew up!" I haven't heard from her since. If she ever reads this, I have one more thing to say to her:

Dear Colleague,

You don't need to grow up; you're great just as you are; you've already grown and you're already up. And you don't need to grow down; you already know how to be down. All you need is to let yourself be you, to continue to grow in whichever way is natural for you, in whichever direction you have the tendency to go, and to know that I have enjoyed knowing you, and being with you on your journey.

Hugs always,
Helen

> We run into different types of people in formal and informal settings, in classes, at conferences, meetings, parties, and wherever people meet one another. Sometimes we interact around business, sometimes play, and sometimes just by accident. Opportunities exist over and over; potential learners are everywhere. We just have to decide when and where we will act on those opportunities.

Keeper of the Keys. Suffice it to say that I believe that our personal philosophy, stored in our *personal knowledge,* is shaped by our *personal knowing and enhanced by reflective knowing.* How we link our personal philosophy with our practice is affected by multiple ways-of-knowing as discussed in previous chapters. From my experience, facilitating the growth of others is not difficult as long as I remember a few prerequisites.

First, I believe that as long as others show interest, there *will be* opportunities to facilitate learning. I just need to be aware that sometimes opportunities come when I least expect them. This means that I have to decide what I want to do when the opportunity exists. Sometimes it is important to put aside the original objective for interacting with another person and take advantage of the *"teaching-learning"* opportunity. I've discussed this issue of communication in previous publications (Erickson, H., 2006b, pp. 307-317) and will revisit it briefly below.

Grasp the opportunities when they come your way.

Second, I also have to decide whether I have the resources needed to facilitate another person at that point in time. It is okay to recognize another person's readiness and to respond by seeding future learning or simply affirming the other person. Remember the MRM assumption that people have an inherent drive to grow; sometimes all they need is an affirmation that their thoughts are worthy, and that they can learn and grow.

We have to take care of ourselves, so we have the resources we need to do our own life-work. Sometimes that means that we have to set priorities. There are times when we simply can't do all that needs to be done; we have to choose where we dedicate our own energy. When this happens, I try to be honest and inform the other person that I care about what is happening to him or her, but right now I need to take care of myself.

These are the times when it is important to be able to assess adaptive potential. Impoverished people can't wait without becoming more impoverished, so they usually get first priority, but not always. Remember, we're setting priorities, so we also have to consider the options, and to be aware of the cost-benefit ratio. That is, we have to be aware of how much time and energy will be required to intervene in comparison to the potential benefit. We can stimulate curiosity and/or initiate exploration without expending many resources. We are just *opening doors*, creating an environment so that those who wish to take the next step feel supported and encouraged rather than defensive and threatened.

Remember, *"Not now"* doesn't mean no or never; it just means not now.

Third, I also believe that it is okay for nurses to differ in what they believe and how they practice, assuming that they practice within the context of Nursing's Scope, Standards and Code of Ethics. I know that some nurses want to stay "connected," to be in a network with others who have different beliefs, but they just don't agree with the MRM philosophy. It is important to reinforce their worth, to stay open to what they have to say, and to be willing to learn from them.

We need diversity in Nursing, and we need to learn how to benefit from the strengths of those who are different from us. We can only do this if we value their orientation as worthy, important, and significant to the practice of Nursing. I like to think about it as fruit salad. It wouldn't be much of a salad if all we had were apples! We also need oranges, bananas, grapes, strawberries, etc. We need diversity if we want to grow and become more fully who we have the ability to be.

Diversity makes us stronger.

Fourth, and perhaps most important is that whenever there are those who want to learn, there are things to be learned from them. Even as we facilitate others to grow and become more fully who they have the ability to be, we too have an opportunity to learn and grow. We need to remember that there is a continuous input-transput-output process that occurs between two people, providing each with an opportunity to learn. The degree to which learning occurs, however, is the individual's responsibility. If we can stimulate interest and curiosity, *and create a safe environment,* many will take the next step and initiate exploration of their beliefs and how they relate to those embedded in the MRM model.

Remember, the long-range goal is growth.

Initiate Exploration

Being Mindful

Cognitive facilitators. Bruner's discovery model suggests that it is important to ensure that the "content to be learned" is broken into small pieces, and that the facilitator use techniques that will encourage learning, a bit at a time. Since a philosophy includes a *personal way-of-knowing that has implications for other ways-of-knowing,* it is important that the teacher assure learners that there are no right or wrong ways to view the world, and that their views are valued and respected, even when they differ from the teacher's. When we work with clients, we talk about "seeding" (Erickson, H., 2006c, p.18; 2006d, pp. 372-373) or a way of initiating growth in another human being. Seeding goes hand-in-glove with stimulating curiosity and interest. It can also be used to initiate exploration. Seeding is similar to Bruner's ideas about breaking content into small units and encouraging learning a bit at a time. The difference is that with Bruner's model, there is specific content to learn, and with seeding, the learning is often about a *way-of-knowing* rather than specific content. That is, *what is to be learned is about a way of knowing about oneself, one's personal beliefs, and how one views their life roles.* This includes the person's role as a professional. It is important that learners feel safe to express their thoughts and feelings and to explore alternatives.

Bruner also talks about the teacher being cognizant of the learner's motivation for learning—that the teacher's goal is to facilitate the learner to move from being concerned with pleasing another person (i.e. extrinsic reward), to learning for one's own sake (i.e. intrinsic reward). Specifically, we want learners to explore their own philosophy, and *to be curious and to wonder* about their own inner knowing. We also want them to think about how their beliefs about people are related to their beliefs about Nursing.

Since a philosophy is something that evolves over time, we don't have to be concerned about whether or not they have assimilated new information at first exposure. Instead, we have the leisure of seeding and directing learning, two strategies which help students assimilate what is consistent with their current schema of the world, reframe or accommodate what they choose to change, and deepen their personal ways-of-knowing. It also helps them have the time to discover ways to incorporate the knowledge acquired from other sources (i.e. ways-of-knowing) with their philosophy. Our goal is to help our mentees be open to explore their inner knowing and discover how it came to be. We do this by nurturing a relationship which enhances security and freedom from threat—one that encourages self-exploration of their beliefs, attitudes, values, and intuition.

> When aiming to facilitate others in deepening their personal understanding, encourage them to explore what they already know, but aren't consciously aware of knowing.

Communications and relations. Relationships are seated in communication. Since our aim is to enhance a sense of security and freedom from threat in our learners, we can assume that our communications with our learners are important.

Communication consists of our verbal statements and voice tones, as well as our body language (Erickson, H., 2006b, pp. 302-317). Communication is ongoing between two people; it cannot be interrupted by another, and it cannot be discontinued once it has started. According to Paul Watzlawick (1967), we are communicating even when we are unaware of our behaviors. Communication is not just verbal; it includes our attitudes and our behaviors. When another person *perceives* that we have communicated with them, a message *is received and encoded* no matter what our intent.

Communication is tricky because we aren't always aware of how others perceive us, or how they are encoding the messages *they think* we have sent. This problem is compounded by the fact that we often send messages on purpose, sometimes without thinking about how the recipient might experience both the verbal and nonverbal components of the message. Communications can become murky and problematic. While we might think we have been clear in our communication with another, we never know for certain how that individual has experienced the interaction.

Yet, communication is the basis for a relationship. Without the awareness that we have the potential to affect others through our words, tones, and body language, we can't be effective in our communications *with them*. We must be purposeful if we are to help people mobilize the courage needed to learn about themselves and their effect on others.

> Without awareness of our potential impact on another human being, we lack clarity in our vision to be facilitators of our students' learning, and we will have difficulty facilitating them as they try to clarify their personal knowledge, recode and extend it. We need to learn to be *mindful,* so we can be purposeful.

Reflexivity. *Awareness* of our potential effect on others *reminds us* that as educators, *our students are our clients*; teaching is our professional practice. This means that every time we interact with students we have an opportunity to facilitate their growth. We also have an opportunity to learn from our interactions. Being aware of these opportunities empowers us to be purposeful and proactive in our work with them, and it reminds us that we can learn by *reflecting on our work* with students.

Chris Johns, who coined the word, *reflexivity*, describes it as "the impact of past experience on the present: the present turning back on itself to reflect on the way it has evolved from past experience" (Johns, 2004, p. 4). Chapter 14 more fully explores reflexivity, reflective knowing and its importance in learning about self and self in relations to others. According to him, "Being mindful is the quintessential nature of reflective practice. It is the ability to be aware of self, within the unfolding moment, without judgment. It is as if I am a witness to self, mindful of how I am thinking, feeling and responding" (Johns, 2002/2010, p. 2).

> Being mindful then is being "conscious and intentional with one's presence and being in the moment…" (Johns, 2004, p. viii). Being mindful is a necessary ingredient if we wish to facilitate students to initiate exploration of their beliefs.

Facilitate growth

I've discussed ways to facilitate growth in earlier publications, particularly Erickson, H., (2006d, pp. 346-391). I'll not repeat that work here other than to say that the premises or assumptions that apply to the practice of MRM with a client are relevant no matter who the client might be. That is, the premises that contribute to the relationship between nurse and patient also contribute to the quality of the relationship between faculty and student. Specifically, these include *unconditional acceptance, presence, intent, affiliated-individuation, nurturance* and *facilitation,* and are discussed below.

Unconditional acceptance

Previously, I stated the following about unconditional acceptance:

> *[N]urses who unconditionally accept the worth of their clients would likely demonstrate an interest in their well-being and show compassion for their human state. The consequences of experiencing Unconditional Acceptance are: a sense of worth and dignity, trust in the provider, the discovery that one's Self is what is important, the ability to listen to one's inner voice, and the initiation of a natural self-healing process.* (Erickson, H., 2006e, p. 342)

Since *our students are our clients,* we can extrapolate from this discussion and the basic premises of MRM. That is, unconditional acceptance of our students means that we recognize them as worthy human-beings, with an inherent need for dignity and a drive toward growth. It means that we recognize the difference between the behaviors of a person and their inherent worth as a human being.

Unconditional acceptance seems so simple, yet it is one of the more difficult concepts to teach and to learn. Most people learn at a very young age that there are *behaviors* others label "good" or "bad." Too often, no distinction is made between the behaviors and the human being. When this happens, it doesn't take long before children learn to link their worth as humans with the descriptors of their behaviors. Often, they aren't informed that *doing bad things* doesn't make one *a bad person,* so they make assumptions, and learn that they are either good or bad. The person and the behaviors become one; they are good or bad, depending on how they behave.

They haven't necessarily learned the moral reasons behind the adult's comments, nor have they had opportunities to explore alternative ways of thinking about the *bad* behaviors. Having learned that there is good and bad, they are soon able to transfer their knowledge, and things like taste, smell, look, feel, and sound are good or bad.

Paradoxically, what we learn about ourselves is often what we apply to others. As educators, we need to explore our beliefs about the human being, determine where they came from, and how they serve us today. When we try to teach this to others, we must have a clear understanding of our own beliefs before we can fully appreciate the worth of another. Take, as an example, the following statement, made by a registered nurse, who had returned to school to earn her baccalaureate degree. This comment was included in her course evaluation report.

> *Unconditional acceptance has freed up my emotional energy so that I can better care for the needs of the patient. For example, there are a number of chemically-dependent patients on my unit. There is a very cynical culture among the nurses toward these patients. Leaving this judgment behind (unconditional acceptance) removes the burden from my shoulders.* (Dawn Krasue, 2009, Metropolitan State University, Student Self-evaluation)

Unconditional acceptance of a human does not mean acceptance of inappropriate behaviors. Nor does it mean that we never provide feedback to learners about their ability to meet course or program objectives, or even our expectations. It does mean, however, that we need to be sure that we try to understand *what motivates the behaviors* before we act. It also means that we try to be constructive and growth-directed in our feedback and critiques, and that we are mindful of the other person's need to be treated respectfully, to retain a sense of dignity, and to have a positive learning experience. The same holds true for others we interact with in informal settings.

But it is not always easy to live by the premises of unconditional acceptance. As humans, our own needs sometimes interfere; we lose track of how we want to interact with others. Let's revisit the situation I discussed earlier in Chapter 5, as I talked about *pacing the learning of others.* I provided a story about Doreen, sitting with her mother who was dying, and her interactions with Ann, a nurse assigned to her for the shift. You may remember that Doreen perceived that Ann was preoccupied with the room, the equipment, and seemed unconcerned with her patient. As Ann seemed to be "monkeying" with an empty catheter bag rather than attending to her mother, Doreen became irritated. In my description I stated the following:

> *As she approached the young nurse, she noted that she was sitting on the floor! What nurse sits on a dirty floor and then goes and takes care of*

other patients! What was she thinking? And then she noticed that she had her face in her hands. WHAT WAS SHE DOING?

As you remember the story and review these comments, you can imagine that Doreen was preoccupied with her own situation and impending loss. When the nurse entered the room and interacted as described, Doreen immediately made some conclusions about this nurse. She concluded that she was not concerned with her mother's comfort, but with the equipment and her patient's vitals.

Doreen was not concerned with Ann as a human, but as *a nurse* who had a power base—someone who had the potential to affect her mother's well-being. She labeled her behaviors and then made assumptions about the follow-up behaviors to support her initial interpretations. Doreen's perceptions of Ann were *conditional*. This is not uncommon when we perceive that the behaviors of others have the potential to affect us.

Unconditional acceptance of another human is very difficult sometimes, particularly when we don't perceive that we have the power base to control our own lives. This case reminds us that it is important to be mindful of our basic beliefs about people. When Doreen paused to note that Ann had her hands over her face, she tapped into her repertoire of knowledge. Although her first reaction was consistent with her conditional judgments, she was able to reconnect with Ann's humanity and unconditionally accept her as she presented herself. When she did this, she was able to remember that Ann's behaviors were not motivated by how she perceived Doreen's mother, but by her own life experience.

This is true most of the time; people often behave in ways we don't understand, approve of, or even like. When we try to understand their behavior before we react, we will discover that most of the time, other persons' behaviors are motivated by their own needs.

We always have choices about our own responses. If we aim to facilitate growth in others, we do not need to personalize their behaviors. Use of unconditional acceptance as a way of interacting with learners is not always easy, but we can always try. When we remember, we are able to connect with others in a *transcendent way.*

> When we are mindful, we are able to go beyond the limits of the here and now to connect with another in a way that transcends the moment. As a result, we both learn from the experience.

Presence

It is much easier to consistently use presence with learners than it is to consistently unconditionally accept them. On the other hand, when we purposefully use intention, we are much more likely to unconditionally accept others for who they are and what they can become. *This is because presence requires intention.* That is, presence requires conscious, cognitive processes (Erickson, H., 2006b, pp. 309-313). Individuals who use presence have to consciously center themselves, so they can direct their energy and focus on the other.

Intentionality

The concept of intentionality has already been mentioned as a prerequisite of presence. In that situation, intentionality is used to initiate a relationship between teacher and student. Intentionality is also used to direct and reinforce learning.

When we direct our intent toward facilitating the growth and well-being of another, we go beyond our own perspectives. The interaction becomes focused on what the other person says, means, needs, and what will help them realize their self-potential. It does not mean that we *intend* that our learners will learn specific value, beliefs, or even content. Instead, it means that we will intend to help our learners explore their personal knowing, consider what they *know to be true*, how they came to acquire their *knowing,* and why it is important to them.

Sometimes these *discoveries* surprise the learner; they come unexpectedly, as though they spring from a source unknown to the learner. Yet, these discoveries come from the individual's own repertoire of knowing, stored deep within their Self.

Bruner and colleagues describe it like this: "The triumph of effective surprise is that it takes one beyond common ways of experiencing the world….Creative products have this power of reordering experience and thought …" (Wood, Bruner, & Ross, 1976, p. 22).

Setting the intent that we will facilitate others to grow is often filled with surprise.

Affiliated-individuation

Affiliated-individuation is another way to think about unconditional acceptance, presence and intentionality. Affiliated-individuation (A-I) is the need to be dependent on others while simultaneously maintaining independence. Educators need to remember that learners have to perceive that they are *safe to be both connected to the educators at the same time that they feel safe to explore their own beliefs and to know or not know what is important to professional practice*—beliefs and knowledge that are sometimes different from those of the educator. This is the essence of A-I in the teaching environment.

Nurturance

We nurture people by unconditionally accepting and purposefully sending intent to facilitate their well-being. We also nurture them with strategies which we purposefully use to enhance their sense of self-worth. Nurturance most often occurs when the learner perceives that the teacher is *available*. This doesn't mean that the teacher is ready to drop everything and respond to the student's needs or be available at all times. It means, instead, that the teacher communicates interest in the learner's needs and uses presence when with the student. It also means that the teacher affirms the student's questions and conveys that they are important, respected, and have merit.

Being available is a matter of perception more than anything else. It is not measured by what we do, but *what we try to be.* When others perceive that we care about them, that we want to help them to learn and grow, *and that we are available* to help them achieve their goals, they feel nurtured.

Facilitation

Often, *the perception that we are available* is sufficient to facilitate learning. Many are able to utilize this *sense of supportive affiliation* to help them help themselves. This doesn't mean that no effort is necessary on the part of the teacher. Indeed, if we want learners to explore their personal knowledge *and their personal way-of-knowing,* we have to stimulate interest and curiosity and initiate the process, as described above, as they progress. Sometimes we have to structure and sequence learning, and we always have to reinforce learning and provide feedback, as needed. Knowledge can only be integrated if there is knowledge to be built upon.

> *We should be clear about what the act of discovery entails. It is rarely, on the frontier of knowledge or elsewhere, that new facts are discovered in the sense of being encountered. Discovery, like surprise, favors the well-prepared mind.* (Bruner, 1965/1971, p.82)

FINAL CONSIDERATIONS

Throughout this chapter I have continuously reflected back on the basic premises of MRM, linked them to the work of Bruner, and added my own thoughts as I have discussed how educators can facilitate others to learn the basic premises of MRM. You may have noticed that I have not discussed how to teach the content *per se*. That is a related, but different issue. Anyone can take the MRM books, divide the content, and teach it, and they can do this with some assurance that their students will learn the content. Since the philosophy is a part of the MRM paradigm, teachers can help students learn that, too, and students can learn it without difficulty. After all, it isn't really that complex when evaluated at the superficial level. Suffice it to say, then, that teachers can teach, and students can learn what has been taught.

That doesn't mean that students will learn how to think about what they have learned, or that they will be able to apply it. If we want learners *to be able to think about what they have learned and to apply what they think about,* then time has to be invested in facilitating them to explore their own philosophy and compare it with that of MRM. Furthermore, until they have compared *and* analyzed the similarities and differences and thought about the implications of both, they will not be able to apply the theory and paradigm. While they may be able to apply individual concepts and aspects of the paradigm, purposeful, proactive application of the theory and paradigm require acceptance of the MRM principles and basic premises.

Specifically, until learners have adopted the basic principles of MRM, they will not be able to proactively apply the theory or paradigm. Thus, this chapter was dedicated to issues related to facilitating understanding of the philosophy, a prerequisite to teaching the theory and how to apply it.

SUMMARY

This chapter discussed factors of consideration for educators—formal or informal—who wish to help others learn the MRM philosophy. I included three phases in the teaching-learning process and provided some thoughts on how to stimulate interest and curiosity, initiate exploration, and facilitate learning. I concluded that this chapter is not about teaching the content of MRM theory; it is about facilitating others to explore their own personal knowing, so they can determine whether MRM is an appropriate theory for their practice. Finally, I stated that a nurse who does not identify with the MRM philosophy will not be able to proactively apply it to practice.

The following chapters build on this work. They provide more specific directions for facilitating students under various conditions. Some relate to the clinical area, some to class design. The last chapter in this book describes the life journey of one nurse who has been facilitated through application of some of these methods. Her work illustrates how important it is for faculty to be mindful of students as humans entering the educational system not as a blank slate, but as a full reservoir of knowledge and experience, waiting to be guided in discovering new knowledge that will help them further their life goals.

CHAPTER 7

FACILITATING THE MODELING AND ROLE-MODELING PROCESESS

Sharon Rogers and Helen L. Erickson

"It is right that philosophy should be called knowledge of the truth…we do not know a truth without knowing its cause." Aristotle, *Metaphysics*

OVERVIEW

The purpose of this chapter is to provide the educator with some tips on facilitating the novice student's acquisition of knowledge needed to practice Modeling and Role-Modeling. We start with a brief overview of the use of the language and proceed to a discussion of the key issues encountered in the teaching-learning environment. Data interpretation and analysis are discussed briefly. We conclude with a discussion about the use of creative, individualized interventions and the potential pitfalls.

USE OF THE LANGUAGE

Background

The terms, *Modeling* and *Role-Modeling* are often confused with the common use of the words. In the conventional use of the term *role-modeling* one demonstrates appropriate behavior and attitudes to another individual. When applied to the academic setting, the faculty's aim is to facilitate the student to learn by observing the expert. For example, a faculty member who wears appropriate attire to class and clinical settings is role-modeling professional expectations of attire for his/her students. Within this context, *modeling* is the performance of these behaviors.

> Generally, the concepts *modeling* and *role-modeling*, defined as setting examples and/or acting as exemplars, can be done with or without purpose and/or intent.

However, these terms, originally coined by Milton Erickson (cited in Erickson et al., 1983/2009, pp. 84-85; p. 94), are defined differently by Erickson, et al. The aim of modeling and role-modeling as used by Erickson, et al. is not to set an example or to be an exemplar. In MRM, the term *modeling* does not mean demonstrating a behavior and *role-modeling* does not mean setting a good example. Instead, it is to facilitate the growth, adaptation and healing of another human being. This orientation will be discussed more fully below.

> Within the MRM theory and paradigm, both concepts are processes, based in the theory and paradigm and performed with purpose and intent.

Construct Clarification

Modeling

The assessment of a client's world-view and the interpretation of the data acquired during assessment is the *modeling process*. It starts with our first interaction with an individual and concludes with an understanding of that person's perspective of their circumstances. Our aim is to learn how clients describe their situation, what they expect will happen, their perceived resources, and life goals. As we listen and observe, we interpret the information acquired using the constructs embedded in the theory. More simplistically, Modeling is the process we use to build mirror images of our clients' worldviews. These worldviews help us understand what they perceive to be important, what caused their problems, what will help them, and the roles they wish to perform in their lives.

Role-Modeling

Role-modeling is defined as

> *...the facilitation of the individual in attaining, maintaining, or promoting health through purposeful interventions. These interventions are planned based on the data analyses....Role-modeling cannot occur until the nurse has modeled her client's world and has aggregated and analyzed the constructs of that world.* (Erickson, et al., 1983/2009, p. 95)

Role-modeling is both an art and a science. The art occurs as the nurse plans and implements creative, individualized interventions that will facilitate the individual's movement toward health. "The science of role-modeling occurs as the nurse plans interventions with respect to her theoretical base for the practice of nursing" (Erickson, et al., 1983/2009, p. 95). As noted by N. Frisch and L. Frisch (2006) Role-modeling proposes that nursing interventions be guided not by the nurse's abstract perceptions of what the client needs, but by the model that she has formed of the client's world-view.

This orientation to nursing is very difficult for some nurses to accept. Many have been educated and socialized to think that the nurse knows what is best for the patient and that nursing is the implementation of skills and techniques. This view is not congruent with MRM.

In their original work, Erickson, et al., 1983/2009 noted the following:

> *Role-modeling is, in our minds, the essence of nurturance. It is the basis for the predictive and prescriptive component of nursing practice. Role-modeling requires an unconditional acceptance of the person, as the person is, while gently encouraging and facilitating growth and development at the person's own pace and within the person's own model.* (p. 95)

Remodeling

In her work with male incest offenders, Scheela (1992) coined the term *remodeling* to help her clients understand the purpose of behavioral-change interventions she implemented with this population. The primary author found that her students often better understand the term *remodeling* first, and are then able to grasp a clearer understanding of the term *role-modeling*.

Scheela's (1992) research participants described the process of remodeling this way:

> *the offender's world falls apart, the offenders take on the project of remodeling themselves, tearing out the damaged parts, rebuilding themselves and their relationships and their environments, doing the upkeep to maintain the remodeling that has been accomplished and, for some, eventually moving on to new remodeling projects.* (p. 10)

While a detailed description of Scheela's (1992) work is not appropriate for the purposes of this chapter, the use of the concept *remodeling* can be a useful tool for working with clients who have a large reservoir of negative developmental residual. Our goal with Role-modeling would be to facilitate the client in the exchange of negative residual for positive residual, or to remodel their residual.

It is important to know, however, that there are many times when nurses facilitate clients' growth, development and adaptation without focusing on the reworking or remodeling of negative residual. For more specific information, the reader is referred to an earlier publication that addresses these issues in detail (Erickson, H., 2006a).

FACILITATING STUDENTS' LEARNING

Assessment of clients' needs occurs during the process of modeling (discussed in detail in Erickson, et al., 1983/2009, pp.116-160). Sometimes however, nurses acquire new information, and therefore, a new understanding of the client's view of the world as they implement previously planned creative, individualized interventions. When this happens, it is important to assure the student that it is safe and appropriate to change strategies based on the new data.

The Primacy of Subjective Data

When using MRM, the student's primary concern is to focus on valuing and affirming the client's perspectives, no matter how strange or inappropriate they may seem to the student. Sometimes nurses think that their client's don't understand, are confused, or that their perspectives are irrelevant to the situation. Nevertheless, when using MRM, the client's perspective is primary. While the client's perspective may seem obvious, we can never tell exactly what an individual is thinking without first asking. An example of this used by the primary author follows:

> *The importance of personal perspectives is well-illustrated by a little boy in a Kenny Rogers' song that I often play for my students when trying to teach this important concept. In this song, the boy spends the afternoon throwing a baseball in the air and swatting at it with his bat. Through the afternoon, he swings and swings without ever hitting the ball. When the song states that he heads into the house, I stop the song and ask my students what the little boy is going to say. Invariably, the students respond, "I'm never going to be any good as a baseball player," or something to that effect. When I restart the song, the little boy says, "Even I didn't know I was that good a pitcher!"*

You never know for sure what another person is thinking unless you ask. Furthermore, when they tell you, that is where you start with interventions, no matter how strange or inappropriate they may seem.

Many examples of the effectiveness of starting with the client's perspective can be found throughout this book and in earlier publications (Erickson, H., 1984, 1988, 1990a, 1990b, 1990c, 2002, 2006a; Erickson, et al., 1983/2009; Kinney & Erickson, H., 1990). Many more could be included here, but at this point one example, offered by the primary author of this chapter, will suffice.

A Level 1 student, minimally acquainted with MRM knew that it was important to validate and affirm the client's world-view. When she took report, she learned the elderly man for whom she would be caring that day was extremely confused and had been somewhat combative during the night. Entering the client's room, she was somewhat anxious about how to approach this confused man, but was determined to model his world. She started by asking him the standard cognition/orientation questions.

When she asked him where he was, he told her he was in the middle of the ocean, alone in a boat. When he told her this, she did not make an effort to orient him to time, place, and situation. Instead, she said, "That must be very scary to be out in the middle of the ocean all alone in a boat with no way to get back to shore." The man nodded his agreement with that obvious statement. The student continued, "What if I get in your boat with you? I will give you an oar and I will take an oar, and we will row back to shore together." The client readily agreed to this arrangement.

The student did not get in bed with him, but lowered the bed rail and held the client's hand as both of them diligently "rowed" to shore. The student consistently encouraged the client to keep rowing, and continually reported that she too was working hard at rowing.

After a few minutes of steady rowing, the student reported she was beginning to see some shore birds in the sky, which indicated they were nearing land. The patient was also able to see these "imaginary" birds. Soon after this, the student began to study the horizon and reported she was quite certain she could see land. The patient agreed that he, too, could see a distant shoreline. Shortly, the student made a bumping sound and movement and said, "I think we're here!" The client agreed and immediately knew he was in the hospital and explained his condition to the student. Of course, he needed a little coaching to remember date and time. This simple intervention by a novice nurse had facilitated her client's emergence from a world of confusion into the world that we generally consider reality. [1]

In the above example, it was appropriate for the student to approach the patient, listen to what the client was saying, interpret, analyze and plan an appropriate intervention. It is also important for the student to continue to make observations to determine the effectiveness of the intervention. This student used classic pacing and leading strategies to facilitate her client to move from feelings

---

[1] This was a clinical experience related by the primary author when teaching at The University of Texas at Austin.

of danger to feelings of safety (Erickson, H., 2006b, pp. 351-388). Without first pacing her client, she would have had difficulty leading, as demonstrated by the previous nurses.

Faculty as Expert and Learner

Ideally, the faculty member has a sophisticated understanding of the situation, including the client's physical status. It is important to ensure that the client is safe and the student has correctly assessed the situation. It is also important since each clinical case serves as a source for continued learning. At a later time, the faculty member can use this story, along with the theoretical underpinnings, to help students grow in their understanding of MRM.[2] Faculty and students can also use clinical experiences as a way of learning about themselves and their profession. This latter issue will be further addressed in Chapter 14 where Chris Johns discusses Reflective Practice.

Discovery Learning Implications

Learning to Know

As discussed earlier in Chapter 5, there are many commonalities between the use of MRM and Bruner's Discovery-Learning methods. The major difference is the focus of attention. With MRM, the client is an individual with health care needs while the client in Bruner's Discovery-Learning methods is the student. Both aim to reinforce learning as it occurs, facilitate growth, and support ownership of new knowledge as it is acquired.

It is important for faculty to remember that students facilitated to learn through Discovery-Learning techniques often own all the knowledge they have acquired. In doing so, they forget that the faculty was the first to use the language, present the ideas, or even suggest interventions. In essence, they often consciously forget the faculty's assistance in the process of assessment, data interpretation, and intervention planning.

When this occurs, students truly "own" the entire learning experience; it is vital that faculty allow them to do this, so that they can *learn from learning* and learn how to jump the gap from *learning to thinking* as described in Chapter 5. Faculty members need to understand that they have achieved their goals as educators; they have facilitated their students to learn not only words and techniques, but also attitudes and behaviors.

An example of such an event, reported by the primary author follows:

---

[2] This interpretation is based on a discussion between the primary author and one of her faculty, M. Weitzel, at The University of Texas at Austin during her doctoral program, 1992.

A student I was supervising in clinical was assigned to care for an extremely confused, combative elderly lady, one morning. Family members had been with her all night and were exhausted, but were reluctant to leave the care of their loved one to this obviously novice student. So the student, the family members, and I held a brief hallway conference. I explained to the family (and the student) that their loved one was probably confused and acting-out because her safety and security needs were not being met. I assured the family that this young student was adept at meeting the safety and security needs of her clients,[3] *and that I would supervise her closely to be sure that all was going well.*[4]

The family left and the student and I had a brief discussion about the aims of intervention, including building a trusting relationship. The student did very well with her client; she was able to remove the Posey belt and the client was well-oriented and happy with the care she received. Later that day, the student breathlessly approached me in the hall and said, "Dr. Rogers! Dr. Rogers! I need to tell you something!" I stopped and allowed her to share with me the breaking news.

She said, "After the family left, I finally figured out that my patient's safety and security needs were not being met. So, I worked hard to build a trusting relationship with her and my intervention worked!" I commended her on her insight[5] *and encouraged her to keep up the good work—a validation of her view of the situation.*

At this point, any attempt at reminding her of my part in the analysis and planning would have confused her and possibly robbed her of what she had learned in this process.

Three Essential Considerations

While there are many sophisticated aspects of Modeling and Role-Modeling, three essential features are important for the educator who intends to

---

[3] Some nurses may be saying, "But we never enter into the client's delusions or hallucinations." Think about this: If someone constantly challenged your view of reality and diligently worked to 'orient' you to their view of reality, would you become healthier, or more frightened and dis-eased? If the healthcare provider cannot understand that another human might have a different reality, who can? Understanding is the beginning; helping people move into a healthier reality is next.

[4] The faculty member recognized that many confused patients (elderly or not) deal with unmet safety and security needs as delineated in Maslow's Hierarchy of Needs, linking the assessment, data interpretation and analysis, intervention, and outcome to the theoretical underpinnings that students are just beginning to understand.

[5] The student had learned that comfort follows need satisfaction.

facilitate students who are using this framework in their practice. We call them the *Primary Source*, *Question*, and *Intent*.

Table 7.1 Factors that facilitate and impede data collection.

	Primary Source	Secondary Sources	Tertiary Sources
Beneficial Factors	•Knows own needs and preferences best. •Only one with his/her experiences and world-view. •Only one who really knows what his/her experience is in the present. •What the client says about his/her needs is the most accurate perspective of those needs.	•May know the needs and preferences of the client very well. •May have a similar world-view or be able to describe the client's world-view. •May have some idea of the current situation. •Can provide information about the relationship and the client's condition that the client does not necessarily have.	•Objective information (lab tests, x-rays, etc.) can be very helpful. •Some HCPs may be able to share strategies that have already worked to meet the client's needs.
Interfering Factors	•Some circumstances may limit the client's ability to communicate effectively.	•May have a different agenda than the client. •May have a very different world-view from the client without an understanding of either the client's view or the difference between the two worldviews. •May see the current situation very differently than the client.	•Often has a different agenda than the client. •May have a very different world-view from the client. •Probably sees the current situation very differently than the client. •May have a personality clash with the client. •May not understand the client's need to have his/her needs met. •May have bought into negative attitudes of other HCPs. •May not approve of the client's lifestyle and/or factors that have led to the current illness. •Often have important power bases that affect the client's well-being.

The Primary Source

First, assessment and data collection must be thorough and accurate with a constant awareness of the client's role as primary provider of information. Family members and close friends often serve as important secondary sources of information, but the chart and reports made by other health care professionals must be considered tertiary in nature (Erickson, et al., 1983/2009, pp.170-171).

Often, during report, students hear very negative assessments of the person they will be caring for. They hear words like "difficult," "uncooperative," "mean," "nasty," or worse. We tell our students to accept evaluations of that nature with the understanding that they are hearing from a tertiary source who usually does not know how to model the client's view of the world. Students need to understand that they may, and usually will, find a very different person once they have done their own assessment and data collection. Table 7.1 (above) delineates some of the beneficial and interfering factors related to data collection from various sources.

During the process of interpreting and analyzing data for the purpose of planning individualized interventions, the client should be included whenever feasible. This is important because the concept of Self-care Knowledge (SCK) is embedded in MRM. According to MRM, SCK is defined as follows:

> *The personal understanding of what is needed to help us grow, develop, or heal. It includes awareness of personal needs and goals, as well as strengths, capabilities, characteristics, values and liabilities. It also includes recognition of what is not needed* (Hertz, & Baas, 2006, p. 98).

This means that clients know, at some level, what has made them sick, and they also know what will comfort them and facilitate healing at that particular time.

The Primary Question

First version. While the original book on MRM (Erickson, et al., 1983/2009) provides detailed information about the assessment process, questions to ask oneself, and things to consider, we have found that many students find the details overwhelming. Therefore, the primary author of this chapter recommends a single question that has proven to be very valuable for novices. It is, "What can I do *with you*, today, to help you feel better?"

This question taps into the client's self-care knowledge and provides direction for the novice as he or she learns to interpret and analyze more complex data. Whenever a student is having difficulty dealing with a patient, invite the student to describe the situation and then ask, "Have you asked 'the question,' yet?" In Rogers's experience, the answer to this question is almost always an embarrassed, "No."

The word "yet" is used in the query to the student as it acts as an *embedded command* (Erickson, H., 2006b, pp. 373-374), informing the student of our expectation that "the question" is always part of a complete assessment. This gives the student an opportunity to complete the assessment before we further discuss the client's needs. It also ensures that the student will remember to ask this question when doing assessments in the future.

Alternative version. Sometimes clients are unable or unwilling to respond to "the question" in a meaningful way. This may indicate trust issues and/or that the client wishes to be cared "for" rather than "with." In this situation students may ask, "What can I do *for you*, today, that will help you feel better?" This version of "the question" almost always elicits a meaningful response.

Dissonance with MRM. Occasionally, a student has asked "the question" but has failed to make any serious attempt to meet the need the client has expressed. Sometimes the student simply doesn't agree that the client's subjective perspectives are "right." Other times, they have misinterpreted the data or are worried about reactions from other healthcare providers.

At this point, it is necessary to facilitate the student's review of the premises and philosophy of MRM, and the data including data interpretations and analysis. These processes must include the client's response and consideration of why the student chose to ignore the client's SCK. Finally, an effective intervention, comfortable for all, can be planned.

Two brief examples demonstrate the effectiveness of asking the above question and meeting the client's needs based on his or her reply to this question.

> *One student came to the authority, quite shaken because her client's response to "the question" had been, "Take me outside to smoke." The student could not believe that I would support her in facilitating such an unhealthy behavior. I explained, "Right now, we meet the client's needs. Later, we can worry about healthy lifestyle choices." The student took the patient in a wheelchair downstairs to the smoking area several times while we were on the floor. When the nurses saw this "extremely difficult" client become a cheerful, pleasant woman, they eagerly took turns taking her downstairs to smoke when they took their own smoke breaks.*

Often students are forced to revise "the question" to meet the needs of the situation. Usually, this is because the charge nurse does not understand or agree that the primary source of information is the client, or that nurses facilitate people in need-satisfaction. Instead, they are focused on treating the disease or controlling the situation. Usually, they have a philosophy of care consistent with the Totality model discussed in Chapter 2. A case example follows to illustrate the importance of attending to the primary source of information, acquired by directly asking clients what they need.

One student was told by her primary nurse that her client had repeatedly refused to ambulate, and it was the student's mission that day to get this generally healthy, postoperative woman ambulating. The primary nurse added, "She's going to want you to give her a bed bath. Don't do that! It would just be buying into her needs."

With all this in mind, the student explained to the client that ambulation was essential to her healing process, and went on to ask, "What can I do with you, today, to make it possible for you to ambulate?" The woman replied, "Well, every morning the nurses have me sit at the sink and take a sponge bath, and by the time I finish doing that, I am so tired that I just crawl back in bed and don't want to get up again." The student responded saying, "What if I give you a bed bath, let you rest 20 minutes, and come back in after that to help you ambulate?" The woman agreed that this sounded like a good plan.

After her bed bath and 20-minute rest, she got out of bed with minimal assistance and ambulated around the unit repeatedly. Of course, the nurses were very interested in the student's strategy, but since she had expressly disobeyed the instructions of the primary nurse, she just had to shrug her shoulders and act mystified. The student knew that by facilitating the client's ambulation the client would be discharged the following day. If that had not been the case, we would have worked harder to help the nurses understand that "meeting needs" leads to client cooperation. However, experience informs me that this is much more difficult to do than it is to talk about. As indicated above, this is usually due to differences in philosophies of nursing and human nature.

The above story also provides an example of how students can not only pace, but lead clients as they ask *the question.* Usually, the question is open-ended, without direction. However, in some cases, as indicated above, it is helpful to include a directive in the question, so that the client can be clear about the intent. Clearly, the student wanted to help her client ambulate; yet, she was willing to listen to what the client knew she needed in order to be able to take this step. This is a good example of affiliated-individuation, a requisite of a trusting nurse-client relationship, as described in the first Aim of Intervention (Erickson, H., 2006c, p. 322; Erickson, et al., 1983/2009, pp. 170-186, p. 190, p. 197).

Student safety

At this point, we need to reiterate that as educators, our students are our clients. We need to remember that *students have to know, beyond any shadow of doubt, that they are 100% safe with faculty* before they will implement interventions that are outside the norm of what is usually considered *acceptable student nurse behavior*. They need to know that faculty will support their creative decisions and will even commend, encourage, and facilitate such behavior. This does not mean that we will not evaluate them, or that we will not identify limitations. It simply means that they are safe with us and can depend on us to respect them, treat them with dignity and fairness. This issue was discussed at length in Chapter 5 when we discussed Bruner's Discovery-Learning methods.

To create an environment which enhances the students' sense of security, we try to model their worldviews as they relate to the academic setting, and understand their expectations. We've learned from experience that students often view their relationship with faculty as untrustworthy and dangerous; they often expect punitive reactions from faculty when they do not do what the faculty perceives as *appropriate nursing behaviors*. More problematic is that they don't always know what the faculty think *is* appropriate.

We try to change these views and expectations, facilitating their learning by teaching them the basic concepts of MRM, and telling them stories about the accomplishments of previous students, and then using positive reinforcements described previously in Chapter 5.

Intent: Intervention Aims

The third essential consideration in implementing MRM is the role of the "Aims of Intervention." The aims are distinguished from intervention goals because they address *intent* rather than objective outcomes.

Delineated by Erickson, et al., (1983/2009, p.170), the aims of MRM interventions are:

1) Build trust,
2) Promote client's positive orientation,
3) Promote client's control,
4) Affirm and promote client's strengths,
5) Set mutual goals that are health-directed.

The MRM Aims of Intervention are discussed at great length in the original work and enlarged upon in Erickson, H., 2006c, pp. 321-322. In the latter book, a sixth Aim, *Prepare Self,* has been added. This Aim is to remind the reader that the nurse is an important component in the nurse-client relationship, and therefore, must be proactive in self-care actions.

Table 7.2, reproduced from the latter book, serves to refresh our understanding of the Aims of Intervention in MRM and their relations with MRM strategies, principles, goals and modalities.

Table 7.2 Relations among Aims of Intervention and MRM strategies, principles, goals and modalities. Reproduced with permission, *Modeling and Role-Modeling: A View from the Client's World,* p.322. Cedar Park, TX: Unicorns Unlimited.

AIMS	STRATEGY	PRINCIPLE	GOAL & MODALITIES
Prepare self	Establish a Mind-set	We have to take care of ourselves first, so we can facilitate the well-being of others.	Increase self resources through meditation, self-hypnosis, centering, Walker & Kinney techniques. (Erickson, H., 2006, Appendices A & E). Set the stage with Intentionality, Unconditional Acceptance. Use hypnotic techniques, guided imagery, client-selected alternative therapies to build relationship.
Build trust	Creating a nurturing space	The nursing process requires that a *trusting* and *functional* relationship exist between nurse and client.	Decrease adverse stimuli and enhance healing stimuli. Use Presence, Intentionality, Unconditional Acceptance to maintain and enhance relationship. Use hypnotic techniques, guided imagery, client-selected alternative therapies to nurture growth.
Promote positive orientation	Create a nurturing space	A-I is dependent on individuals perceiving they are acceptable, respectable, and worthwhile human beings.	Promote self-worth, dignity and spiritual awareness. Use hypnotic techniques, healing touch, therapeutic touch, reiki. Maintain Presence, Intentionality, Unconditional Acceptance to deepen the connection; encourage client self-care knowledge.
Promote perceived control	Facilitate the story	Human development is dependent on individuals perceiving they have some control while experiencing affiliation.	Facilitate clients' sense of intra and interconnectedness, enhance Self-awareness. Use empathy, Presence, Unconditional Acceptance and purposeful Intentionality to create a safe environment. Use healing touch, therapeutic touch, reflexology, hypnotic techniques to mobilize and build resources and enhance awareness of Self-care Knowledge with inner voice.
Affirm and promote strengths	Nurture growth	There is an innate drive toward holistic health that is facilitated by consistent and systematic nurturance.	Facilitate dynamic, adaptive mind-body-spirit holism with Self-knowing. Maintain Presence, Intentionality, Unconditional Acceptance to maintain and enhance a safe environment. Use communication and selected hypnotic techniques, guided imagery in conjunction with selected energy therapies to mobilize and build resources, enhance Self –knowing and develop Self-awareness.
Set mutual goals that are health-directed	Nurture growth	Human growth is dependent on satisfaction of basic needs and facilitated by growth-need satisfaction.	Facilitate healthy problem-solving and coping. Maintain Presence, Intentionality, and Unconditional Acceptance to further enhance sense of affiliated-individuation. Use communication techniques and guided imagery to facilitate goal-setting.

Data Interpretation and Analysis

Background

Before addressing specific interpretation and analysis strategies, it is important to remind the reader that client needs are always the first and foremost concern in practicing Nursing from the MRM perspective. "It is assumed that all behaviors are motivated by needs and that needs are biophysical, social, psychological, and cognitive in nature" (Erickson, H., 1990a, p. 15).

It is also important to remember that all actions are self-care actions. "The choice to be dependent, not perform one's own daily life activities is a self-care action" (Erickson, H., 1990a, p. 14), even when we, as nurses, view this behavior as non-beneficial for the client.

Critical Thinking

Simplistic analysis. As discussed earlier, having novice students ask the question, "What can I do with you, today, to help you feel better?" is a very effective assessment tool. While clients' responses to this question are usually quite straight-forward, the student needs to interpret and analyze this response with the patient in order to affirm that the client has understood the question and responded in a manner that will lead to *beneficial interventions*. Beneficial interventions are those that meet the clients' needs, facilitate them to grow, adapt, and/or heal. To illustrate this, two very similar stories will be shared.

> *The first story is about a student in one of my clinical groups. When she asked her client the question, the client responded, "I want you to do whatever it is you have to do, and just leave me alone the rest of the time." The student interpreted this response as being very honest and straight-forward and determined that the client needed some solitude. According to the report she had received at shift change, she had learned that this client frequently complained about frequent, unnecessary interruptions.*
>
> *The student replied, "Okay. I will take your vital signs and do a quick physical assessment, right now. I will then bring your breakfast tray and remove it from your room after you finish eating. After that, I will not need to bother you again until noon. At that time, I will bring your lunch and take your vital signs. After lunch, I will remove your tray and let you have the rest of the afternoon to yourself. But I do need to tell you that you are my only patient, so I will be sitting right outside your door anytime you need me."*

> *The client agreed that this plan was very satisfactory. The student was totally true to her word; she did not even stick her head in the door from time to time to check on the client. When this client was discharged later that afternoon, she pointed to this bored, frustrated student and said, "This young lady is the best nurse in this hospital!"*

Because this student interpreted and analyzed the data accurately, she was able to design and implement creative, individualized interventions. She understood that her client needed solitude and rest. As a result, she drew strong accolades from the client, confirming her professional ability to use critical thinking appropriately.

More sophisticated analysis. The second story is similar, but the interpretation of what the patient really needed, and the interventions implemented by student are very different. Interpretations of the data are more sophisticated; they require more in-depth analysis. The verbatim evaluation related by a client, describing her interaction with a student nurse who cared for her in the hospital is presented below, followed by a discussion of the interpretation/analysis of data.

> *...By that point I had had it with everyone and everything, and I was the nastiest b-i-t-c-h on the face of this universe, and yet she* [the student nurse] *still displayed that very warm loving thing, like—"What do you need; do you need me to get you something? Do you need help out of the bed? Do you want me to . . .?" Very soothingly. I told her I was really grumpy and wanted to be left alone. She said, "Okay, just call me when. . . ." And even with that, she would come back every so often you know, when you say "No," but you really mean "Yes, I want you to check on me." Well, she would come check on me every so often. . . . She saw right through me.* (Rogers, 2002, p.170)

This student had learned in report that the client was very difficult and uncooperative—one that none of the nurses wanted as an assignment. According to the tertiary sources of information, nothing pleased her and she was unwilling to try to help herself. As the student listened to the client's comments, she interpreted "leave me alone" to mean, "I am scared and frustrated to the point of breaking. I do not want you in here if you are going to treat me like the other nurses have been treating me, but I need your presence, if you can help me feel safe." Whether this interpretation was based on an understanding of safety and security needs as discussed in Maslow's Hierarchy of needs, observations of non-verbal cues, or whether it was intuitive, the interventions designed from the interpretation/analyses seemed to meet the needs of this client.

It should be noted that earlier, we referred to the need for *beneficial interventions*. There are occasions when a client might request assistance with an activity that is *not growth-or health-directed* and lacks the potential for learning, building trust, or meeting basic needs. (For e.g., assistance in committing suicide). In this case, the nurse should demur in a very caring manner, continue to assess the client's view of the world and needs, and try to discover an intervention that is growth- and health-directed.

Creative, Individualized Interventions

Designing and implementing creative and individualized interventions consistent with the premises of MRM requires that nurses use multiple ways-of-knowing and multiple types of knowledge, discussed earlier in Section 1 of this book. Here, we pick up on this premise and offer some insights we've gained through the years. We start with intuitive knowing (a type of inductive logic) and proceed to a discussion of the application of several constructs in MRM.

Esthetic Knowing and Intuitive Knowledge

It is important for both students and faculty to value the importance of intuitive knowledge. We often know things we do not know we know. This has been discussed in Chapters 2-4 of this book and previously in H. Erickson, 2006d, p.32; and Erickson, et al., 1983/2009, p. 170-171. Explicitly, in Chapter 4 of this book, *Looking to the Future: Curriculum Implications* the authors state:

> *We believe that Intuition is a type of Esthetic Knowledge. We gain intuition by integrating various types of knowledge, (such as personal, ethical, reflective, and empirical knowledge), recycling through knowledge acquired from the various Ways-of-Knowing, each time gaining a deeper understanding of the essence of nursing. As with other growth experiences, it is not a "once-and-for-all" experience, but a continuous deepening of understanding and knowing—knowing about Self and knowing about others.* (Erickson, H & Erickson, M, 2010, p. 90)

While some may consider actions based on intuitive knowing unscientific, we believe that intuitive knowing is one of the most important tools a nurse can possess. As an example of this, a previously published story will be shared.

> *Mr. Davis had been admitted to the hospital for emergency abdominal surgery a few days earlier. He was now experiencing symptoms of alcohol withdrawal although his family had not recognized that he was an alcoholic. His physicians did not believe in supporting his*

alcoholism with the administration of ethanol to alleviate the withdrawal symptoms, although the nurses had suggested that this would be a beneficial intervention for this particular client. He became increasingly difficult to care for as his agitation and hallucinatory experiences increased.

Additionally, the integrity of his abdominal wound was at risk due to his obesity and constant restlessness. Although he was necessarily restrained, the nurses were increasingly concerned about the possibility of Mr. Davis injuring himself or one of the staff. They were also concerned because he had not slept for 48 hours, and they realized that his physical resources were being exhausted.

Ms. Rose, a young nurse, had followed accepted routine in attempting to orient Mr. Davis as to time and place and refusing to support his delusion that everyone was in severe danger of being swept away in a flood. As the situation continued to deteriorate, she considered the possibility of utilizing a different strategy.

The next time Ms. Rose entered Mr. Davis's room, he pointed to a spot on the wall and frantically said, "Nurse, hand me that knife over there. I need to cut myself loose and get out of here before that flood kills me!" Ms. Rose responded, "Mr. Davis, I see that knife. If the flood waters continue to rise, I will be glad to get it and cut you loose myself. Right now, though, the water isn't even up to the second floor. We're on the fourth floor, and I think maybe the water has quit rising. I will keep close watch on it, though. I even have a boat outside your door, and if the water gets too high, I'll come and get you, and we'll both leave. Until, then, though, why don't you take a nap? I know you're awfully tired."

After that encounter, Mr. Davis slept for 36 hours. When he awakened, he was refreshed, oriented and his recovery was uneventful. (Rogers, 1996, p. 175-6)

It can now be told that Ms. Rose was, in reality, S. Rogers, primary author of this chapter. This event occurred before the theory of MRM had been written. She states,

I must confess that my actions were totally intuitive and flew in the face of all I had been taught about dealing with clients suffering from delirium tremens. When asked what I had done to calm this extremely agitated man, I had to shrug my shoulders in ignorance, like many of my students in later years, for I had been practicing nursing behind closed doors and could not reveal the nature of my "inappropriate" intervention.

When I evaluate this event with what I currently know, I can identify many components of MRM. First, it is important to note that I attempted to soothe this man using strategies that are still used by many healthcare providers. But, he could not be dissuaded that his view of the world was not "reality." So, in desperation, I modeled his view of the world.

I recognized how frightening it would be to be in four-point leather restraints with a flood rising around me. I then intuitively understood that the only possible relief for this man (and those trying to care for him) was to step into his world and try to make it safe for him. I did this by validating his view of the world and promising to save him from the rising flood if it reached the floor we were on. I then suggested he take a nap, since he was obviously very tired.

Stepping into the Client's World. While *stepping into the client's world* sounds like modeling the client's world, it is more than that. It also involves interpretation, analysis, and planning interventions. It has a strong intuitive component, but the more it is implemented the more it truly becomes a cognitive process based on our scientific understanding of human behavior.

In the above story, not only did Rogers model the client's view of the world, but she also stepped into that world and began to understand how truly frightened this man was. As she understood (interpreted) his fear, she was able to plan an individualized intervention that would facilitate a sense of safety.

In another situation, the primary author *stepped into the client's world,* hoping to help a family member through the process of alcohol detoxification and delirium tremens. In that particular situation, she found herself switching between "orientation to reality" and "validation of his hallucinations." She states,

One moment, when he thought his friend's children were lost in the woods close to our house, I said, "No, they are safely at home in bed. Your brain is playing tricks on you because it wants some alcohol so badly." The next moment I wiped away the cobwebs that were falling on him from the ceiling.

In a lengthy reflection on this event and the many pieces of this puzzle that are too numerous to detail here, I concluded that I was using orientation versus validation, depending upon which strategy helped the client feel safest at the moment. This conclusion requires further examination through formal research, but, for the moment, I believe that Role-modeling in this situation involved an intuitive knowing derived by stepping into the client's world.

The stories presented above provide examples of a nurse purposefully creating a caring-healing field (Brekke & Schultz, 2006, pp. 52-61; Erickson, H., 2006f, pp. 424-440; Kinney, 2006, pp. 278-299) with the intent of facilitating coping in clients. As we enter a "*functional, trusting relationship*" (Erickson, et al., 1983/2009, p. 322), we create an energy field (Brekke, & Schultz, 2006, pp. 45-64) that promotes healing and well-being.

Labeling is Destructive. As mentioned in several of the above examples, the need for safety and security is essential for well-being and healing in our clients. It is important to help students understand that the behavior of many of our "difficult," "non-compliant," and confused clients is driven by the failure of healthcare professionals to meet their safety and security needs. When call-lights are not answered, when nurses refuse to tell clients what medications are being administered, when nurses tell clients, "That's not how we do it here," the client becomes increasingly fearful and uncooperative (Rogers, 2002).

The client, who in an earlier story referred to herself as a "b-i-t-c-h," asked her physician to discharge her home even though she was still suffering from a paralytic ileus. When asked why she wanted to go home even though she was still so sick, she looked at her interviewer as though the interviewer was out of her mind and said, "I was sure that if I stayed in the hospital, the nurses would find some way to kill me!" (Rogers, 2002, pp. 309-310)

Adherence versus Compliance. The MRM model calls for the use of the word *adherence* rather than *compliance*. The implications are that the client is involved with setting the goals for their care. When we talk about *non*-adherence, we have to revisit the original, mutually-set goal (Erickson, et al., 1983/2009, pp. 170-177) and reevaluate the situation. When we discuss non-compliance, we only have to consider the nurse or doctor's goals for care. It should be noted that these are usually done within the Totality model and are directed at the cure or control of disease, not the health, growth and adaptation of a human being.

Adaptive Potential and Maladaptive Coping. Another group of clients who warrant consideration of need status are those we see in the healthcare system often referred to by staff as "frequent flyers." Another way to think of them is to consider them as in maladaptive coping; some are impoverished, some are not.

Some of these clients are truly ill, but seem to seek health care more often than necessary, while some of these clients report problems and symptoms that elude the most sophisticated efforts at diagnosis. Many of these clients show-up at the emergency room or clinic on almost a daily basis to get their love and belonging needs met. If nurses can recognize this and role-model for the patient an alternative strategy for getting these needs met, their visits will diminish. One of the LVN to RN students of the primary author asked for help planning a strategy to help a client who frequently visited the emergency room (ER) where the nurse worked. The client was asthmatic and visited the ER almost daily, but usually did not need such sophisticated care as provided in the ER.

The LVN knew that the young woman had no children, was not employed, and had no friends or family in the area other than her husband. Together, the faculty and student designed a plan for the student to expand her knowledge of the client's world-view. Part of this assessment would include trying to discover what this woman "dreamed" of doing. As this LVN proceeded, she learned that her client's dream was to work with children. As part of her intervention, the student suggested that her client might volunteer at a nearby daycare center. Weeks went by without an ER visit by this client.

Finally, she stopped by one evening just to chat. She said she had not had an asthma attack in weeks. She also shared that she had "had the idea" of volunteering at the nearby daycare center and had eventually become a full-fledged employee. She had learned to get her psychosocial needs met within the system, rather than crossing over to the physiological system (Benson, 2006, p. 253; Erickson et al., 1983/2009, pp. 75-83; Walker & Erickson, H., 2006, pp. 67-94). She moved from using maladaptive coping to adaptive coping, a state in the Adaptive Potential Assessment Model (APAM) which will be discussed more thoroughly below.

Although this client stated that *she* had conceived the idea of volunteering and never mentioned the nurse's part in her growth, at some level, she knew the nurse was somehow involved in her idea. This is why she returned to report her situation.

> When clients "own or co-own" the plan, it is much more effective than when we, the nurses, try to own it.

Empirical Knowing

The Adaptive Potential Assessment Model Revisited

The Adaptive Potential Assessment Model (APAM) (Erickson, H., 1976; Erickson, H., & Swain, M., 1990; Erickson, et al., 1983/2009, pp. 82-84) is an extremely valuable tool in helping students model the needs of their clients, and in turn, plan strategies that will facilitate the movement of the client to a healthier location on the APAM model. Using the APAM model requires an understanding of Selye's General Adaptation Syndrome (G.A.S.) (Selye, 1976) and Engel's human responses to stressors (Engel, 1962). While this understanding is a necessary underpinning, the APAM model is much more holistic in nature that either Selye's G.A.S. or Engel's human responses to stressors (Erickson, et al., 1983/2009, pp.75-81). The APAM, reproduced here in Figure 7.1, is described more fully in Erickson et al., 1983/2009, pp. 75-83, and expanded upon by Benson, 2006, pp. 250-266).

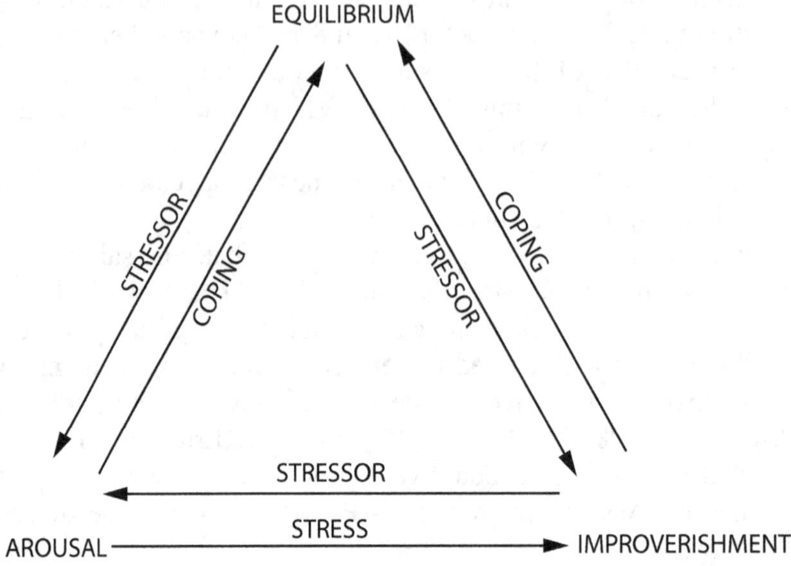

Figure 7.1 The Adaptive Potential Assessment Model.
Reprinted with permission. Erickson, et al., *Modeling and Role-Modeling: A Theory and Paradigm for Nursing,* 1983/2009, p. 82. Cedar Park, TX: EST Co.

Accordingly, persons in an *arousal* state have experienced a stressor(s) within the past 72 hours. These individuals have a high potential for mobilizing the resources needed to contend with those stressors (Erickson, H., 1990. p. 17). The state of arousal in a client is marked by feelings of tension and anxiety without feelings of fatigue, sadness, and depression. Often, the motor-sensory behavior of the client is elevated, vital signs are elevated, and verbal expressions of anxiety are elevated. The bottom right corner of APAM is labeled *Impoverishment*, and is the stress state that should be of highest concern to nurses. When in Impoverishment, the client may express marked feelings of tension and anxiety with feelings of fatigue, sadness, and depression. While verbal anxiety, motor-sensory behavior and vital signs may be elevated, as the client moves closer to total Impoverishment these parameters will diminish until death occurs. One effective exercise for clinical students is to mark their client's position on the APAM at the beginning of their shift and then again at the end of the shift. This facilitates the student's ability to identify stressors and distressors and the resulting stress, the client's coping resources (internal and external), and interpretation of the client's adaptation to the situation.

Discussion of the student's interpretation of the client's needs and how the planned interventions moved the client to a healthier plane are great material for post-conference. In one of these post-conference experiences, the primary author and her students were discussing the placement of a client who seemed somewhat impoverished, but was very close to arousal in much of his behavior. When this question was posed to Helen Erickson, she responded, "Remember, each stage can be thought of as being in a continuum" (Erickson, personal communication, 1994).

"Stretched - Out" APAM
(Corners of the Triangle)

High Level Health & Well- Being		Health Within Illness
	EQUILIBRIUM	
Full Frontal Attack With All Resources		Conservative Withdrawal
	AROUSAL	
Protective Withdrawal		Complete Depletion
	IMPOVERISHMENT	

Figure 7.2 Rogers' version of APAM for clinical students use.

Based on this discussion, the tool, shown in Figure 7.2, was developed. This model is largely self-explanatory, but some of the terms will be addressed for clarity. Health Within Illness is a difficult concept for some healthcare providers to accept. But many individuals are able to attain a state of healthy equilibrium in spite of illness. Possibly, this is seen most often in those with acceptance and healthy adaptation to chronic illness, but it can be seen in acute disease states as well. Clients who are in a high-level stress state experiencing multiple stressors are sometimes demanding and even "difficult," but they require little attention from nurses unless assistance in receiving a needed resource requires healthcare provider intervention.

The client in Conservative Withdrawal still has some resources (internal and/or external) available, but he/she needs someone to facilitate access to those resources. We always tell our students, "These individuals are just waiting for the right student to come along and discover what type of assistance they need." The client in Protective Withdrawal has used all resources knowingly available and has largely given-up on finding that nurse who can facilitate recovery. In fact, this client is truly protecting himself or herself from the biocidic attacks of healthcare professionals (Halldorsdottir, 1991).

The distance between Conservative Withdrawal and Protective Withdrawal is quite small, and students are very adept at moving clients from Protective Withdrawal to Conservative Withdrawal and up into a healthier state of Arousal. Complete depletion leads to death, but even at this end of the Impoverishment continuum, nursing care using the tenets of MRM can lead to healing.

Developmental Theories

Developmental theories that drive our understanding of patient needs in MRM are significant, but discussion of those theories will be brief in this chapter. For more discussion of these theories refer to the original authors. For an understanding of how these were integrated and expanded to create a comprehensive model that includes relations among developmental theory, needs status, loss and grief, and ability to cope, see Erickson et al., 1983/2009 (pp. 78-83, 121-122, 154-160, 177), and M. Erickson, (2006a, pp. 225-229).

Background information. Engel (1962, cited in Erickson, H., 1976) discussed psychological development in health and disease. While Engel espoused the general idea of a mind-body connection, his understanding of this relationship was very rudimentary, compared to our understanding of psychoneuroimmunology (PNI) today. Piaget's (1969) research related to cognitive development also provides important information related to the developmental residual of our clients. As we think about all these developmental theories, it is important to note that the chronological age of a client does not always match the developmental age and stage of that client. This will be discussed further in this section.

Erikson (1963) developed the most comprehensive model of psychosocial development, describing the stages, tasks of development and residual that emerges across the lifespan. Erikson argued that development is discontinuous, and is epigenetic. This means that there are specific starting and stopping points of each stage, and that the human has the ability to work and rework each stage throughout the lifespan. The latter concept is extremely important in MRM as it implies that people always have the potential to grow and become more fully who they are intended to be.

Developmental Issues in MRM. Margaret Erickson (2006b) expanded and revised Erik Erikson's model of development. Her aims were to include psychosocial development of the fetus and a last stage that represents the dying process (p. 128), and to modify Erikson's premises to be consistent with MRM. M. Erickson's discussion of developmental processes is extremely important for faculty who wish to teach MRM.

Negative residual can exist at any of the stages discussed by the above theorists, but perhaps the one we see most in our hospitalized clients is that of trust vs. mistrust, a task that is worked on in the stage of infancy. If the infant does not receive the needed love and care that should be provided by parents or substitute caregivers, that individual deals with a negative residual of mistrust throughout his/her lifetime.

Often, this mistrust is made evident in the healthcare client through non-adherence to a prescribed regimen, being difficult and demanding, and/or downright nasty. Needless to say, with these clients, the first Aim of Intervention, creating trust, can be time-consuming, but is almost always rewarding.[6] In conclusion to this section, it must be noted that establishing a client's negative developmental residual is one of the most important steps in data analysis and interpretation. As nurses, we must understand why a client seems to be acting like an infant or a two-year-old. Simply stated, they are working on issues of trust and autonomy, even as they try to work through their chronologically appropriate life-stage tasks.

Integrative Knowing

As the reader has seen, MRM-based interventions are not what we might commonly describe as *textbook interventions*. Instead, each intervention was designed to meet the needs of a unique client in a specific situation. This is the essence of Role-Modeling. No two humans are the same even though all humans have many commonalities. No two people perceive things exactly alike although many of us think alike, and no two people have the same life-experiences—each of us is on our own journey. As a result, interventions need to be *tailored* (Erickson, Milton,[7]) for each individual. We need to use multiple ways-of-knowing, integrate them and create personalized interventions.

Greater detail on how to meet specific needs at various stages of life can be found in H. Erickson, 2006g, pp. 325-345; we do not intend to repeat that work here. However, we would like to discuss a few creative, individualized interventions that are easy for students to understand and use.

Textbook versus Individualized Care

In one facility where the primary author of this chapter taught clinical students, the standard student care plan asked the student to list several textbook

---

[6] Finch's work (1987) with a sample of hospitalized medical-surgical patients showed that there was a significant relationship between length of stay and mistrust measured as a negative developmental residual. There was no significant relationship with trust residual.

[7] The reader interested in Milton Erickson's work will find this reference as a beginning. There are many wonderful publications by him and about him that can be found through a Google search of Milton Erickson or by going to the Milton Erickson website, www.**erickson-foundation**.org. For the curious reader, Milton Erickson was H. Erickson's father-in-law and mentor and M. Erickson's grandfather.

interventions and describe how those interventions had been implemented. Instead, she asked students in her clinical group to list one or two textbook interventions and describe why those interventions were not appropriate for their client.

The students loved this exercise, and at the end of the semester were in general agreement that they had not cared for a "textbook" client during the entire semester.

Reframing

Reframing, a technique developed by Milton Erickson, and incorporated into MRM by H. Erickson and others (2006a, p. 19, p. 120, p. 373, p. 480) occurs as we change the language to create what is viewed as negative to a positive perspective (Erickson, H., 2006b, p. 372). It is defined (Erickson, H., 2006a) as a "communication technique that facilitates a change in perception of an event, situation, condition, and so forth" (p. 479). Too many of our clients see their illness as punishment from God or a nameless higher power. Students become very adept at helping clients see their current situation as an opportunity for growth and potentially helping others in the future.

Most people are not able to reframe life experiences on their own; if they could, they would have already done it. They come to healthcare providers because they need help. Often, little is required to facilitate reframing.

Imagery and Relaxation Techniques

Guided imagery and relaxation are two techniques discussed by several authors in respect to MRM in H. Erickson, 2006a (pp. 101-2, pp. 298-9, pp. 314-322) that can be sophisticated and used in complex cases; they can also be simplified and used by novices in some cases. If clients are not too impoverished, they usually respond fairly well. The primary author provides the following example:

> *One semester, I had a group of students who were each required to implement an individual teaching project for a client. We were on an orthopedic unit where many of the clients had issues with pain control. One of the students decided to teach one of these clients an imagery/relaxation script that he could implement for himself when she (the student) was no longer available to help him with the script. She repeatedly practiced the script that she had selected; her husband served as her pseudo-client. By the time she was finished practicing, she was relaxed and fluent.*
>
> *Once she was ready, she asked to be assigned to the most difficult pain-control client on the unit. The nurses said, "You really don't want to*

try this on this man. No matter what we give him or how we reposition him, he screams that his pain is a 10 on a scale of 1 to 10!" The student said, "That is exactly the kind of client I want to implement this with." So, she accomplished standard care with him in the morning, taking vital signs, doing a complete assessment, giving him a bed bath, doing her best to establish a trusting relationship. Then, in the early afternoon she and I entered her client's room. The student had already asked him if he would be willing to learn a unique method for controlling his own pain, and he had eagerly agreed.

The student first asked the client about his level of pain, which, as usual, he described as "10." She then darkened the room, pulling the drapes and turning off all lights. In a very soft, soothing, monotonous voice, she began by taking the client through a relaxation script. Visually, he began to appear less anxious and distressed. Then, she said, "Okay, now I want you to think about your pain as a red rubber ball." The client nodded his assent to this direction. The student said, "I want you to let that ball get bigger and bigger." Once again, he nodded his assent. She said, "Is your pain getting worse?" He nodded. She then said, "Now, I want you to let that ball shrink down to the size it was a minute ago. Does that help?" The client nodded. "Now, shrink it as small as you possibly can." The room remained totally silent for quite some time, then the client nodded that the ball was very small. "Okay, now throw it away as far from you as you can," which the client physically did.

Before we left the room, the student reminded the client that he could now implement this technique for himself anytime he needed comfort. She also asked him about his current pain on a scale of 1 to 10, and he made a zero with his fingers, not wanting to break the magic of the moment.

We know that novice students can use such techniques and are often successful. There are many other techniques which can be included in their repertoire of skills and strategies that facilitate people to take control of their own life and to enhance their ability to heal and grow. However, to ensure the safety and well-being of clients, it is important for faculty to acquire a level of sophisticated knowledge about the use and actions of both guided imagery and relaxation techniques.

FINAL NOTES

We would like to end this chapter with two reminders for faculty. First of all, students are far more imaginative in developing creative, individualized interventions than we might imagine. Generally, that is because we have socialized them that it is okay to be creative, as long as we use data to support decisions and our interventions are always growth-directed. Secondly, students must know beyond any shadow of doubt that they are safe in implementing these creative, individualized interventions. This, however, places the responsibility for safety of clients and students on the faculty. While faculty members have always recognized their responsibility to the patients being cared for by students, many do not think about the risks students take when encouraged to be creative and holistic in their plans of care. According to Halldorsdottir (1991), there are five basic ways to be in a relationship with another person.

Ways-of-Being With

Drawing from a secondary analysis of two earlier qualitative studies, Halldorsdottir identified examples of caring and uncaring encounters in hospitals. Her first study involved interviews with nine former patients. The second study entailed similar interviews with nine former Nursing students. The five modes that Halldorsdottir (1991) identified are (a) *life-destroying* or biocidic, (b) *life-restraining* or biostatic, (c) *life-neutral* or biopassive, (d) *life-sustaining* or bioactive, and (e) *life-giving* or biogenic.

The biocidic mode of *being with* another is the most inhumane and is represented by all forms of violence. While any form of physical abuse belongs in this category, it also includes dominance and depersonalization. Also part of this mode is hardheartedness or cold-heartedness. The biostatic mode includes insensitivity or indifference that results in discouragement or uneasiness in the other. It can involve imposing one's will on another, fault-finding, anger, blaming, or just being unfriendly. The biopassive mode of being with another is perceived apathy—inattention to patients and their specific, individual needs. While biopassive nurses may be very concerned with and effective at task performance, they express no concern for the patient as a person. The bioactive mode "involves benevolence, good will, genuine kindness and concern, beneficence, and kindheartedness. It is protecting life, relieving suffering, keeping promises, respecting the other, and acknowledging the other's human-hood" (Halldorsdottir, 1991, p. 43). The biogenic mode of being with another is the most cogent to this current discussion. This mode is "represented by healing love" (p. 44). The life-giving presence "restores well being and human dignity" (p. 44). It is hardly necessary to add that if all nurses were aware of their bioactive and biogenic presence with patients, all nurses could be healing nurses, even in the face of terminal illness.

Implications

We contend that it is important to discuss the potential philosophical diversity and ways-of-being that students encounter with faculty, peers and clients. They need to be able to understand how important relationships are in life, and specifically, in professional practice. They should know that people do not always share philosophies, but they will *always* act on them. When students are taught to practice from a holistic paradigm, they need to understand that some faculty (and later on, some charge nurses) will not understand what they are doing, and will declare that they are practicing inappropriately; sometimes they are accused of practicing outside the professional code.

We cannot protect our students from these experiences, but we can prepare them for such events. The best preparation beyond learning the basic ethics of Nursing is to help them learn the language embedded in their chosen theory. It is equally important to help them learn how to use assessment and interpretation tools, and to plan appropriate interventions and research designs.

A story, related by Sharon Rogers, illustrating this point, follows:

> *A student who had learned about MRM during a Level 2 clinical rotation decided to implement what she had learned during her pediatric rotation. She was caring for a child, 8 or 9 years old, who had intractable abdominal pain. He had been through every imaginable test and no medical diagnosis had been reached; he was scheduled for an exploratory laparotomy that afternoon.*
>
> *When the family left together for lunch, this student went into this child's room and said, "Why do you think your tummy hurts so badly?" With this question, her little client poured out a horrific story of constant, unrelenting abuse at home. The student eagerly went out to the nurses' station to share this story with her clinical instructor and the charge nurse. Both of them were horrified, not by the little boy's story, but by the fact that this student had stepped so inappropriately out of her role as "student nurse" to elicit this information.*
>
> *The little boy proceeded to the operating room, and the clinical instructor tried to get the student removed from the Nursing program. Had a very influential person with a holistic philosophy not been available to step into the breach, this student would have been expelled from the program.*

Proactivity. When students learn the language of a Nursing theory, including relationships among concepts, they are able to describe how they interpret data, what relationships they have identified, and justify their intervention decisions. Without the use of the language, they have no way to communicate their observations.

Consistent with this, it is imperative that they also learn how to interpret the data and analyze relations among them. These skills help them demonstrate their ability to use critical thinking skills. Finally, students also need to learn to use research findings derived from testing various aspects of the theory, to help them plan appropriate interventions. Without the use of critical thinking and research findings, unorthodox and individualized interventions may appear to be arbitrary and without direction—landmarks of unprofessional behavior. Armed with a Nursing theory consistent with their basic philosophy, students can learn how to be proactive. They have the potential to be Nursing's leaders.

SUMMARY

This chapter has discussed several of the basic components of the MRM theory and paradigm and described how faculty can use it with undergraduate students. The use of intuition and novice strategies has also been included to help faculty teach this part of the theory of Modeling and Role-Modeling to student nurses.

The faculty-student relationship was also addressed. We proposed that students learn best when the focus is on their growth and ability to know at multiple levels. Pacing or validation and affirmation of their world-view is important if we, as faculty, wish to lead them to discover their potential as professional nurses. Finally, when faculty members facilitate students to learn by discovery, they can anticipate that their students will want to "own" what they do and what they know, even though you know it was your idea and suggestion. When this occurs, faculty should be gratified that they have successfully mentored one more group of young nurses; they have successfully fulfilled their responsibility to society.

CHAPTER 8

FACILITATING PERSONAL KNOWLEDGE DEVELOPMENT

Carolyn K. Kinney

'Learning' is, most often, figuring out how to use what you already know in order to go beyond what you currently think. There are many ways of doing that. Some are more intuitive; others are formally derivational. But they all depend on knowing something "structural" about what you are contemplating—how to put it together. Knowing how something is put together is worth a thousand facts about it. It permits you to go beyond it. (Bruner, 1984, p. 183)

OVERVIEW

For almost 25 years, I have implemented versions of the teaching-learning strategies described in this chapter, using them successfully in courses in undergraduate, RN-BSN completion, Master's and doctoral programs. The outcomes for the learners and for me as their teacher have been overwhelmingly positive, enlightening, and rewarding. The purpose of this chapter is to describe how this approach was used to facilitate graduate students' learning by discovery as proposed by Bruner and presented in detail in Chapter 5 of this book.

As indicated in the Bruner quote above, the goal is to help students learn how to put together what they previously knew and are now learning, so that they can go beyond what they currently *think*. One student, I'll call Mary, is forever etched in my memory as an exemplar of the type of self-discovery, heightened sense of self-awareness, and deepened understanding of holistic nursing that can be facilitated through this strategy. My personal experience with Mary is provided as an example and is intermixed with a formal discussion of the theoretical background of my work.

PROVIDING THE STRUCTURE FOR DISCOVERY-LEARNING

Some students are initially uncomfortable with what they experience as ambiguous expectations or a lack of straight didactic information, and a few are never able to appreciate the type of learning opportunity the approach provides them. However, the large majority are surprised with how energized they feel as they have self-discoveries. Subsequently, many embrace the fact that they had the opportunity to learn how to think and to express themselves in ways that had not been allowed in previous educational settings. The notion that they have intuitive and personal knowledge that can be brought forth and expressed as worthwhile information is empowering. This connection to their own personal knowledge gives them a renewed enthusiasm for nursing and their role as a nurse. I have used this approach to help students form a foundation of personal knowledge upon which subsequent learning opportunities can be built. To begin, we start with their beliefs.

Starting with the Student's Belief System

Consistent with the Modeling and Role-Modeling premise that starting with the client's perspectives (modeling the client's world) and providing an environment that nurtures self-expression and growth is critical to successful nursing care, similar principles can be implemented in the educational setting through application of strategies compatible with Bruner's discovery-learning theory (Bruner, 1966). Bruner posits that learning be viewed as a process of personal discovery where learners draw on their own past experiences and existing knowledge to discover concepts and relationships and new truths to be learned. The goal is to guide students in recoding old knowledge and integrating it with new knowledge to build their own unique and personal base of knowledge. This knowledge-base then serves as a foundation for future knowledge building in a spiral-like learning process (Bruner, 1967). Bruner describes the process of teaching a subject as beginning "with an 'intuitive' account that is well within the reach of a student and then circle back later to a more formal or highly structured account, until, with however many more recyclings are necessary, the learner has mastered the topic or subject in its full generative power" (Bruner, 1996, p. 92).

Setting the Stage for Discovery

Based on Bruner's framework and educational strategies, an active discovery-learning approach is recommended to help students develop an understanding of holistic philosophy. By starting with an assignment that taps into their intuitive knowledge about the subject, learners are supported in exploring their unique perspectives and their personal world-view. This process facilitates students in bringing into their conscious awareness and putting into their own words their intuitive personal belief systems, their personal knowing (Carper, 1978).

To set the stage for the course, on the first day of class I provide the typical overview of the course by guiding students through the course objectives, learning activities and expectations. While doing this, I emphasize the course's educational philosophy, and highlight learning activities and educational premises, as outlined in Table 8.1. For example, I stress that in this course students and faculty are partners in learning, that students will have opportunities to learn more about themselves and become more aware and comfortable with what they know, and that self-discovery is key to learning. For this course in particular, I emphasize the value of becoming aware of one's personal philosophy and provide a brief introduction to philosophy, in general, and Nursing philosophy, in particular.

Table 8.1 Relations between Bruner's Discovery Methods and teaching activities.

Bruner Strategy	**Premises**	**Instructor Activities**
Create a predisposition for learning by providing a nurturing environment.	Students and faculty are partners; • honest and thoughtful dialogue is an expectation; • being open to learning more about one's self provides a foundation for being receptive to others; and • learning is life-long for faculty and students; we continually learn from each other.	For this specific course, I: • emphasized that a collaborative faculty-student relationships is desired; • initiated the learning experience by explaining that the teaching/learning philosophy is based on the belief that learning is a mutual endeavor and is a life-long process;
Build an initial structure or scaffold for learning.	Faculty members are responsible for providing relevant information and learning opportunities with the goal of facilitating learning.	• provided a description of what is meant by philosophy and Nursing philosophy, and the value to Nursing; • explained that all of us have a philosophy; • expressed understanding that articulating our philosophy can be a real challenge; and
Provide opportunity for self-discovery, exploration, and creativity.	Faculty are responsible for relevant information and learning opportunities that facilitate learning; and students, responsible for their own learning, can plan their schedule of study using predetermined deadlines.	• assigned a written project titled: *My Personal and Professional Philosophy* following the criteria outlined in Table 8.2.

To reinforce the value of self-examination and being thoughtful and intuitively aware as nurses, I include didactic information during the early class sessions about reflective practice as described by Schön (1983). Specifically, I provide a brief overview of Schön's work related to successful reflective practitioners in practice-based professions. (I highly recommend using Christopher Johns' work to help students understand reflective practice.)

Table 8.2 An example of a class assignment.

A. Course objectives:
Upon completion of this course, students will be able to:
1. Articulate their personal and professional philosophies.
2. Articulate how their personal philosophy informs their interpretation of Nursing's discipline and practice.

B. Content of the paper:
1. Write a clear description of your own personal philosophy. Be brief and use your own words. This section provides the basis for the remainder of the paper.
2. Provide explicit statements regarding your definition or description of the four Metaparadigm concepts of: person, health, environment, and nursing. This section provides the opportunity to increase clarity in your views and understanding of each of these concepts.
3. Describe how you believe the four concepts are inter-related in your practice experiences. This section gives you the opportunity to articulate your thoughts about your nursing practice model; that is, using your own words, you are to describe how you believe these concepts relate and how these relationships influence your practice of nursing and/or how you would like to practice nursing.
4. Summarize what you have written and provide conclusions pertaining to your philosophical beliefs and your philosophy of nursing practice. Indicate any inconsistencies you have discovered between your beliefs and your actions and behaviors. This section gives you the opportunity to focus on what you have discovered about yourself, your world-view, and your nursing philosophy. Openly and honestly critique yourself as appropriate, indicating areas you are satisfied with and those which you would like to improve.

C. Paper Format:
1. Use an appropriate formal paper writing style with the exception that you are expected to write in a first-person, narrative style, using a conversational tone.
2. Follow a standard outline for a formal paper including an introduction, summary, and conclusions.
3. Limit the paper to a total of five word-processed double spaced pages.
4. A reference list is not required. However, if the ideas or work of anyone other than yourself is included, you are to use appropriate APA referencing and citation.
5. Correct grammar, spelling, and consistent writing style are expected.

Present your ideas, beliefs, and views thoughtfully and coherently. Build progressively and logically from one section to the next and be as clear as you can about how your thinking has developed and progressed.

The ultimate success of a discovery-learning approach requires the purposeful and intentional creation of an environment that supports students' sense that it is safe for them to engage in self-discovery; one that nurtures individual self-expression and promotes a sense of self-confidence and fosters an ability to trust their own knowledge and wisdom. Moreover, by experiencing a safe learning environment, students' attitudes of inquiry and exploration are stimulated, thus enabling them to engage more fully in the learning process.

Teaching/learning Strategy

While a variety of teaching-learning strategies may be used to accomplish the desired outcome of facilitating students' articulation of their personal and professional philosophy, I use an inductive self-discovery approach, building on strategies consistent with Bruner's educational theory. Table 8.2 provides an example of a course assignment used to guide learning.

This process is described more completely below as I discuss Mary's experiences with discovery-learning. While Mary stands out, she represents countless numbers of other nurses with whom I have had contact over the years. She impressed me with her sincerity and compassion based on contributions she made in class, her written work, and conversations I had with her outside of class.

The following, written in italics, is a brief description of what transpired as Mary, a first semester graduate student, experienced discovery-learning. I have inserted analytical statements to help the reader understand the importance of Mary's experience and my part in it.

AN EXEMPLAR OF LEARNING

Mary's Story

From her nonverbal behavior, I interpreted that Mary was conflicted about what she was hearing. Appearing both eager and hesitant, she sat in the front row and made eye contact with me, listened carefully and nodded her head at times, yet at other times she sat back in her chair with folded arms and furrowed brow. When I asked the students if they had questions, concerns, or responses to what I had been discussing, Mary quickly volunteered that what I'd said about what we would be doing in this course brought up a recent experience and she'd like to share it. She told of wanting to care for her clients as people and how difficult it was when she was not supported by other nurses in spending the time with them that she felt was needed. She gave a poignant account of Mrs. P. who had metastatic breast cancer and was suffering severe bone pain. The woman's family lived too far from the hospital to come see her regularly. Recently, Mrs. P. had received several letters, but due to her pain medications was unable to focus her eyes to read the letters. Mary offered to sit with her and read her letters for her. When other nurses found out what Mary was doing, she was criticized for getting too involved.

My first response to Mary was to thank her for speaking up in class and sharing her experiences. Next, I acknowledged that her wanting to see her clients as people with multiple needs, as more than just their medical diagnosis or someone with a health problem, was an excellent example of practicing from a nursing perspective, and a holistic perspective in particular. I emphasized that rather than limiting her care only to a medical perspective, she was helping her client maintain a connection with her loved ones and this, in turn, could have a positive effect on her healing process. By recognizing and acting on her belief that family support is an important aspect of a person's holistic well-being, she was being true to her nursing philosophy even though, at that time, she may not have thought about it in those terms.

Confirming the Focus of Learning

As I made these points, I watched for confirmation from Mary that I had understood her thoughts and feelings about the situation. She nodded in enthusiastic agreement and said, "All I was doing was what my client needed me to do and I felt discounted by the other nurses and criticized for neglecting my *work*." According to Bruner's learning theory, the goal of teaching is to facilitate learning by providing appropriate learning experiences and stimulating critical thinking skills rather than simply transmitting knowledge. In other words, the focus is on what is learned rather than on what is taught.

I went over to Mary, gently touched her arm, looked directly in her eyes, and said, "Mary, you were being the best nurse you knew how to be and were responding to your client's holistic needs. You <u>were</u> doing your work." I stood by her for a few seconds and then said that if it was alright with her I would like to turn to a related aspect of what she had experienced and pose a question. She smiled and nodded assent, so I proceeded, saying, "It is very difficult to do what we believe our clients need when we ourselves do not feel supported by our colleagues." I then asked her to explore what she would like to have happen if this type of situation were to occur again. She admitted she was at a loss as to what to do, but felt it was important that nurses work together and not against one another. I confirmed this as an appropriate expectation from one professional to another, and as professionals we have the responsibility to *practice in this way; that is, to respect each other as human beings with needs and expectations. I then said to her that "On some level you do know what to do; it is a knowing that is within you and I'm confident you will discover what you know but don't know you know." I paused for a few seconds to let this idea sink in and then asked her if she had anything more she'd like to share. She appeared very thoughtful and contemplative, yet smiled again and responded, "No, not right now." I said, 'Okay then, I'd like to open up the discussion to input from others" and invited the other students to join in.*

Many experiences were described by other students and the discussion continued for many minutes. Where possible, I brought to their awareness how what they said reflected their personal philosophical perspectives and that each person had both a unique, yet often at the same time, a shared understanding of what was being discussed. As the discussion was coming to a close, I looked at Mary and noted that it was understandable to have a sense of sadness about 'the restrictive and callous healthcare environment.' I choose these words intentionally because Mary had used them earlier and I wanted to be sure she knew I'd heard her and understood how she experienced the environment. I emphasized that it is also important to realize that as professionals we can and do have the ability and responsibility to change the environment. When we acknowledge the human needs in others, we are better able to address those needs from a holistic perspective and, in turn, increase the likelihood that everyone's needs will be addressed, especially our clients'.

I turned to the class as a whole and said that "Through our work in this course and the discoveries all of you will make, we can help each other learn ways to make a difference in the healthcare settings in which we work and with the people for whom we provide care." I added that there would be many more similar and different discoveries made by everyone in the class. I emphasized that it was apparent that everyone was already learning much about themselves as a result of the discussion and I was eager to see what else they learned and discovered as they wrote their papers.

Mind Set of the Educator

As mentioned above, the goal of Bruner's approach to teaching is to facilitate learning by providing appropriate learning experiences and stimulating critical thinking skills rather than simply transmitting knowledge—that is, to focus on what is learned rather than on what is taught. Adding to this general goal, it is recommended that the educator keep in mind that a major purpose of this assignment is to mentor students in their thinking about the value of holistic philosophy and to recognize that one's beliefs serve as a basis for nursing care. Through careful handling of this assignment, educators can lead-by-example and provide compassionate, accepting, and sensitive support and encouragement to the students.

> *Mary came to me after class and revealed that the Master's program was a last resort before she abandoned Nursing all together. She admitted she was conflicted about what she wanted to do about her future, and was initially skeptical about the value of writing her philosophy and the purpose this would serve. She acknowledged she was now curious about the assignment and was enthusiastic about what she would "come up with." She added, "Thanks for being so understanding."*

Course Objectives

There are three specific educational objectives for the course assignment shown in Table 8.2 above. These are shown in Table 8.3.

Table 8.3 Educational objectives for student assignment.

a. This assignment provides a vehicle for teacher and learner to engage in an exchange regarding the student's philosophical beliefs and beginning ability to acknowledge and articulate his/her philosophy of Nursing.
b. The students are given the opportunity to tap into their intuitive and personal knowing, and bring into conscious awareness their personal philosophy, and how their beliefs influence the way they think about nursing and nursing care.
c. The teacher is given the opportunity to provide comments that validate students' perspectives, offer alternative views where appropriate, and create a fertile environment for continued exploration and learning—that is, set in motion the spiral of learning proposed by Bruner.

> *Mary's paper was exquisite. She provided a clear and thoughtful description of her personal philosophy and was very candid about how she had gradually lost sight of why she had become a nurse. She discovered that how she thought had a strong influence on the way she acted. She provided examples of times she believed she had been true to her philosophy and revealed ways she had not. She recognized that she is responsible for supporting other nurses in ways she wants to be supported by them and indicated this as one of the most important discoveries she had made in writing her paper. She further acknowledged that being able to view colleagues holistically was equally important as viewing our clients holistically, and at times more challenging.*

During the class session when the papers were due, Mary volunteered to share her thoughts and indicated that as she wrote her paper she came to realize she had, too often, let others and situations constrict the way she practiced nursing. She had lost connection with her beliefs, particularly about the importance of treating others with dignity and compassion, including her Nursing colleagues, regardless of whether they had the same values or looked at the world the same way she did. She vowed to remind herself regularly about how important it is to stay committed to her clients, be supportive of other nurses, be true to herself and her beliefs, and not let unsupportive circumstances dictate how she practiced nursing.

Evaluation of Students' work

The grading outcome is primarily based on students' ability to address the topic, express themselves clearly and logically, and meet formal paper requirements. It is important to provide written input and feedback to the students that encourages self-expression and self-discovery, validates their personal views, confirms their right to their views, and encourages them to openly express themselves. It is recommended that criticism or judgment of the students' views as right or wrong is not compatible with the goal of the assignment and is to be avoided. It is appropriate, however, to bring the students' attention to inconsistencies in their thinking and actions or where their beliefs do not translate directly into their described behavior. The long range goal is to encourage students to engage in continuous self-evaluation and critique and develop a comfort with and appreciation for the value of an ongoing reflective practice (see Chapter 14).

Becoming a Reflective Practitioner

The best way I know to describe the shift in students' thinking that occurs as they engage in the self-examination of discovery-learning is that they see themselves *becoming reflective practitioners*. I use 'becoming' intentionally because reflective practice takes…well...practice. Students know this. As Chris Johns (Chapter 14) explains, reflective-practice "…takes time and hard work" (p. 328). Students showing a desire to be more reflective, mindful, and purposeful in their practice also acknowledge this change will not happen overnight. The intellectual and emotional stimulation of examining one's self, and how one's world-view provides the basis for one's approach to life and one's life-work, serves as a stimulus for the *beginning of this becoming.*

Regardless of whether or not students fully embrace self-discovery and self-reflection, it is important to model their world and acknowledge to them that you recognize the challenge of self-examination and reflection that comes with discovery learning. As described previously, creating a nurturing environment where students are given permission to learn at their own pace is critical to their comfort and success with this type of learning experience. This is even more important for students having difficulty with this way of thinking and being.

To facilitate students' ease with this process and help them be more mindful and reflective in their nursing practice, I remind them that each person's perspective has value. I encourage students to be gentle with one another and to treat each other's ideas and views with respect as each shares what they are learning. I explain that this type of sharing enables them to learn from one another and gives them the opportunity to expand their world-view as they hear what their peers are learning.

To plant the seed for future learning, I try to say in as many ways as I can that *we are all teachers and learners*. When each of us, in our role as students, becomes more comfortable with reflecting-in-practice and sharing what we learn, we become teachers for each other and the resulting knowledge-building and collective wisdom is enhanced for all. The reflective process becomes a dance among self-discovery and development of personal knowledge, experiencing positive reinforcing for being willing to share discoveries, and reaping the benefits of mutual learning and self-reflective practice.

Learning to Learn

Mary stopped by my office several times during the remainder of her program. Each time she told me she would always remember what she learned from me, that she was continuing to develop and evolve how she thought about herself, nursing, and her role as a nurse, and she gave examples of how she passed on her new knowledge and new ways of thinking to others in subsequent classes. She was especially pleased with the idea that life would continue to provide her with learning opportunities, and that she would continue to grow in mind, body, and spirit—as a person and a nurse, and in her ability to care for her clients from a holistic perspective. She acknowledged that she was now comfortable with remaining open to and welcomed those possibilities.

Just prior to graduation, she made an appointment to see me "so she could be sure I was there." She wanted me to know that often she would ask herself, "How would Dr. Kinney handle this?" That awareness and that connection was a part of who she had become. I reinforced this idea and said that she would always be a part of me. As we said good-bye she handed me a package that contained a framed poem she had written.

Table 8.4 Mary's Poem

Students will come and students will go,
The knowledge you share allows them to grow.

You reach out your hand and touch their heart,
Encouraging words of wisdom to them you impart.

A caring compassion illuminates from you,
As teacher, as mentor and "role model" too.

Personal 'aha's" for students there truly are many,
All are made possible with your help Dr. Kinney.

Although students will come and students will go,
The knowledge you share means more than you know.

EVALUATION: IMPORTANT COMPONENT OF DISCOVERY-LEARNING

There are three aspects important to the concept of evaluation. The first addresses the faculty's evaluation of the student, the second is the student's self-evaluation, and the third is the faculty's self-evaluation and growth. I have briefly addressed the first above; here I will address the latter two.

Student's Self-Evaluation

When students learn by discovery, self-evaluation is ongoing. That is, students are constantly evaluating what they are learning, making decisions about its merits, and considering how such knowledge relates with what they already know. As they make decisions, they acquire new personal knowledge *and* new ways of knowing. In Mary's case, her poem provides evidence that her self-evaluation affected both of these, knowledge and knowing. It is noteworthy that as the poem progresses it reflects that she was able to move from knowledge to wisdom and develop an awareness of where this wisdom comes from—that is, she recognizes that the 'ahas' (as she describes it) she experienced originated from ***within*** her. Her poem confirms that through the process of articulating her own philosophy she was facilitated in uncovering her own wisdom and connecting with her own humanity and the humanity of others.

Faculty's Self-evaluation and Growth

When faculty engage in continuous self-evaluation, their own growth is promoted and their effectiveness as teachers is significantly enhanced as well. Each time I think about the multitude of students like Mary that I have taught over the years and I pause to read her poem, the 'aha' for me is the power and beauty of connecting with others as people, and the realization that in doing so we all grow in our ability to be human and we are all the better for it. I recognize that through my own comfort with being a learner as well as a teacher, I continue to know more about myself and the ever expanding sense of who I am. Seeing the growth in my students meets my Generativity needs (Maslow, 1968) and gives me hope for and confidence in the future of Nursing. Experiencing my own growth as a teacher and a person gives me a renewed sense of my own life's purpose.

Guidelines Only

I believe that each teacher has his/her own style; therefore, I share my thoughts and approaches as guides rather than as the only or even the best way. After 25 plus years in academia, I can say with confidence that teaching by discovery-learning has been my most satisfying and rewarding type of teaching experience. Each time I use this approach, it provides my students and me the stimulus for going beyond (Bruner, 1983) what we currently think. I have grown personally and professionally and have relished the personal and professional growth I've seen in my students. It is my hope that what I've offered here will provide some tools to help you have an equally rewarding experience.

SUMMARY

This chapter presented a teaching/learning strategy I have used to facilitate graduate students in developing their personal knowledge. The structure for this strategy, based on Bruner's (1967) Discovery-Learning theory, is provided and includes: Starting with the Students' Belief System and Creating a Nurturing Learning Environment; Setting the Stage for Discovery; Teaching/Learning Strategy; and Components of Evaluation. An exemplar case is inter-mixed with my description of the strategy with the goal of providing a direct application and making the process easier to follow.

CHAPTER 9

SYNTHESIZING KNOWLEDGE

Margaret Erickson and Da'Lynn Kay Clayton

For, after all, all that any training is to do for us is: to teach us how to train ourselves, how to observe for ourselves, how to think out things for ourselves. Don't let us allow the first week, the second week, the third week to pass by—I will not say in idleness, but in bustle. Begin, for instance, at once making notes of your cases. From the first moment you see a case, you can observe it. Nay, it is one of the first things a Nurse is strictly called upon to do: to observe her sick. (Nightingale, 1915, p. 49)

OVERVIEW

Nurses have difficulty linking Nursing theory, practice, and research in a meaningful way. In this chapter we build on Donald Schön's (1983/1991, 1987) scholarship studying professional practitioners and offer a model for nurses who wish to facilitate nurses in learning how to think about relations among theory, practice and research.

In this chapter, we will discuss a course we have taught that helps students to jump the gap from knowledge to practice, using the analysis-synthesizing process of individual cases. We will also identify factors conducive to a good learning environment. We will explore how Nursing students are taught to think and learn about learning. Next, we will explore and discuss the steps of process: presentation of cases; identification of important case phenomena; conceptual labels for the relationships between the phenomena and development of a conceptual model depicting the relationships between identified concepts. We will discuss the relationship between the process and the development of a conceptual framework that supports continuity in practice by linking knowledge with practice.

Throughout our discussion we talk about implications of teaching students how to create a knowledge base, using discovery-learning methods. Finally, we present a few of our serendipitous discoveries acquired through using these methods and a few factors that faculty might consider if they wish to adopt a course like the one described in this chapter.

THINKING ABOUT LEARNING AND LEARNING TO THINK

Background

Interested in the structure of *reflection-in-practice,* Schön concluded that professionals are "susceptible to a kind of rigor that is both like and unlike the rigor of scholarly work and controlled experimentation" (1983/1991, p. ix.). He describes this as a research methodology where the client becomes a case for analysis—one that can be reflected upon for the purpose of learning. In other words, each client may be viewed as a unique case study, rich in data that can be examined and extrapolated from to create practice models that can be applied to an individual as well as to groups. He described this as an *N of One* practice methodology.[1]

While Schön (1987) has discussed the importance of professionals understanding and reflecting on their experience with individual clients' world experiences, Johns (1995, 2002, 2004, 2009) has done extensive work on the importance of the nurse reflecting on his/her own experiences while nursing others.

We believe that it is both important and necessary for the nurse to reflect on both the clients' experiences as well as his/her own in order to achieve a holistic perspective and, ultimately, facilitate optimal nursing care.

Through a process of case analysis and synthesis, developed by Helen Erickson (1982, 1985) with the help of colleagues,[2] students can be facilitated to learn how to "reflect" on their own and their clients' experiences. These reflections can then be used to build a rich knowledge base grounded in clinical experiences, identify concepts to be researched, and articulate practice-based theories which facilitate caring and healing nurse-client relationships.

Thinking About Learning

The importance of nurses understanding how personal and philosophical beliefs guide Nursing research and practice was discussed in the Section 1 of this book. We agree with the tenets presented in these chapters; we believe our

---

[1] Per conversation with Helen Erickson who enjoyed a semester-long workshop under his mentorship while at The University of Michigan, Ann Arbor.

[2] Our approach is based on a Socratic method of learning, described by Bruner as a Discovery-Learning methodology of teaching. The course was first developed at The University of Michigan (U of M) in 1985 by Helen Erickson, PhD, RN, AHN-BC, FAAN. It was later taught at the University of South Carolina and The University of Texas at Austin. Appendix D provides a condensed version of a teaching manual prepared in 1986 by Erickson for the faculty at U of M.

fundamental principles and beliefs provide the philosophical framework for our practice and, therefore, affect the nursing care provided. Since the movement for Nursing to be scientifically-based, nursing care is often guided by the positivist scientific view and process.

Although many nurses intuitively reflect on their own experiences with clients, the use of reflection as an important aspect of nursing practice has only recently been identified in the literature (Johns, 1995, 2002, 2004, 2009). Prior to Johns's work, Schön (1983/1991, 1987) stated that professionals should reflect on their practice to discover the essence of their profession.

Concurrent with Schön's work, stimulated by her own combined clinical and academic experience and Schön's mentorship, H. Erickson led faculty at The University of Michigan in the conceptualization, development and implementation of a course designed to help students reflect on their practice, so they could rethink and recode knowledge acquired through academic and clinical experiences. Through a process we call "Synthesis," students are given the opportunity to learn to *reflect* on their clinical experiences in a way which allows them to understand the uniqueness of individuals, to *synthesize* what they've learned, and to *integrate* it with knowledge acquired through their formal education. Using this approach, students achieve greater insight which can be used to guide their practice.

Implications

While educators typically challenge students to provide *patient-centered* caring, students often have trouble *understanding* the personal needs of each client because they have not been taught how to critically think about the human as a unique individual. Although they may have been taught that each person is unique, many have not been taught how to jump the gap from learning to thinking (Bruner, 1965). As a result, they are unable to understand the implications of the *individual's unique perspective*.

We think it is essential that nurses learn how to think about clients as individuals—each uniquely different from any other human being—at the same time that they think about how their clients are like others. When they do this, they are able to apply knowledge that is truly person-centered, focused on individual needs, and scientifically based.

Philosophical Considerations

Nurse educators traditionally encourage deductive thinking processes first, emphasizing the importance of students being able to memorize and apply information and facts. Dependent upon educators to "*teach*" them, students often assume a passive role. Subsequently, they often have less enthusiasm for the subject, experience difficulty retaining and applying knowledge, and have difficulty thinking about what has been learned to what might be possible. Or as Bruner might say, they have trouble jumping the gap from learning to thinking.

Our philosophy and belief systems not only guide our professional practice, but also determine our orientation to education, how we facilitate students to learn, and the instructional methodologies we use. As educators, we (the authors) believe knowledge is best acquired by Socratic methods, described more specifically in Chapter 5 as Bruner's Discovery-Learning Methods (Bruner, 1965).

Retroductive Thinking

The course we describe is taught in the senior year in conjunction with other Nursing courses. We start by guiding students through a process which helps them explore their clinical experiences and existing knowledge. In the course of this journey they gain insight, discover facts, patterns, relationships and new truths. This process is somewhat different from that usually used by nurse educators. We build on knowledge acquired deductively, but emphasize the importance of inductive reasoning, too.

While most students are taught retroductive reasoning, we think they are usually taught how to use deductive thinking first with inductive reasoning as secondary. This is contrary to the natural way of learning about new phenomena. As described by Erickson, H., (1985):

> *As children we see the world inductively. For example: a child learns that a furry animal, with four legs, a tail, and the ability to bark is a dog. The child brings many different pieces of information together and creates the image of a dog. As we get older and enter the educational system we are socialized and taught to learn deductively.* (p. 22)

In other words, as we grow, instead of inductively bringing bits of information together to create a concept or image, we are taught to be deductive and to use what information we have learned, and apply it. Rather than identifying bits of information and looking for relationships among them, we tend to look for evidence of something we already *know about*, and find the bits of information that support our premise. Unfortunately, this type of thinking allows, and even encourages us, to overlook other bits of information important to understanding the uniqueness of an individual—information that might help us discriminate among situations that look very much alike.

> Our aim as teachers is to facilitate students through a retroductive process which *starts with inductive* reasoning and then moves on to deductive reasoning.

Learning to Think

Significance of Learning to Think

Immersion. Through the "Synthesis" course, students are helped to explore and examine what they already know, but haven't deconstructed, synthesized, or integrated to a higher level of knowledge. Using the N of One Method, they assume an active role in learning as they immerse themselves in their experiences. During this process students discover that there is more to their client's experience than first observed, *and* that there are commonalities among clients which they can use to provide sophisticated person-centered caring. They gain insight into the importance of looking at each client as an individual while also learning how people are *alike in their differences.*

Discoveries. More specifically, students are taught to deconstruct client experiences so that they can *discover an individual's unique nature and lived experiences,* and then they are taught to use deductive thinking to look across cases and *identify how people are alike.* As they learn to recognize individual phenomena within a case, they gain confidence in their ability to see each person as a unique human being. And as they learn to *put together bits of information* to create a new "whole," they gain confidence in their ability to develop critical thinking skills and to transfer knowledge. These retroductive thinking processes, focused on *inductive processes first* followed by deductive processes, help students become active participants in the learning process. They also help them jump the gap from learning to thinking.

Ownership. Interacting with their environment, students use their senses to collect data which is then organized and labeled. Knowledge gained is based on the students' experiences and interactions with their environment and is grounded in a personal framework. Since it is owned by the learner, it is more meaningful and easier for them to apply in their nursing practice. Students using the N of One approach discover how to be true to the essence of the client and to Nursing. Furthermore, because their practice is congruent with their philosophy, it allows the student to maximize their potential.

> Many important nursing interventions are not articulated and it is not always clear to the nurse how the care they are giving affects client outcomes. Utilizing a retroductive process, students bring together the different ways-of-knowing to create integrative knowing, a higher level of cognitive processing. This, in turn, creates a new knowledge base which can be used to guide their Nursing practice. Nurses are also able to articulate the care they are giving and to link those interventions to client outcomes.

Limitations of Aggregate Data

Case studies, a clinical version of the *N of One Method,* previously used by nurses was abandoned for seemingly "higher level" scientific methods.

> The notion that nurses should do post-facto reflection on their nursing experiences started with Nightingale in the 1800s and continued as a means for learning how to think about Nursing. In the 1960s it was abandoned for acquiring knowledge by way of scientific methods.

Variations Among People. While we recognize the value in aggregate data, we also realize that knowledge is vastly limited if we cannot apply it to an individual, or provide care to individuals on a case-by-case basis depending on the individual's personal situation. Let us take for example the "normal temperature" of the human being. For the majority of people (70%) a normal temperature is 98.6 degrees. However, 30% of the population has either a higher or lower temperature than that considered normal.

If practice is based on the assumption that the normal temperature is 98.6 without any variation among individuals, nurses would not know that a person who normally runs a base temperature of 97.0 is febrile at 98.8 degrees.

Scientific Methods. Thorne, Kirkham, and McDonald's (1997) methods of *Interpretative Description* further support the idea of developing Nursing knowledge based on a person's perspective and the importance of aggregating data. They emphasize that nurses must be able to take that knowledge and apply it back to the individual. Today, Nursing has a respected body of knowledge, scientifically developed and validated, wherein data derived from individuals was aggregated. Nurses are learning how to think. This course was designed to prepare novices to follow this path.

We present the course specifics below, describing how we taught it. Following that, we provide an example of student stories with phenomena, concepts, and models derived by groups of students.

COURSE SPECIFICS

Establishing an Environment Conducive to Learning

Preliminary Planning

Prior to beginning the journey of self-discovery, it is imperative that the faculty member create an environment perceived by the students to be safe and growth-oriented. This is true in both formal and informal educational settings. In either case, the instructor needs to consider the students' predisposition to learning; how they will structure, sequence, and reinforce the learning; and how they will evaluate what has been learned. It is important that the learner and the educator undertake the process together, and that it is based on a trusting, interactive relationship.

The teacher's attitude of unconditional acceptance of the student as a human, open and vulnerable, is crucial. Students need to know that they are safe if they are to be able to undertake self-disclosure, express feelings, share experiences, articulate beliefs, and gain insight and knowledge regarding their case examples. Only when they feel safe are they comfortable with telling their stories, exploring for uncovered phenomena, and reflecting on their clients' lived experiences.

The educator who chooses to use the N of One method has an advantage if they philosophically support key concepts in MRM including unconditional acceptance, nurturance, client as primary data source, growth and development across the lifespan—concepts consistent with Bruner's Discovery-Learning methods. Positive feedback from the teacher, described in Chapter 5, is designed to help students gain insight into their personal and professional experiences.

> The educator facilitates students in learning how to think independently rather than focusing on thinking as the educator thinks and being congruent with the teacher's thinking or understandings.

Structuring and Sequencing Learning

We structured and sequenced the content so it would remind students of the knowledge they had acquired in other courses and help them frame their knowing differently. Learning was carefully paced to ensure that students could be successful in this phase of the course which was designed to help them *learn how to think about their practice.* Our goal was to open the door to alternative ways-of-knowing and to facilitate active and direct learning.

We wanted the students to embrace discovery of what they already knew (but did not know they knew), to recode past learning so they could conceptualize and contextualize their Nursing practice. We believed that it was important for Nursing students to be able to take these steps, so they could link knowledge with practice after graduating from Nursing school.

Phase One: Predisposing Factors

Reframing Expectations. The first phase of the course is designed to "open the door to alternative ways of learning" and to contextualize future learning. Since most nurses have *learned to learn* through deductive processes, the first consideration is to plan teaching strategies that will motivate the student to "let go" of deductive learning habits, and to adopt a freedom that allows and supports discoveries. This often creates anxiety in students. They are socialized to learn what the teacher wants them to know and to ignore or compartmentalize other observations.

For this course, we used the first few classes to teach students that there are alternative ways to learn, and to reinforce their learning of retroductive processes. We set the stage by reviewing Bloom's taxonomy, explaining that they will learn how to synthesize in this course, but first they will revisit clinical cases to gain new insights about their clients and/or their relationship with them. This might mean that they will start at the beginning of Bloom's taxonomy, but they will soon *discover* that what they have learned helps them understand higher levels of knowledge differently.

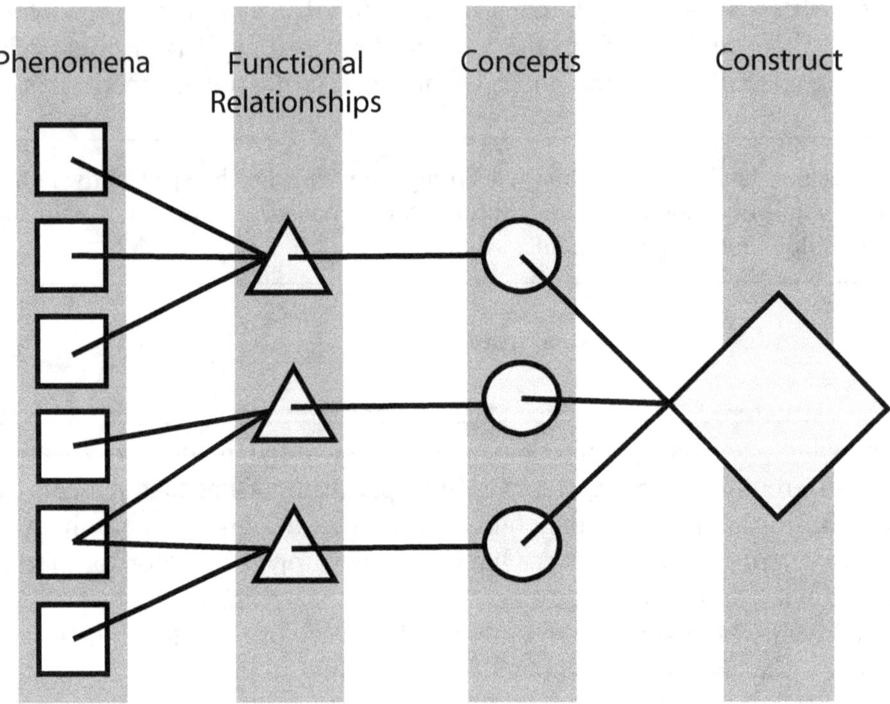

Figure 9.1 Visual aid used to help students understand relations among phenomena, their functional relations, concepts, and constructions. Reprinted with permission, from Erickson, H. (1985) *Synthesizing Clinical Experiences.* Ann Arbor, MI: The University of Michigan, Biomedical Communications.

We used visual aids similar to those shown in Appendix D to help them understand our intent. For example, we wanted to be certain that they understood the differences among phenomena, concepts and constructs, so we used a visual aid similar to Figure 9.1 (above) as we described concepts and constructs commonly found in Nursing literature.

We also wanted to be certain that they understand that Nursing is based in a relationship, so we used a visual aid such as the one shown in Figure 9.2 as we described the impact nurses have on their clients, and vice versa. It is not just a one-way street.

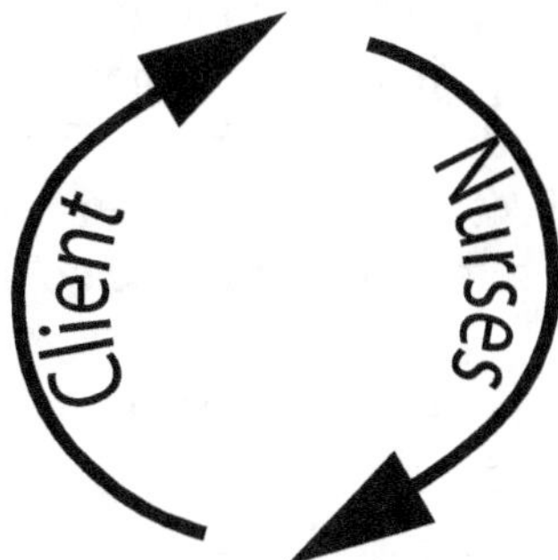

Fig 9.2 Relationship between nurse and client. Reprinted with permission from H. Erickson, unpublished manuscript.

Contextualizing Expectations. As we build on the notion that Nursing is relationship-based, we also want them to remember that they are interacting with clients not only as humans, but also as professionals. We review the Nurse Practice Act and compare it to the state's Medical Practice Act, the ANA Social Policy, Nursing's Code of Ethics, and other Nursing documents to help them contextualize what they are going to *discover*. These documents help them clarify differences among the professions—an important step in learning how to discriminate among cases.

Evaluating Learning. We conclude this unit with an open-book quiz. Students are asked a few essay questions designed to help them integrate what they have learned. They must contain their responses to a half page per question, and must write in their own words. Specifically, we want them to be able to define and differentiate phenomena, concepts, constructs, conceptual frameworks, and a theory; to explain why they need to learn to label and articulate phenomena and find relations among them; identify the levels of theory development; and the relationship between theory and practice.

We use the open-book essay approach since it is a means to "guide" discovery and encourage integration of knowledge. While students can read the content found in books and their notes, they cannot write about what they have learned unless they have incorporated and integrated it in their minds.

Feedback to the quiz is provided during the following class. This reinforces learning and encourages students to move on to the next phase of the class—exploration of their cases. They need to know that the faculty thinks they have learned sufficiently before they can take the risk of examining their past clinical experiences. When we find students who are not ready to proceed, we set aside additional time to explore with them what they need in order to be successful.

Phase Two: Initiating Learning

Framing the Experience. The second phase of the course is designed to help students explore and tap into their knowledge base, acquired through multiple ways of knowing, and to think about what they learned and what else there is to be discovered. We set the stage for their exploration by first explaining (again) what they will be doing for the rest of the course.

Table 9.1 Activities students experience in the synthesis process, the purpose for the activities, and expected outcomes.

	Activity	Purpose	Outcome
Individual cases	Write case stories.	Reflect on case to "remember" the details.	Case story written in detail, including rich inclusion of phenomena.
	Identify phenomena in individual cases.	Identify the "details."	Explicate phenomena key to understanding the story.
	Link alike phenomena.	Interpret symbolism of "detail."	Chunk information so it can be labeled or identified as a *concept.*
Across cases	Identify "alike" concepts.	Identify similarities across cases.	Describe similarities in cases.
	Explore differences in phenomena across cases.	Explore differences in cases by comparing differences in phenomena that create "alike" concepts.	Explain differences in cases.

Table 9.1 describes the activities that each student will undertake as they move through the phases of exploring individual cases, examining their own set of cases to find commonalities, and across multiple cases to create a practice model. Table 9.1 also shows the purpose for each of these activities, and the anticipated student outcomes.

Next we provide an example drawn from the literature discussed in Appendix D, p. 433, (i.e. the Teddy Bear Method) and explain how nurses came to this practice model. Students are then informed that as they initiate their own case analysis *they will make discoveries*, they will *be surprised* at what they find, and *that all discoveries are important*.

Initially, learners are asked to write about three to four cases from their clinical practice. They are told that they should select cases that "just pop into their mind" and that they should *not* try to find cases that are alike—that will only hamper their learning. Instead, they are encouraged to trust their *personal knowing*, to let their stories emerge. They are also advised that at first sight there may appear to be no similarities in their cases, but *they will discover* that all cases have something in common even though they may be talking about an infant in intensive care unit, an older gentleman who falls and fractures his hip, and a mother giving birth.

The Format. They are encouraged to write about their cases as if they are writing in personal journals. We encourage them to write details, to describe what was seen, smelled, heard, observed, and felt. We want them to begin to see the phenomena rather than to label the concept itself. We also tell them that each case will take one to three pages, usually no more, but sometimes less.

Enhancing Discovery. Our work as educators is to help students remember how to be inductive in their thinking. This can be a challenge as we often use concepts when describing a case. For example, if a student wrote "Mrs. Jones was grief-stricken when I walked in the room" they would be asked to explain how they knew that Mrs. J. was grieving and why did they say she was "grief-*stricken.*" Questions such as: "How do you know Ms. J. was grief stricken?" "Please provide more details," or "What phenomena were present that let you know that Ms. J. was experiencing feelings of grief?" may be helpful.

When the student enriches the sentence to "Mrs. Jones was huddled in her blankets, her tear-streaked face turned towards me, and she sobbed quietly after she heard her diagnosis," a much clearer picture emerges. The latter statement provides significant details and information that the student will use later in the process as they begin to cluster related phenomena.

No Blank Slates. We have noted that many students have difficulty getting started. When this happens, we simply ask them to talk aloud, to tell us a story about a clinical experience. Many have said that they don't have any stories. When this happens, we ask them if they were in the clinical that week. When they affirm that they were, and we ask them how long they were there, they always say six to eight hours. We can then ask them to tell us what happened in those hours. Sometimes we have to ask, "What else did you see?" "Why do you think that?" "How did you feel about that?" and other questions that help students tell their stories. Bottom line: no one really has a blank slate; everyone has stories. They just have to be reassured that their stories are worthy, that they are what we want them to tell, and that they have important information to *discover*. It should also be noted that these stories are usually told in front of the entire class; everyone listens, everyone learns, and everyone grows when this happens. It should also be noted that students cannot tell their stories, or explore their nurse-client experiences unless they feel safe and know, without doubt, that their faculty respect them, will guide them, and will understand their vulnerabilities.

Finally, it is also important to note that students often choose to discuss traumatic experiences, or deal with personal issues and concerns that have impacted their ability to provide care, caused them anxiety, stress, or personal suffering. Often, they are hesitant at first, but the story pours out when the instructor *listens*. It is essential that the teacher understands that students may be vulnerable and need to have their feelings (sadness, anxiety, frustration, etc.) validated so they can proceed.

Phase Three: Identification of Relationships

Identify Phenomena. After they have been written, students explore the cases to discover and identify the phenomena. They are encouraged to do this by listing the phenomena on a sheet of paper, chalk board, or some other erasable surface. The learner may find it helpful to first highlight or underline all phenomena in their story before transcribing them into a list.

Phenomena Clustering and Concept Formation (Within a Case). Once the phenomena in individual cases are identified, the next step is to help students explore how phenomena, within a case, are linked with one another, how the phenomena create concepts, and what they want to call the concepts. Students rarely have difficulty with this step. They are usually able to identify multiple linkages without difficulty. Sometimes they are puzzled and think that a phenomenon relates to more than one concept (see Figure 9.1 above). When this happens, we tell them to leave it in their model for the time being; that they will sort it out as time goes by.

Clustering is based on an individual's sense of logic, intuition, and personal understanding. Aggregate of data (i.e., the phenomena) must hold together. There must be more than two phenomena to support a conceptual label; not all phenomena have to be used.

As students begin to label the concepts, they may struggle with what conceptual label best fits the phenomena they have identified. It is important to remind students that they may identify different phenomena that represent the same concept. For example, in the two cases presented below, both clients experienced loss of physical health and body image. Their losses were very similar. In another case, a patient may have experienced a different kind of loss. A death, losing a desired job or promotion, relationship, ideal, etc., can all be perceived by an individual as a loss. The important thing is that there are outcomes to loss. We want the student to understand that these linkages exist between concepts, and they exist across groups of people.

Feedback as a Way to Learn. During this phase students may want to discuss the process with their faculty as they try to match the phenomena with the correct conceptual labels. To encourage the students' interpretation of the relationships among phenomena, questions such as those shown in Table 9.2 might be asked:

Table 9.2 Leading questions that help students find linkages among phenomena.

What did you see (hear, smell, feel) here?
What do you think is going on?
How do these relate or connect to each other?
What else do see?
Are there any other phenomena that are related to this group?
When you bring these pieces together what image, picture, or thought comes to your mind?

Across Cases. Next, students are asked to look across their cases and, based on the concepts identified, pinpoint commonalities and differences among them. During this step students learn that although the concept may be the same or very similar, different phenomena may be present within an individual case. When this happens, they are encouraged to revisit their cases, decide if they want to alter their findings, or perhaps, find new linkages. They are reminded that each concept formed has to have at least two phenomena, preferably more, to create a concept, *and* each concept has to be labeled.

Model Development. After concepts are identified, it is time for students to contemplate how these concepts relate with one another both within their individual cases and across them. Most learners need at least six to seven concepts to develop a conceptual model based on the conceptual linkages; however, working with more than 12 to 13 concepts is challenging to most learners. They have to explore questions such as those shown in Table 9.3.

Table 9.3 Rhetorical questions for students as they think about their concepts and their relations with one another.

Do the concepts show a sequence in time?
Which concept(s) come first?
Are certain concepts predicted or outcome concepts as a result of interactions among other concepts?

This part of the process may require that students spend time discussing relationships among the concepts with their faculty member. The relationships among the concepts create a beginning practice model which they can use in practice. When they are finished with their practice model, they write the final section of their paper explaining what they have learned in this step of the process.

Practice Implications. The final section of the paper is designed to build on what they have learned. Students are instructed to think about their practice model and to discuss the implications of what they have discovered. They are expected to be able to describe their model, explain how they would change their practice based on what they have learned, and/or to support what they did.

Maintenance and Direction. With all students, as we reviewed their papers, we used feedback to show support and validate their learning. Examples of our comments included "Great Job!", "Good insight!", "I would love to have you be my mother's nurse?" and "I wonder what else you will discover." (For additional comments, see Table 9.4).

Table 9.4 Comments that help Students in the Discovery Process.

How insightful!	Interesting information.	What did you see? Hear? Feel?
Good for you!	Good description.	More details please
Keep up the Good work! This is a good start. Tell me more.	How did you know this? How can you describe this?	Great start. Can you build on this?

We think it is important to reinforce learning and encourage further discoveries so that students will have the courage needed to further explore personal knowing, and to discover what is unknown and sometimes perceived as threatening.

We also, carefully, try to avoid negative feedback. For example, comments written in red ink are often perceived as criticism and may cause students distress. If the ink is black, blue or another color perceived as supportive or positive, the comments are more likely to be perceived as a critique or helpful versus critical in nature.

Evaluation. Faculty responsibilities are to read, comment, suggest, reinforce, and direct learning at this time. Criteria for grading must be provided in advance so that students will be clear about faculty expectations. We grade on presentation as well as reasoning used throughout the paper. It is important to remember to provide positive feedback which includes direction for future learning, so that students will continue to learn during the remainder of the course. Suggestions for positive evaluations can be found in Chapter 5. It is also important for faculty to complete grading of the papers before students are expected to proceed to Phase Four. Without a clear understanding of where they stand in the class, they are not certain about their own *thinking processes.* Faculty feedback ensures them that they are *learning how to think* and that they simply need to continue in order to be successful in jumping the gap from learning to thinking.

Faculty Trepidations. Some faculty members find this step difficult, at first, but soon learn how to be efficient and enjoy their own discoveries. Not only do they have to read, critique and grade student papers in a short time, they also have to search for commonalities among student papers. This is because the next phase of the course requires that students be grouped together to repeat the process they have just completed. Unless faculty are committed to this method of facilitating learning, they may not be willing to invest the time necessary to provide feedback, as indicated here. This is further discussed below when we talk about the limitations of this course.

Phase Four: Creating a Group Practice Model

Comparing Stories. During this phase of the course, students work in groups. While they are provided class time for group activities, faculty needs to be clear that they will also need to work together outside of class time. They are advised that they will repeat the aggregation across the cases they have just completed. This time, however, they will work with other students. They are informed that commonalities were found among the students' concepts, and that they would be grouped accordingly. The groups are then organized, and they are advised to start by sharing their stories, concepts, and models with one another. Following that, they are expected to find commonalities across their cases and to be able to explain the differences based on variance in their concepts and/or constructs.

As students share their stories with classmates, they begin to discover that there are more commonalities than differences among people. Furthermore, many of the differences can be explained by the variance in the shared similarities. For e.g., the individuals' abilities to cope, the nature and number of their losses, the degree of support they have, their perception of control, etc. The same or similar concepts may be present in different ways at various stages—that is, how one exhibits loss, sadness, trust, or control may depend on their developmental stage.

For example, feelings related to loss of control will be demonstrated differently at the stage of Autonomy, Intimacy, or Generativity. A toddler who does not want to leave lies down on the floor and has a temper tantrum. The 39 year-old business executive in the hospital, after a heart attack, yells, "Give me the phone! You can't tell me I can't call the office. I have work to do." The 70 year-old states, "What do you mean I cannot get up and walk? Don't restrain me. I'm not going to fall." Although these phenomena are different, the concepts are the same. That is, the people are all feeling a loss of control.

An important "ahha" occurs when students realize that despite the differences in clients' chronological ages, developmental stages, disease processes, etc. common conceptual issues exist throughout the life span. This insight is important as students begin to think about cases as a complex of concepts versus phenomena, the first step towards the development of a group conceptual framework.

Model Presentation. We have handled the last part of this class in different ways. Our favorite version is to require that students create posters illustrating their group practice model and the implications, and include research questions derived from examining the model. When we use this version, other students are invited to attend the poster session, offered in the School of Nursing during regular class time. Students are graded not only on the succinctness of the model, the appropriateness of their research questions and references drawn from the literature which support or refute their work, but also on their professional demeanor during their poster presentation.

An alternate version of this requirement is to simply have students, as a group, write a paper that includes the above criteria. We believe that students enjoy the first version more, share in the responsibility more equally, and gain a greater sense of pride in what they have accomplished than they do when they write a group paper.

In all cases, we know that students often rediscover why they went into Nursing during this phase of the course. Their passion for nursing is rekindled as their understanding of the nurse-client relationship is enhanced. Several students have tested relationships found in their personal model in subsequent research classes; others have returned to graduate school to further their understanding of what they had learned.

For example, one of our students completed a version of this course in graduate school, and then published her model (Lee, 2006). She described the process as a catharsis. Lee stated, "Discovering my model of nursing care helps me see more clearly the importance of caring for my patients as individuals" (p.19). Much to our joy, several former students have talked with us, years later, about their experience in this course and what they learned.

AN EXAMPLAR

Case Examples

Two case examples provided by students will be used to demonstrate the synthesis process described above. These are reproduced here exactly as presented by the students.

> ***Sally*** *was admitted to the Labor and Delivery unit accompanied by her husband and mother. During admission, I asked if she had a birthing plan. Her husband stated that their plan included subdued lighting, a quiet environment with gentle music playing; Sally's mother and husband would assist with breathing exercises. There were to be no intravenous solutions or pain medication. She wanted to do a "completely natural" birth. I replied saying, "We'll do everything we can to support your plan. I'm going to let you rest now. Let me know if you need anything." Sally smiled and said quietly, "I'm fine. I'm sure it will go well. We've planned for his birth." Lights were turned down, music quietly played, ice chips were provided. Sally was encouraged to rest. Her husband and mother took turns gently rubbing her back.*
>
> *As the evening progressed, Sally's contractions became more painful. Using her call light she cried out, "I need to see my nurse. It hurts so bad." I arrived and asked how I could help. I noticed that Sally was diaphoretic, clutching her stomach, and rocking back and forth in her bed, and crying, "I can't take the pain anymore!" I suggested some interventions which supported Sally's birthing plan: a change in her position in bed, a cool washcloth for her forehead, back massage, and a relaxation technique. Sally yelled, "I don't want any of those things! I want something for this **** pain!" Her husband leaned in close and said "Honey, you know you don't want any medication. Remember, we agreed to do it naturally." With tears running down her face, she yelled, "Get out of my face and out of my room. Give me something for pain now!" Taking her hand gently, I quietly said, "I know you are in a lot of pain right now and I will call the doctor and have him get you something so you are more comfortable." Sally clung to my hand and said, "It just hurts so bad! Help me!"*
>
> *The doctor arrived a few minutes later. Sally chose to have an epidural. She received relief and was easily able to deliver a healthy baby boy. A short while later, Sally called for me and said, "I'm sorry I had to have an epidural and was so difficult. I felt everything was out of control and I really hurt. You helped me and listened to me. You were there for*

me." As I left the room, Sally was gently stroking and talking to her new baby. Her mother and husband were smiling at the bedside.

***Evan**, a 69-year veteran, was dying. He had liver cancer with metastasis to his lungs and was always gasping for air. He had been hospitalized for several weeks. His family all lived out of state. The staff asked me to see him as he had "this crazy idea that his family can take him home. What if he dies along the way?"*

Upon entering the room I noticed a tiny, cachexic gentleman huddled in his bed coverings. I introduced myself and pulled up a chair along the bedside, so we could be at eye-level. I quietly asked, "How can I help you?" Slowly, in a faint, whispery voice he answered, "I'm dying. I want to go home and be with my family. I don't want to take my last breath here, alone. I've been told that I can be transferred to a nursing home close to my home in Colorado, but it will take a week to make arrangements." Teary-eyed, he said, "I don't think I have that long. My family said they'll come get me." Leaning towards me, reaching for my hand, he said, "Everyone says I can't go home until a bed is available in the nursing home and an ambulance can take me there. Can't you please do anything? You're my last hope."

I told him that I would do what I could to help him get home. I explained that his doctor might not agree to his discharge and he might need to sign out against medical advice. He smiled at me and seemed to straighten up in his bed as he said, "So what is he going to do to me? Refuse to admit me to the hospital in the future?" We spent the next hour discussing preparations for his trip home: how the family planned to transport him; the comfort measures needed for the long drive; who would be making the trip with him, and other necessary arrangements. I told him I'd make the necessary arrangements and contact his family immediately. His family happily agreed to come, saying, "We're so glad he's coming home. This is where he should be. We'll leave right away. It'll take us about 12 hours to get there. We'll bring the motor home, so he'll be more comfortable on the trip home." I arranged for medication and oxygen, so Evan could be comfortable on his trip home. The Doctor agreed to send him AMA.

I returned to see him later that afternoon. His face lit up with a smile, he motioned to the chair for me to sit down and thanked me for helping him. His family arrived early the next morning. He greeted them with a big smile when they entered his room. I asked if there was anything else he needed. He replied "No, I am all set and ready to go."As I gently and carefully helped him out of the wheelchair into the motor home, he squeezed my hand, and thanked me again, "for letting me go home." I learned a few days later that Evan had died quietly and peacefully, surrounded by his family, on the way home.

Table 9.5 Case one, Sally's birthing experience.

Phenomena	Concept
*Crying: "I can't take the pain anymore; yelled "I don't want any of those things, I want something for this **** pain!"; sorry I had to have an epidural; was so difficult; everything was out of control; I really hurt*	Loss
Cried: "I need my nurse."; "It hurts so bad", Diaphoretic, clutching her stomach, and rocking back and forth, tears running down her face she yelled, "Get out of my face and out of my room. Give me something for pain now; said "It just hurts so bad! Help me!"	Distress
Accompanied by husband and mother; asked if she had a birthing plan; Sally's mother and husband would assist with breathing exercises; husband and mother gently rubbing back; "You were there for me"; mother and husband were smiling at the bedside.	Perceived Support
Plan included subdued lighting, a quiet environment with gentle music playing; There was to be no IV or pain medication; wanted to do a "completely natural" birth; "I'm sure it will go well. We've planned for his birth"; smiled and said quietly; chose to have an epidural.	Perceived Control
"I need my nurse"; clung to my hand; "You helped me and listened to me; You were there for me."	Connection
"I'm fine"; relief from epidural; You helped me and listened to me.	Need Satisfaction
Asked if she had a birthing plan; we'll do everything we can to support your plan; going to let you rest now; Let me know if you need anything; Lights turned down, music quietly played, ice chips were provided. Sally encouraged to rest; how I could help; suggested interventions that supported Sally's birthing plan; taking her hand gently, quietly; know you are in a lot of pain right now and will call doctor and have him get something so you are more comfortable.	Nursing care
Easily able to deliver a healthy baby boy; gently stroking and talking to her new baby; mother and husband smiling at the bedside	Positive Client Outcome

Table 9.6 Case two, Evan goes home.

Phenomena	**Concept**
Dying; liver cancer, metastasis to lungs; always gasping for air; hospitalized for several weeks; cachexic;, family all out of state	Loss
Smiled at me and seemed to straighten up in his bed; "So what is he going to do to me, refuse to readmit me to the hospital in the future?"; spent the next hour discussing preparations needed for his trip home; " I am all set and ready to go."	Perceived Control
My family said they'll come get me; spent the next hour discussing preparations needed for his trip home; family happily agreed to come. "We're so glad he's coming home. This is where he should be. We'll leave right away. It'll take us about 12 hours to get there. We'll bring the motor home so he'll be more comfortable on the trip home." Surrounded by family on the way home.	Perceived Support
Huddled in his bed covering; slowly, in a faint, whispery voice; "I'm dying. I want to go home and be with my family. I don't want to take my last breath here, alone...told that I can be transferred to a nursing home close to my home in Colorado, but it will take a week to make arrangements"; Teary-eyed said, "I don't think I have that long; Everyone says I can't go home... Can't you please do anything? You're my last hope."	Distress
Leaning towards me; reaching for my hand; His face lit up with a smile; he motioned to the chair for me to sit down; thanked me for helping him; squeezed my hand; thanked me again	Connection
Greeted them with a big smile; He replied "No I am all set and ready to go"; "for letting me go home."	Need Satisfaction
I introduced myself and pulled up a chair along the bedside; at eye-level with him; quietly asked "How can I help you?"; told him that I would do what I could to help him get home; comfort measures needed for the long drive; told him I'd make the necessary arrangements; would contact his family immediately; arranged for medication and oxygen so could be comfortable on his trip home; I returned to see him later that afternoon; asked if there was anything else he needed; gently and carefully helped him out of the wheelchair into the motor home.	Nursing Care
Doctor agreed to send him AMA; died quietly and peacefully, surrounded by his family on way home.	Positive Client Outcome

Data Aggregation

Tables 9.5 and 9.6 (above) illustrate the phenomena extrapolated from the above cases, the interpretations, and the concepts created from articulating the phenomena.

Figure 9.3 shows a model drawn from data articulation. Figure 9.4 shows an alternative interpretation of relations among the data. While the two models are very similar, Figure 9.3 illustrates what happens *within the client, with a suggestion of nursing actions* (i.e., nurse and client connect and nurse facilitates client in meeting needs) while 9.4 specifies the nurses' behaviors from the clients', depicting an interaction between nurse and client. For example, nursing care provided with intent to meet client needs results in connection between nurse and client. This results in client's perception of support and control, which then affects his/her ability to cope with distress, resulting in a positive client outcome.

Figure 9.4 illustrates the nurse-client relationship shown above in Figure 9.2

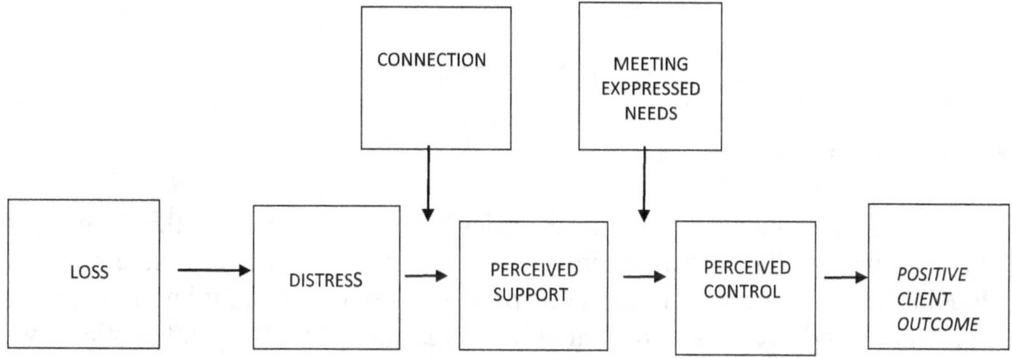

Figure 9.3 Model created by students from data articulation.

Either model is appropriate, depending on the students' focus. It should be noted, however, that students are more likely to derive a model such as the one illustrated in 9.4 if they have had opportunities to discuss their model with others, and if they have been encouraged to work in groups.

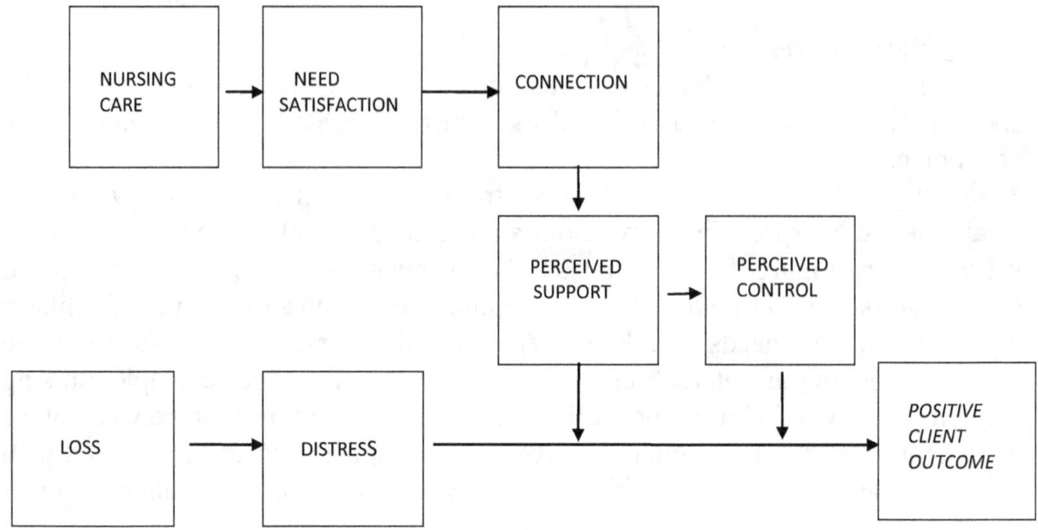

Figure 9.4 Alternative model created by students from data articulation.

POSTSCRIPT

Faculty Discoveries

We have made several discoveries as we have taught this course. As students undergo the Synthesis process, they learn how to better understand and Model the client's world. Through this process, they gain insight into their clients' experiences and feelings. This, in turn, helps them in future interactions with clients as they have begun to learn that behaviors, words, and interactions are an outcome of the clients' needs and experiences.

Synthesis allows the learner to discover how to focus on the responses and not the symptoms (ANA Social Policy Statement, 1983). Students who have taken this course are able to be more holistic in their practice, have a greater understanding of the client's world-view, and are able to understand their clinical experiences at a conceptual level.

As nurses, we often find it difficult to not personalize patients' feelings, statements, or reactions. When feelings or experiences are labeled and understood at a conceptual level, students are more objective. As students learn to think about their clinical experiences from a conceptual perspective, it allows them to de-personalize the experience, be more purposeful in their assessments, and plan therapeutic interventions to achieve desired outcomes. Finally, with the development of a theoretical framework they can now articulate to others how and why they are implementing their holistic nursing interventions.

Another discovery that students make as they experience the synthesis process is that conceptual models and theory can be useful and help them in their professional practice. As teachers, it is a pleasure to watch students grow as they learn to think about their practice and future nursing interventions from a conceptual model rather than random cases and experiences. Finally, teaching the Synthesis class enlightened the educators on the value of using Inductive and retroductive teaching methodologies.

Serendipitous Finding

A somewhat unexpected finding has been reported by nearly all faculty members, known to us, who have taught this course. Although the course is taught to undergraduate students with minimal clinical experience, many have had traumatic experiences which they have been unable to examine, or discuss with faculty or other appropriate persons. Yet they need to, so they can find meaning in their experiences.

Most students come to us without first experiencing the depth of pain and suffering they will witness as student nurses. Often they experience loss of life without an opportunity to reconcile their own feelings. The majority of students are able to adapt, but on occasion, there are some who need additional help.

Many times, students are unaware of these feelings; they have learned to wall them off. Some have said that they had decided that they just needed to pretend that it hadn't happened, to distance themselves and move on. Others had questioned whether or not they were "cut out" for Nursing. When this happens, we assure them that their feelings are normal, shared by others, and that it is very important to address them. We will further discuss this group in the next section of this book. This chapter is about those who are able to accommodate and assimilate their experiences and move on without detaching from the source of their pain—their clients.

Faculty considerations

There are a few factors for faculty to think about before launching a course like this. First and foremost is that faculty must be comfortable with the process and philosophical assumptions underlying the course. Students often share stories that are emotionally challenging and not only require careful processing by faculty, but also support and insight (see Chapter 13). Faculty members who hold a wholistic or Totality view of Nursing are sometimes focused on pathophysiology and tasks related to practice; some think that this type of learning is a waste of time. It is important for faculty to discuss the philosophy behind this course before deciding who should teach the course.

Next, time is needed for faculty to assist students with the process, and students need adequate time to go through the multi-leveled process, build on previous learning, and acquire new ways of thinking. This journey cannot be done in a short period of time. For example, some faculty members have indicated that this can be done in a two week course. Our experience indicates that it cannot; it requires several weeks for the ideas and concepts to be explored, examined, identified, connected and most important, integrated.

Like a beautiful garden, ideas and the creation of new integrative knowledge requires that the gardener plant seed, provide nutrients, weed-out things that are not helpful/useful and give time for growth to occur. Despite these limitations, we feel that the Synthesis class is one of the most important classes nurses can experience.

SUMMARY

This chapter described a course developed to help students learn how to think about their practice, conceptually. Our aim is to help them understand that phenomena are usually related, their relationships create concepts, that concepts can also be linked to create constructs, and that relations among concepts and/or constructs provide nurses with a greater understanding of their practice. Students discover that client behaviors, previously perceived as independent or erratic, and often framed as unimportant, are linked and have meaning. Understanding them can help nurses be purposeful in their practice and prescribe care effectively.

Most important is that we aim to teach students how to learn and how to think about what they are learning—lessons which can serve them throughout life. Feedback from many students confirms that they have accomplished this latter goal. Most students who take this course learn how to jump the gap from learning to thinking, described by Bruner as an important skill needed to continue learning, even in the absence of formal education.

CHAPTER 10

EVALUATING STUDENT GROWTH

Ellen Schultz

The mere way in which a thing is said or done to patient, or probationer, makes all the difference...I have been in positions of authority myself and have always tried to remember that to use such an advantage inconsiderately is—cowardly. To be sharp upon them is worse in me than in them to be sharp upon me. No one can trample on others, and govern them. To win them is half, I might say the whole, secret of "having charge". (Nightingale, 1915, pp.15-16)

OVERVIEW

The American Association of Colleges of Nursing and the National League for Nursing support the development of faculty through publication, seminars and conferences. A host of topics offered through these sources includes theories of teaching-learning, the use of innovative strategies to create positive learning environments, and the incorporation of technology in teaching and evaluation. Other literature also provides a wealth of research findings, conceptual papers, and practical tips on teaching-learning processes.

In total, the literature and other sources of information indicate that teaching has changed from the didactic presentation of content to teaching-learning as a process. The first emphasizes *what to teach*; the latter *how to teach.* The first focuses on the teacher and the second focuses on how the teacher can facilitate the learner. Concurrently, with changes in the focus from a didactic to a process approach, the evaluation of students has also evolved.

Many levels of evaluation are crucial to the educational process including evaluation of student learning, peers, programs, and self-evaluation of teaching effectiveness. Students, faculty colleagues, program and university administrators, accrediting agencies, healthcare facilities and society are all stakeholders to whom faculty may be accountable in the evaluation process. While all aspects of evaluation are important in Nursing education, this chapter focuses on the evaluation of student learning with an emphasis on the use of evaluation to facilitate the student's growth. More specifically, this chapter discusses the basics of evaluation processes and describes evaluation methods used by faculty who adopted the Modeling and Role-Modeling (MRM) theory as the foundation for their educational programs.

FACULTY REFLECTIONS AND PLANNING

Defining the Process

The evaluation process is complex. It isn't something that happens after teaching content or concepts; it is something that is thought through in advance. It should be planned and developed in conjunction with the teaching-learning process. This means that Nursing faculty needs to understand the components of the evaluation process, and they need guidelines for thinking about it, shown in Table 10.1.

Table 10.1 Components and their definitions, guidelines, and related faculty considerations.

Components (Worral, 2003)	**Definitions** (Worral, 2003)	**Guidelines** (Nitko, 1983/2007)	**Considerations** (Moskal, 2003)
Audience	Those for whom the evaluation is being done.		
Purpose	The reason that the evaluation is being initiated.	Identify the desired learning outcomes and the behaviors that represent the achievement of the objectives.	By completing the performance assessment, the student should have a valuable learning experience, and the faculty an evaluative experience.
Questions to be asked	Measurable, specific questions related to the purpose.	Provide opportunities for assessment that meet students' needs.	The behavior being assessed should reflect an activity that is valued in clinical practice and is consistent with real situations.
Scope	Sets limits on how much or how many will be evaluated.	Consider the limitations of assessment strategies, remembering that they represent only a sample of students' behaviors.	•Assessment should be free from bias; •The activity being evaluated should not examine unintended variables; all elements should relate directly to the objectives.
Resources	A realistic estimate of materials, equipment, people, facilities and time needed.	Employ a variety of measurement techniques to evaluate learning outcomes.	

Three authors who offer valuable insight for faculty are Worral (2003), Nitko (1983/2007), and Moskal (2003). Worral indicates that there are five components involved in the evaluation process. Each should be considered as faculty plan for and carry out the strategies specific to their program. Nitko provides guidelines for faculty to keep in mind during the planning and implementation phases of these processes. Since Nursing is a practice profession, it is also important to think about how to evaluate performance. Moskal offers several factors which provide insight in this area. The relations among these can be seen in Table 10.1 (above).

The evaluation process provides the information needed to determine the extent to which educational objectives have been met—information needed to determine the students' readiness to progress.

Remembering the Context

Metropolitan State's School of Nursing evaluation process was developed to be consistent with the University's mission and the School of Nursing's philosophy, as discussed in Chapter 4. Table 10.2 below, illustrates the relationships among program philosophy, outcomes, course objectives and evaluation strategies. The examples are from the curriculum at Metropolitan State University undergraduate program which is based on the Modeling and Role-Modeling Nursing theory. Several student self-evaluations, submitted at the end of the Fall, 2009 semester by RN-BSN completions students are included throughout the text. More details about evaluation strategies are provided later in the chapter.

Faculty members demonstrate their commitment to their selected Nursing theory through the way in which they engage with students, not only in the teaching process, but also in the evaluation process.

Table 10.2 Relationships among Philosophy, Outcomes, Objectives and Evaluation Strategies.

Philosophy	BSN Outcome	Course Objectives	Evaluation Strategies
As a practice profession, Nursing serves society through knowledgeable and humanistic caring directed toward healing in the human health experience. We value self-care as an essential component of nursing practice and personal development.	Practice holistic nursing care directed toward healing in the human health experience for diverse populations.	Utilize critical thinking skills in applying knowledge of clinical decision-making process, including aggregation and interpretation of data, pattern analysis and implementation of the Aims of Intervention.	Case Study Assignment: Students write a developmental history on a client; complete data collection; aggregate, interpret and synthesize data; develop nursing diagnoses; and plan interventions based on the Aims of Intervention.
	Engage in holistic self-care practices.	Articulate insights gained through participation in self-care/self-healing activities.	Self-care Assignment: Students asses their self-care needs (self-care knowledge), identify what they will do for self-care during the semester and what is required to do it (self-care resources), implement the plan (self-care action), and reflect, through journaling, on the experience.
	Practice professional Nursing that is grounded in current evidence from multiple ways-of-knowing.	Explore the use of therapeutic communication, relaxation, imagery, therapeutic touch, and promotion of spiritual well-being in providing holistic nursing care.	Online discussion forum. Case study discussion and application of interventions. Online quiz.

DEFINING THE FOCUS

Spiral Learning

Student evaluation is the process of gathering data, placing value on the findings, and making judgments based on them. Information obtained through the evaluation processes serves to inform students and faculty about the students' growth and their readiness for the next phase in their professional development. It results in the identification of the strengths and weaknesses of the students. "It involves collecting data to determine if what is observed is different than what is expected" (Hayes, 2007, p. 410). It also provides the faculty with data regarding what is needed in the next phase of education. The two, past accomplishments and future learning needs, are interactive and ongoing. Worral (2003) describes it as a "process within a process–a critical component of the nursing process, the decision-making process, and the education process…Because these processes are cyclical, evaluation serves as the critical bridge at the end of one cycle that guides direction of the next cycle" (p. 494).

> It is important for faculty to remember that students learn from their interactions with them. What they learn will affect how they think and what they are interested in learning in the future.

The Responsibility and an Opportunity

A Belief Statement

As faculty members consider how to design evaluation strategies and tools to carry out their plans, they must consider their personal philosophy. As Erickson states in Chapter 3, "Personal philosophies affect what faculty believe students should be taught and how they should be taught. Personal philosophies are often the unspoken, unwritten, underpinnings of the curricula" (p 73).

This suggests that faculty members who have identified a single Nursing theory as the foundation for their curriculum have the *responsibility* to consider how to incorporate the theoretical concepts and related philosophy into their evaluation processes. It should permeate all aspects of the program. Implementation should not be limited to teaching students how to apply the theory to their Nursing practice; it should also guide the interactions between and among students and faculty, set the tone for the milieu of the learning environment, and influence the teaching/learning/evaluation strategies and the processes utilized.

According to Hayes, "The roles of evaluation depend on what that something is that is being evaluated and on whose standards or values the results will be analyzed. Therefore, the role of evaluation is situational and specific" (2007, p. 410). Hayes makes an important point when identifying the "something" that is being evaluated and the "standards" of evaluation. While it is anticipated that student performance will be evaluated in Nursing education, assessing student growth is of equal importance. Evaluation data collected can be used to advise students about progress made in achieving course outcomes and in meeting their goals for personal growth. The standards for judging the data will differ if the focus is on student growth rather than on performance.

That is, it is not appropriate to use only multiple-choice exams with the intent of practicing for the NCLEX if the Nursing program is based on a holistic nursing theory which emphasizes the role of the nurse as facilitating growth in clients. Since students *are* the faculty's clients, concepts of holism should be applied to student evaluation as well as included in the teaching-learning process and the content of the curriculum.

> Faculty members who have purposefully selected a theoretical framework as the bases for their curricula have a responsibility to consider how to teach such content and how to incorporate it into their evaluation processes.

Worldviews

At the heart of Modeling and Role-Modeling theory is Model of the World. This concept was originally described in relationship to the client. Understanding the client's model of the world or the client's perspective gives a nurse the foundation to develop nursing interventions that are unique to the client. Nurses utilize therapeutic communication skills to elicit the client's story and personal perspective. Students also have their individual models of the world both in terms of their personal lives and their role as students; students are the faculty's clients.

Growth

The focus of this chapter is the evaluation of student growth. Therefore, it is important to consider the characteristics of growth. Erickson (2006a) identifies several characteristics of growth. Growth is a "positive change that occurs when our needs are met" (p. 327). At times difficult to recognize, growth is gradual and elusive. Growth is unique to the person. "No one can know what another person needs in order to grow; it is very personal knowledge" (p.329). Following an overall design, growth is ordered. Finally, growth is contextual. Students learn within a specific learning environment and have a perception of their role within that environment. These characteristics further support the need for a variety of strategies that capture the complex nature of the student and the learning experiences. Table 10.3 provides examples of ways to support and assess student growth based on the characteristics described above.

Table 10.3 Characteristics of growth and strategies for faculty support and Assessment of growth.

Characteristics of growth (Erickson, 2006a)	**Strategies for support and assessment of growth**
Growth is a positive change, occurring when needs are met.	Provide a learning atmosphere that supports students in finding ways to have learning needs met as holistic persons.
Growth is gradual.	Offer multiple opportunities for assessment and evaluation during the educational program that will document student growth over time.
Growth is unique.	Offer various tools for evaluation to capture the personal ways in which growth is demonstrated.
Growth is ordered.	Provide structure in the learning environment to support the "predictable" aspect of the growth process.
Growth is elusive.	Assist students to identify ways in which their needs are being met. Support reflection on self-care knowledge.
Growth is contextual.	Assess the learning environment. Provide evaluation experiences that encourage students to reflect on the learning environment.

Linking Philosophy to Practice

Faculty members who embrace the MRM theory use the Aims of Intervention and concepts of nurturance, facilitation and life-time growth and development to implement their evaluation plan. The Aims of Intervention help remind faculty of their intent and what they aim to happen as they work with students. The concepts guide the implementation of their strategies. For example, "Nurturance fuses and integrates cognitive, physiological, and affective processes" (Erickson, et al., 1983/2009, p. 48). In the evaluative process, this means that the student is viewed as holistic. The cognitive, physiologic, and affective aspects of the person are seen as interacting dynamically. Therefore, evaluation strategies are directed toward the multiple interacting subsystems.

> Nursing faculty who integrate a holistic nursing theory such as Modeling and Role-Modeling have a sound rationale on which to base their strategies for evaluating student growth.

Aims of Intervention

The MRM Aims of Intervention serve as reminders for faculty as they plan and implement their strategies. Designed to provide a framework for nurses to plan interventions for clients, the universal nature of the aims makes them applicable in the teaching/leaning process. Schultz (1998) previously described how the Aims of Intervention are used to guide the process of student advising. This chapter builds on that work. The Aims of Intervention can also be used throughout the implementation of the evaluation process, particularly since the Metro State evaluation process is designed to facilitate student growth.

Table 10.4 provides linkages among the Aims of Intervention and suggested evaluation strategies used at Metro State University. Specifically, the MRM Aims of Intervention are to build trust, promote positive orientation, promote client control, affirm and promote strengths and set mutual goals that are health-directed (Erickson, 2006a). Each is described briefly below. For more detail, visit the work of other authors in Erickson, (2006b), Erickson, et al., (1983/2009), and Schultz (1998).

Table 10.4 MRM Aims of Intervention and evaluation strategies.

Aims of Intervention	**Evaluation Strategy**
Build trust	Establish an interactive interpersonal relationship. Understand the student's model of the world through active listening. Evaluate according to the plan and criteria presented to students at the beginning of the term. Provide accurate, honest feedback based on evaluative data. Utilize open and direct communication.
Promote positive orientation	Ask students to reflect on past accomplishments as part of self-evaluation. Help students build upon past accomplishments as a basis for demonstrating new learning. Assist students to project into the future as successful holistic nurses. Model the student's world.
Promote Control	Clearly outline the processes and criteria for evaluation. Provide options such as learning contracts which allow students choices in how they will be evaluated. Assist students in selecting evaluation strategies that are consistent with their needs and learning styles. Promote negotiation strategies. Direct students to resources that facilitate gaining control.
Promote strengths	Expect students to include reflection on strengths in self-evaluation. Identify student accomplishments and highlight them. Nominate students for appropriate awards, scholarships, and other acknowledgements. Assist students to relate new learning to concepts and skills that have been mastered.
Set mutual goals	Assist students in developing learning contracts. Encourage students to identify barriers to meeting expected outcomes. Expect students to set realistic goals. Assist students to identify unmet needs that interfere with goal attainment (Schultz, 1998).

Build Trust

When faculty members evaluate students, they make value judgments about the data they collect through various evaluation strategies. This process is more effective if done within a trusting relationship. This can be done by remembering the basic premises of MRM, particularly unconditional acceptance, and the human need for dignity and respect, and growth.

Promote a Positive Orientation

The process of evaluation has the potential to threaten students' sense of self-concept. The two aspects of positive orientation which faculty should consider are promoting self-worth and promoting hope for the future (Erickson, et al., 1983/2009, pp. 180-92).

Promote Control

Students may perceive that they have no control in the evaluation process. Some students believe "no matter what I do, I can't get it right." In order to progress successfully in the Nursing program, students need to have the perception that they have some control in the evaluation process.

Promote Strengths

Faculty must maintain a balanced approach to evaluation that includes the strengths of the student as well as learning gaps. For example, when faculty are concerned about a student action in clinical which jeopardizes client safety, the evaluation could focus only on what the student did that was wrong.

Set Mutual Goals

While faculty are ultimately responsible for planning and implementing student evaluation, the process offers opportunities for students and faculty to work together to set educational goals.

> The Aims of Intervention help faculty to be mindful and purposeful in their interactions with students.

Nurturing Growth and Development

Nurturing, facilitating, and recognizing lifetime growth and development in the teaching/learning process are consistent with servant teaching. Based on Greenleaf's (2002) concept of servant leadership, "the servant teacher recognizes the tremendous responsibility to do everything within his or her power to nurture the personal, professional and spiritual growth of students [while] identifying students' needs and providing developmental opportunities" (Robinson, 2009, p.

11). In order to nurture and facilitate student development, faculty must embrace the concept of unconditional acceptance. When a teacher unconditionally accepts a student, the student is viewed as "a unique, worthwhile, important individual with no strings attached" (Erickson, et al., 1983/2009, p. 255). They learn how be like their faculty, and they jump the gap from learning to thinking.

> *Unconditional acceptance has freed up my emotional energy so that I can better care for the needs of the patient. For example, there are a number of chemically-dependent patients on my unit. There is a very cynical culture among the nurses toward these patients. Leaving this judgment behind,* [i.e., using] *unconditional acceptance, removes the burden from my shoulders.* (Dawn Krasue, Student Self-evaluation, 2009)

When the concept of facilitation is applied to evaluation, the teacher acts as a facilitator, not an effector. Through the ongoing relationship, the faculty member assists the student to "identify, mobilize, and develop his or her own strengths" (Erickson, et al., 1983/2009, p. 48). The faculty promotes student self-reflection and self-critique. In a practicum situation for example, rather than offering a list of clinical inadequacies or taking over for the student, the instructor coaches the student through a procedure by asking relevant questions and assisting the student to connect new learning to concepts that have been mastered.

> The National League for Nursing (2004) has identified hallmarks of excellence in Nursing education. The hallmarks that focus on evaluation promote teaching/learning/evaluation strategies that are innovative and varied. Their aim is to enhance learning for a diverse student population using strategies that promote interaction among faculty, students and colleagues, and strategies that are evidence-based.

DEFINING SPECIFICS

Types of Evaluation

The two types of evaluation described in most texts on student evaluation are *formative* and *summative* evaluation. Evaluation of students occurs both during the process of learning within a course or clinical experience and at the end of the learning experience.

Process or formative evaluation is conducted *during* the learning experience. It measures progress toward an outcome and allows for adjustments to be made, as needed. In clinical settings, for example, process evaluation is often ongoing and provides students frequent and periodic feedback on clinical practice throughout the term, giving students the opportunity to modify behavior as needed (Bourke & Ihrke, 2009; Hayes, 2007).

Outcome or summative evaluation is conducted at the *end* of the learning experience and "measures changes occurring as a result of teaching and learning" (Worral, 2003, p. 499). The focus of summative evaluation is the entire course or clinical experience and the degree to which objectives were met, resulting in the assignment of a course grade (Bourke & Ihrke, 2009).

More specific types of evaluation described by Worral (2003) are content and impact evaluation. **Content evaluation** focuses on what learners have learned during a specific learning experience. The focus is on short-term outcomes and specific objectives. In contrast, **Impact evaluation** is broad in scope, directed toward determining the worth of the learning activity.

The following section provides details about selected strategies used by the Metropolitan State University School of Nursing faculty.

Evaluation Strategies

Foundational to Modeling and Role-Modeling (MRM) theory is the belief that "human beings are holistic persons who have multiple interacting subsystems" permeated by genetic makeup and spiritual drive (Erickson, et al., 1983/2009, p. 44). Faculty members utilizing the MRM theory appreciate the holistic dimension of the students. While a majority of the teaching/learning processes focus on the cognitive dimension of the students, the students bring their holistic selves into every teaching/learning experience. This holistic view supports models which "take an eclectic view on learning, and acknowledge that people learn in numerous different ways" (Van Merrienborr & Paas, 2003, p.17). Different ways of learning call for different evaluative strategies. Even when the teaching is primarily focused on the cognitive dimension, such as a lecture on pathophysiology, the dynamic interactive nature of the subsystems in the holistic person requires that the instructor acknowledge the impact of other subsystems on the learning process. For example, the emotional state of the student will influence what is "heard" during the lecture and what is answered on a written examination.

Because students are viewed as holistic, and because they utilize multiple ways-of-knowing (described in chapter 3) a variety of evaluation strategies should be implemented within a Nursing program. The use of multiple evaluation strategies represents a

> *...shift in learning and evaluation, away from viewing elements that are taught, and from tests that determine if parts have been learned* [reductionism], *to a view of the whole* [holism], *a pattern of inter-related phenomena in which students find a natural way to learn, criticize and evaluate, and become liberated from teacher-formulated behaviors.* (Goldenberg & Dietrich, 2002, p. 303)

Use of a variety of evaluation strategies increases the likelihood that multiple ways of knowing will be evaluated in an individual course or a Nursing program.

> A number of evaluation strategies may be implemented to determine the learner's current knowledge, needs for personal growth, and current learning needs. The strategies chosen should relate to the overall evaluation plan of the Nursing program, the outcomes being evaluated, the complexity and domain of the learning experience, and the characteristics and developmental stage of the students. They should also be consistent with the theoretical model which frames the curricula.

Written Examinations

Written examinations have held an important role in the evaluation of Nursing students. To accurately determine the extent to which students are knowledgeable and can think critically by using written tests requires careful test planning and development. Written examinations are suited to formative and summative assessment. Helpful feedback from tests, taken as part of formative assessment, "provides specific comments about errors and specific suggestions for improvement and encourages students to focus their attention thoughtfully on the task rather than simply getting the right answer" (Boston, 2002, para. 5). Written exams may be appropriate for classroom and clinical evaluation.

Exams can be classified as *norm-referenced* and *criterion-referenced.* The purpose of norm-referenced tests is to compare the achievement of a student with the student's peer group which can produce a rank order of students. Commonly used in national standardized tests, norm-referenced tests are not designed to indicate what a student has learned, but rather how a student compares to others in the group (Bond, 1996; McDonald, 2007). In contrast, criterion-referenced tests determine the student's level of performance in relation to identified learning outcomes. These tests are based on pre-determined performance expectations of the curriculum of a specific Nursing program.

Factors to consider when using written exams include the purpose of the test, content and course objectives to be assessed in the examination, level of difficulty, length of the test, types of items included, format for question presentation, and reliability and validity of test items (Kirkpatrick & Dewitt, 2009; McDonald, 2007). Numerous resources are available to assist faculty to prepare written examinations including books, journal articles, internet sources and the National Council of State Boards of Nursing.

The ways in which examinations are used in a program will, in part, depend on the teaching/learning philosophy of the Nursing faculty. The beliefs of the faculty will influence decisions about issues such as options to retake examinations to achieve mastery, collaborative test-taking, and how and what type of feedback is provided to students. In programs which prepare students for licensure, written tests can serve to build the test-taking skills needed for examinations such as NCLEX.

Concept Maps

Concept maps provide a graphic, hierarchical means of demonstrating the relationship among concepts. The fundamental idea behind concept mapping originates from Ausubel's cognitive psychology in which he describes learning taking place "by assimilation of new concepts and propositions into existing concept and propositional framework held by the learner" (Novak & Canas, 2008, p. 3). Concept mapping has been used as a teaching-learning tool in Nursing education to demonstrate the relationship among concepts learned in a course or learning situation. Concept mapping may be done individually or as a collaborative learning experience with groups of students.

Concept mapping may also be used as an evaluation tool. MacNeil (2007) proposes that concept maps may be used to gather data about what students have learned in a class. Prior to a lecture, students create a concept map related to the primary concepts of the class. At the completion of the class, students complete another concept map and the results are compared. MacNeil found that the maps demonstrated increasing complexity and improvement in relationships among concepts. This strategy, presented as a means of course evaluation, may be used to provide feedback on individual student learning as well as "details on the teaching effectiveness of every week's lecture topics, which the traditional course survey did not" (p. 233). Hayes (2007) recommends the use of concept maps in the clinical setting to promote connecting patient situations with previously learned concepts. Novak and Canas (2008) further state that concept maps "can be as effective as more time-consuming clinical interviews for identifying the relevant knowledge a learner possesses before or after instruction" (p.5).

Portfolio Assessment

A portfolio is a collection of documents that reflects ways in which the students have achieved learning outcomes. Portfolios are appropriate for learning and evaluation in both the classroom and in clinical experiences and may be used for formative or summative evaluation. Portfolio assessment is thought to foster "authentic assessment" in which the context and content of the learning are nearly identical to those of the situation in which they will be used (White, 2004). Growth and learning portfolios are used to assess students' progress, while best-work portfolios demonstrate students' mastery of learning objectives (Hayes, 2007).

The assignments included in the portfolio are intentionally designed to demonstrate achievement in either course or program outcomes. "Focused less on the textbook content and more on thought processes, including discrimination and creativity, use of the student portfolio can demonstrate a wide range of student abilities that can easily complement the student's actual real-time clinical performance" (McDonald, 2007, p.265). When students are given feedback regarding strengths and weaknesses, they can make improvements. Critical thinking is stimulated as students reflect on the work in their portfolio (Kirkpatrick & DeWitt, 2009).

Contained within the portfolio may be a variety of assignments such as case studies, reflective journals, concept maps, and research critiques. In some cases students may select the means through which learning in a content area was demonstrated or a problem solved facilitating student ownership in their own learning and evaluation. Portfolios are a useful evaluation strategy for both students and faculty when the focus is on student growth, especially the components that include reflective activities.

Journal

The process of reflecting on and writing about experiences may be used as a teaching/learning strategy in Nursing courses; for example, when a student explores a newly learned concept, or in clinical practicum when a student reflects on performance. Some of the outcomes of reflective writing are promotion of knowledge transfer, knowledge transformation, analysis and critical thinking about a situation, exploration of feelings, and increased self-awareness (Kirkpatrick & DeWitt, 2009; Nielsen, Stragnell, & Jester, 2007). Journal writing is one of the metacognitive strategies. "A metacognitive strategy is an activity that promotes conscious executive control of one's thought processes. Metacognitive strategies such as reflection on experience and articulation of reflections in either verbal or written form help enhance understanding of phenomena encountered in the clinical setting. This is accomplished by "bringing observations and perceptions to a conscious level for review and analysis" (Ertmer & Newby, 1996, p. 39).

> *I had a revelation in this course—not everyone wants to 'get Better.' All patients have different goals during their journeys. Many medical processionals assume that the patient wishes to be cured. In fact, the goal may be as simple as going home to reconnect with family. It is important for the nurse to develop goals of care with patient input.* (Teresa Cyrus, Student Self-evaluation, 2009)

Journal assignments may be structured or free-flowing. In either case, the purpose, format, and goals of the assignment must be clearly identified (O'Connor, 2006). "The reflective process begins when one returns to the experience, recalls what has occurred, and replays the experience. This is accomplished through four key elements: relating new data to that which is already known, seeking relationship among data, determining the authenticity of ideas and feelings, and making knowledge one's own" (Nielsen, et al., 2007, p. 513). When the evaluation process focuses on students' growth, rather than being limited to performance, students have permission to reflect on the progress they have made on personally-determined, holistic outcomes.

The use of journals for student evaluation is controversial. Some authors believe that if journals are used as evaluative tools and are graded, it may impact truthfulness and the depth of expression of student entries. Grading may also encourage students to write to meet perceived instructor expectations rather than to deeply explore issues. Some of the ways to deal with these issues is to clearly explain the evaluation process with specific criteria, provide feedback that supports student improvement, base comments on data rather than opinion, comment on the learning to be gained from the assignment, and focus on processes and patterns that the student reveals rather than content alone (Hayes, 2007; Kirkpatrick & Dewitt, 2009; O'Connor, 2006). It helps them uncover personal knowledge, and integrate it into their knowledge base used to practice.

> *I find it rewarding to learn more about the theory and reasoning behind why we do the things we do. For example, I would, at times, feel frustrated with clients' behaviors. After taking this course, I have been able to see things more clearly. People are the way they are because of their life experiences; they are only trying to meet their needs. Need deficits drive their behavior. This has allowed me to unconditionally accept clients as they are; I believe I have become a better nurse. Some of the concepts we learned this semester I feel I practiced, but just didn't have a name for them. It is so rewarding when you know why you do what you do.* (Sara Adelmann, Student Self-evaluation, 2009)

Written Papers and Projects

A wide array of assignments falls under the category of written papers and projects. These assignments can demonstrate critical thinking skills, organizational ability, research skills, synthesis of concepts and creativity, as well as writing ability. Written papers may include assignments such as an in-depth exploration of a topic, ways to resolve an ethical dilemma, a policy analysis, or a critical reflection about a patient-care experience.

There are several issues that challenge faculty when evaluating students' papers and other written projects. Guidelines for completion of the written project must be clearly written, including required components, structure, format, length, reference requirements, and process for submitting the paper. Kirkpatrick and DeWitt (2009) identify reliability of grading as an issue and suggest anonymous grading as a strategy to increase objectivity.

Students express the subjectivity in grading papers as a concern. Scoring rubrics provide the criteria and the observable indicators which are used in grading, increasing the objectivity of the grading. Rubrics may be classified as *holistic* or *analytic*. When using the holistic rubric, the evaluator scores the overall process or product as a whole. The analytic rubric allows the evaluator to score individual parts of the assignment and then sum the parts to determine the final score (Mertler, 2001). Scores must then be converted into grades for the assignment.

Performance Evaluation

Practice disciplines such as Nursing rely on performance demonstration as a way to evaluate the application of theory in clinical practice. "Clinical evaluation addresses three dimensions of student learning–cognitive, affective, and psychomotor–and is the most challenging of the evaluative processes. Inherent in this process is the need to demonstrate progressive acquisition of increasingly complex competencies" (Hayes, 2007, p. 420). Students may be evaluated according to norm-referenced or criterion-referenced assessment plans.

Because, by its nature, performance assessment is subjective, attention must be given to ensuring fairness in evaluation. Moskal (2003) offers some recommendations (see Table 10.5) for the development of performance assessments.

Table 10.5 Moskal's (2003) recommendations for performance evaluation.

1. The behavior being assessed should reflect an activity that is valued in clinical practice and is consistent with real situations.
2. When a performance assessment is completed, the student should have a valuable learning experience, and the faculty will have a valuable evaluative experience.
3. The goals and objectives should be aligned with the measurable outcomes of the student performance.
4. The activity being evaluated should not examine unintended variables; all elements should relate directly to the objectives.
5. Assessment should be free from bias.

When performance occurs in a clinical setting, students are evaluated in an uncontrolled setting. Although the criteria for evaluation are consistent, the experiences encountered by students in clinical practice are not. This may challenge the goal of fairness in evaluation. In some programs, simulated experiences are used for evaluation in order to increase consistency among student experiences. The use of a performance evaluation rubric also increases objectivity in grading.

Self-Evaluation

The evaluation methods to this point are those for which the faculty members have primary responsibility. Student self-evaluation is another strategy for gathering data about student progress while fostering critical thinking skills. Goldenberg and Dietrich (2002) describe self-evaluation as "a valuable method to identify students' own strengths, provide guidelines for self-directed learning, act as a vehicle for communication, foster professional growth and learning, and provide teachers with information for summative (end of instruction) evaluation" (p. 306).

Self-evaluation can take a variety of forms including responding to specific instructor questions, rating self on accomplishment of outcomes, journaling about clinical performance, reflecting on learning challenges and personal growth. Self-evaluation is commonly done during or at the end of a course. However, it may be a strategy used at the beginning of a course to provide the student with a basis to make a decision about compatibility with a teaching/learning style such as online education. Whatever the form, self-evaluation should open a dialogue between the student and instructor that provides the students with direction for future learning. When the program or course evaluation process focuses on student growth, self-evaluation will provide opportunities for students to evaluate self-determined goals which reflect their growth over time.

> *The heart to heart relationship/connection was something that really stuck in my head because of the importance that one must be loving, compassionate, and open with oneself in order to, in return, be a loving and compassionate nurse to a patient. One does not happen without the other and that is something we should think about daily.* (Becky Demars, Student Self-evaluation, 2009)

An Analysis of Various Strategies

By integrating a holistic Nursing theory such as Modeling and Role-Modeling into the curriculum and, therefore, the evaluation process, faculty members are encouraged to think beyond performance evaluation to include student growth. Faculty is not limited to "rigid and restrictive guides for evaluation" that restrict student creativity but can "offer a wider range of options, ideas, teaching and evaluation strategies" (Goldenberg & Dietrich, 2002, p. 307).

Written examinations can serve an important role in evaluation in a Nursing program using MRM, but will be used as one of many strategies. In some programs, exams are used almost exclusively. Although the development of valid and reliable exams is complex, the ease of administration and grading as well as students' need to learn to take written exams often serve as rationale for their use. Their focus is primarily on the cognitive aspect. In contrast, **concept maps** highlight students' creativity and visual abilities. They can assess both the cognitive and affective domains. It helps them practice more holistically.

> *I, now, like to ask my patients what they think is causing their problems. Often, I am quite surprised to hear their answers. Generally, the interventions I had in mind change from a medically-based perspective to a more holistically-based approach. It simplifies my work.* (Michelle Coyle, Student Self-evaluation, 2009)

Self-evaluation is an important evaluation strategy from the Modeling and Role-Modeling perspective. Self-evaluation facilitates the access of self-care knowledge or self-knowledge as described in Chapter 3. In MRM, Self-care Knowledge is one aspect of the concept of self-care. Self-care is comprised of Self-care Knowledge, Self-care Resources, and Self-care Actions. Within MRM theory, Self-care Knowledge is described this way. "At some level a person knows what has made him or her sick, lessened his or her effectiveness or interfered with his or her growth. The person knows what will make him or her well, optimize his or her effectiveness or fulfillment (given the circumstances) or promote his or her growth" (Erickson, et al., 1983/2009, p. 254). Self-care knowledge serves as the "basis for one's personal model of the world" (Hertz & Baas, 2006, p. 119). From this perspective, the student serves as a valuable resource in the evaluative process. Not only can the student compare his or her own progress against the course outcomes, but can also identify, at some level, what has impeded growth, if that is the case, and what will help. Self-evaluation requires contemplation and reflection. Journals may be one of the vehicles through which self-evaluation is demonstrated, and can be used to evaluate both the cognitive and affective domains through active student involvement. Guided by faculty questions, students can look inward for answers, to integrate what they are learning with what they already know.

MRM has taught me to delve into the more holistic perspective in caring for my patients. I have learned to be more self-aware and to view the medical world from a different angle—that of my patient. This will enable me to change my perspective of nursing to incorporate mind, body, and spiritual healing. (Dani Yang, Student Self-evaluation, 2009)

Students' Self-evaluation Comments

At the end of each course, students are asked to comment on their learning experience. Several of their comments have been dispersed throughout this chapter. While this chapter focuses on evaluation strategies used by faculty at Metro State University, it is important that these strategies go hand-in-glove with our educational philosophy of teaching. That is, we believe that it is important to focus on facilitating students to learn, as described in earlier chapters in this book. Two additional student self-evaluations illustrating why this is important are shown below.

> *To be able to see past patient behaviors, to understand what their basic needs are...is to truly have a window into their world. Then and only then can we touch, teach, and facilitate healing. What a privilege; what a responsibility.* (Susan Vold, Student Self-evaluation, 2009)

> *The concept from Modeling and Role-Modeling that I have started incorporating into my nursing practice is the idea of being. The idea of performing procedures, yet engaging and acknowledging the presence of my client with intention changed my practice. The idea of a holistic view of the client, body mind and soul, allows the nurse and client to build trust which is fundamental to caring for someone.* (Cynthia Garley, Student Self-evaluation, 2009)

A Case Example

The two types of evaluation and several strategies, discussed above, are demonstrated in the following situation.

> *Ann is a nursing student enrolled in a Nursing fundamentals course that includes both theory and practicum. Students in the course receive a syllabus which lists the outcomes for the course and the types of assignments that will be used to demonstrate to what level the objectives have been met. One of the objectives of the course relates to the use of therapeutic communication skills. The students in this course work with*

elderly residents in an assisted living facility. The director of nursing at the facility has requested that Nursing students come to her facility, knowing that one strong component of the course is the development of therapeutic communication skills. She hopes to assist her staff in developing better communication with the residents.

During the second week of practicum, Ann's instructor, having had the opportunity to observe an interaction between Ann and one of the residents, provides feedback on the skills demonstrated during the interaction. This formative evaluation alerts Ann to areas in which her communication style can be improved. This feedback provides Ann with the chance to develop more therapeutic communication strategies prior to the formal evaluation at the end of the semester.

During the class presentation on therapeutic communication, the benefits of asking open questions were described. However, examples of open questions were not demonstrated by the instructor. During the practicum, Ann's instructor notes that Ann asks primarily closed questions that elicit minimal responses from the client. This content evaluation provides the instructor with information on the degree to which Ann is able to meet the outcome and leads the instructor to consider a different strategy for teaching the specific area of open-ended questions.

At the end of the semester, summative evaluation of communication is demonstrated in a taped interview that is graded based on course expectations. The director of nursing at the assisted living is interested in how the communication that nursing students have modeled has influenced the communication between the residents and her staff. She plans an impact evaluation to determine the effects on her facility.

Constraints on Faculty

There is wide variability in teaching/learning experiences in Nursing. A faculty member engaged in lecturing to over one hundred students could not realistically consider understanding the model of the world of each student that will be evaluated in that course. In contrast, a nurse educator orienting a small group of new graduates, or a clinical instructor teaching eight students in a practicum experience will have more opportunities to know and understand each individual student. In both situations, the instructors must be aware that the student's model of the world is the lens through which the learning experience is viewed. Journals and other reflective assignments also provide insights into the student's model of the world. In situations in which the instructor is able to incorporate the student's model of the world, the learning experience is enhanced for the student.

MRM theory proposes that people are born with an inherent desire to fulfill their potential through the life span. The belief in lifetime growth and development is based on the idea that "if they are given accurate information, emotional support, and assistance for the changes they desire, they will make good decisions for themselves" (Erickson, et al., 1983/2009, p. 46).

Feedback as a Cognitive Facilitator

It is clear that all students do not come to the learning experience with the same potential and not all students will be successful in Nursing education. Nevertheless, when discussing the results of evaluation data, the instructor who integrates MRM theory will clearly present the assessment data. Rather than taking the "you just don't get it" attitude, the instructor may ask the student to reflect on the barriers that interfere with his/her inherent desire to fulfill his/her potential.

> Feedback is an important part of the learning process. Students learn from feedback, and when done properly, it helps them grow as humans and as professionals, and provides the basis for continued learning.

SUMMARY

This chapter described multiple factors related to the evaluation of students at Metropolitan State University, School of Nursing. It described faculty considerations as they planned and implemented a multifaceted, multidimensional evaluation plan based in the Modeling and Role-Modeling theory and focused on facilitating student growth.

It included a description of how faculty members link their philosophy to their practice strategies for student evaluation in Nursing education, described various types of strategies used, and their linkages to the MRM model.

CHAPTER 11

ISSUES FOR A CULTURALLY-DIVERSE SOCIETY

Judith E. Hertz, Barbara L. Irvin, Susan S. Bowman

Today's world is a multicultural one comprised of diverse populations, values and beliefs, with instant satellite and internet communication continually exposing us to the plights and joys of people all over the world. In our personal and professional interactions with others in diverse roles and settings, we have found that Modeling and Role-Modeling (MRM) provides a reliable theoretical framework to guide curricular and practice decisions, no matter where we are located. Therefore, we feel privileged to share, in this chapter, some of our thoughts and experiences using MRM theory with culturally-diverse populations and settings.

OVERVIEW

The purpose of this chapter is to share some of the knowledge and experience of three seasoned faculty who have taught the theoretical underpinnings and application of Modeling and Role-Modeling theory to several culturally-diverse groups of learners:

1) Undergraduate and graduate Nursing students working with and caring for others from diverse cultural backgrounds;
2) Staff nurses, administrators and advanced practice nurses working with and caring for others from cultures different from their own or ours; and,
3) Nursing faculty, outside the U.S., developing a baccalaureate level curriculum based on MRM theory.

The chapter begins with an overview of the Taiwan experience and then contains a general overview of nursing practice from a Modeling and Role-Modeling perspective in a culturally-diverse society. There is a discussion of the major concepts within the MRM theory as they relate to cultural diversity, followed by two sections focusing on issues important to nurse managers and nurse educators. Finally, the chapter deals specifically with MRM as it was applied with Nursing faculty in Taiwan. A model of cultural relevance is presented to show the process and approach used.

THE TAIWAN EXPERIENCE

During the academic year 1995-1996, two of the authors[1] served as invited visiting professors for a large Nursing program located in southern Taiwan. One of the goals for the Nursing program at that time was to expand opportunities for Nursing education at the school, as the decision had been made to add two years of Nursing coursework to the associates program so that students could obtain a baccalaureate degree. The main thrust of our job then was to teach the Nursing faculty about Modeling and Role-Modeling (MRM) Nursing theory and guide them in developing the new curriculum using MRM as the organizing framework.

Although we had prior experience with MRM theory in our teaching, research, and practice, we had never tried to teach or apply the theory with a group of nurse educators in a foreign country, much less live there for an extended period of time. Therefore, we viewed this as an exciting opportunity and eagerly, albeit naively, began our once-in-a-lifetime adventure.

When we arrived in Taiwan, we were immediately immersed in Taiwanese culture and a school with over six thousand Nursing students, facing more than a bit of culture shock! Not only were there several nationalities and cultures represented on the island, the official language was Mandarin Chinese. Fortunately, since we were totally unfamiliar with the language, we were each assigned a translator to help us with our adaptation and day-to-day needs. Each translator was a trusted member of the Nursing faculty who had previously experienced her own culture shock while completing baccalaureate and master's degrees in the United States. These translators, with assistance from the Dean of Faculty and the School Director, were committed to helping us be comfortable, ensuring that our basic needs were met and that our overall experience in Taiwan and at the school, in particular, would be positive for us as well as beneficial for them.

Upon our arrival in Taiwan, we began learning through firsthand experiences and publications about the values, beliefs, and norms of the local people as well as the faculty and curriculum of the Nursing school. We were privileged to share housing with a local Chinese family and to have time to talk to each other in depth on a daily basis. Reflecting back on this experience, we realize we were able to build on our own personal strengths and life experiences as we began to construct a model of the world experienced by the Nursing faculty and people served by nurses around the island.

It is the experience in Taiwan, in particular, coupled with our collective decades of practice and teaching involving students and patients from many

---

[1] Judith Hertz and Barbara Irvin

different ethnic and cultural backgrounds that served as the impetus for writing this chapter.

NURSING PRACTICE IN A CULTURALLY-DIVERSE SOCIETY

Nurses have both the privilege and obligation to "practice with compassion and respect for the inherent dignity, worth and uniqueness of each individual" (ANA, 2001, p. 2). Thus, it is imperative that they truly listen to their clients and discern what is important to them. This openness to the perspective of the client, while recognizing one's own perspective as separate, helps to establish a shared perceptual field in which communication, empathy, conflict, reflection, understanding and validation may occur (Munhall, 1993). Being open to what one does not know, as described by the term *unknowing*, helps nurses avoid premature judgments and remain alert to what clients might be able to reveal to themselves as well as the nurse (Heath, 1998, p. 1055; Munhall, 1993) about what is going on and what might be needed or not needed to help them in a situation to grow, develop or heal. This information, referred to in Modeling and Role-Modeling theory as Self-care Knowledge, includes values, strengths and liabilities (Hertz & Baas, 2006, p. 98).

Learning about clients' self-care knowledge is vital so that nurses can understand *their* perspective of what is going on and help them in health-promoting ways. Without intentional effort to gain trust, through the provision of respectful, culturally-competent and congruent care, this self-care knowledge might not be revealed. Thus (as discussed in Chapter 1), how a nurse views the world and thinks about nursing care is critical for identifying what is needed to facilitate and nurture client health and healing behaviors, or self-care actions.

Being well grounded in a theoretical model of practice such as Modeling and Role Modeling, helps nurses use the theory to guide their thought processes, clinical judgments and nursing actions from the first client meeting through assessment, mutual goal-setting and outcome evaluation. Additionally, having the ability to provide culturally-competent care requires that the nurse integrate knowledge and experience with others from different backgrounds with personal beliefs, attitudes and skills that enhance communication and lead to effective interactions in a variety of multicultural situations (Andrews & Boyle, 2008).

Energy Fields

During the initial period of getting acquainted and developing a relationship to gain understanding of the client's situation, the nurse and client are in relatively close proximity and begin to establish a shared field of energy. If the nurse is accepting, respectful, nonjudgmental and truly interested in getting to know the client, the client will sense this and be more willing to share information than if the client perceives the nurse to be indifferent, distracted, rude, insulting or judgmental. As the shared energy field expands or contracts, the relationship develops with increasing trust, or conflict and mistrust.

In their discussion of energy fields, Brekke and Schultz (2006) use pictures to depict shared energy fields between two persons in positive interaction contrasted with two where the energy exchange is too weak to sustain a balanced interaction. Imagine what this exchange would be like in a multicultural situation in which a client and nurse feel distrustful or resentful of each other for some reason, or where a client overheard two staff members making negative remarks about people of the client's ethnicity just before one of them came into the room to administer a medication and change a dressing?

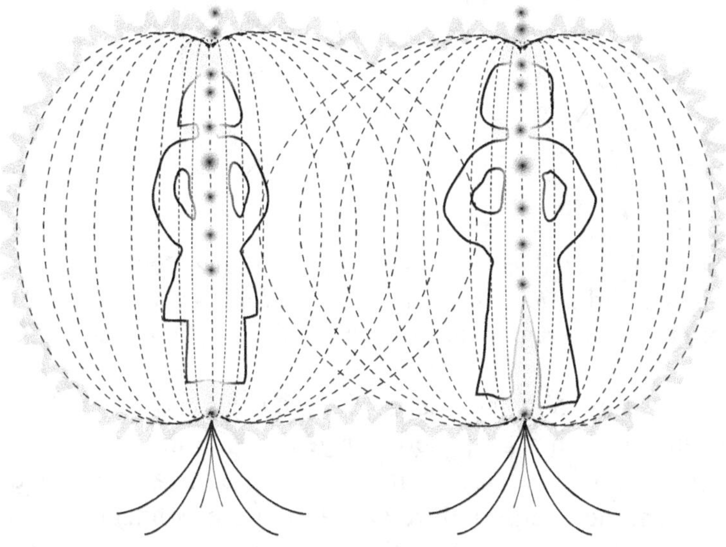

Fig. 11.1 Energy fields and aura of two people positively interacting with one another. Brekke & Shultz (2006). Energy Theories. In H. Erickson (Ed), *Modeling and Role-Modeling: A View from the Client's World* (p. 59). Reprinted with permission. Unicorns Unlimited: Cedar Park, TX.

Citing the quantum physics related research of Martha Rogers (1981) regarding energy fields and nurse-client relationships, N. C. Frisch and L. E. Frisch (1998) describe how the energy field of the nurse and client can influence each other. These authors assert that if we are feeling scattered and fragmented because of what is going on at work or at home, we can inadvertently deplete our energy field. In such times, we are not only in a poor space to help another, we might also take on the sadness, pain, or anger in our client's field, making ourselves vulnerable to negative emotions and illness. Healers are well aware of this phenomenon.

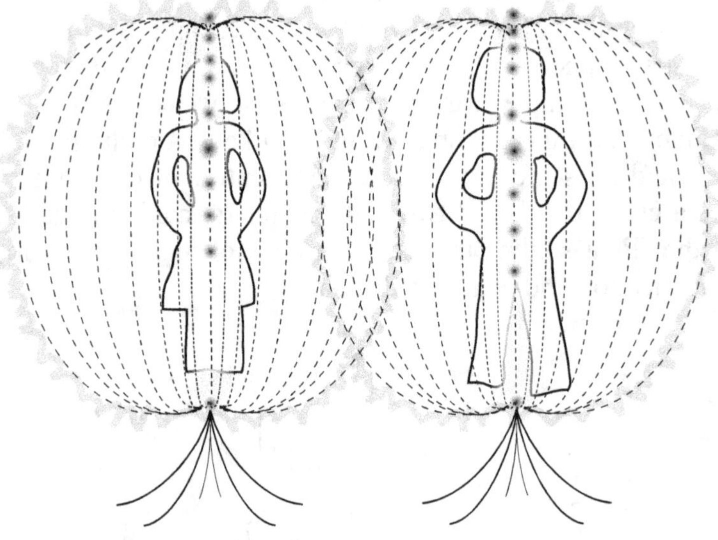

Fig 11.2 Energy fields of isolated individuals. Brekke & Shultz (2006). Energy Theories. In H. Erickson (Ed), *Modeling and Role-Modeling: A View from the Client's World* (p.60). Reprinted with permission. Unicorns Unlimited: Cedar Park, TX

Conversely, we can calm the energy disturbances around us by focusing our thoughts and intentions in a purposeful way. Imagine the difference we can make in a rushed, chaotic or unpleasant situation on a clinical unit if we make a conscious effort to calm the energy before and during our connections with other individuals or groups. This focused attention helps to establish a mind-set and create a nurturing space (Erickson, H. 2006, pp. 313-14).

One of the authors relates a personal experience of attending to her son in a critical care unit following a serious head injury. Since the situation involved continuous intracranial pressure (ICP) monitoring, it was easy for her to see when these pressures went up or down. Most nurses who work in neuroscience units can identify activities that cause increases and decreases in ICP. In this particular situation, physical contact such as touching the boy's arm or hand and focusing calm, caring concern toward him would bring down the ICP. One day, after focusing her attention on her son and bringing the pressure down, this mom became involved in writing a letter to a friend. When she looked up from the letter, she was amazed to see that although she was still maintaining physical contact with her son his ICP had gone back up. Redirecting her attention had also redirected the flow of energy.

During the same hospitalization, the mother and her husband observed that there was one particular critical care nurse who appeared to put forth a high degree of energy. When this nurse was in the room there was a sense that he "took up a lot of space," even though his physical size was not excessive. On the nights when this particular nurse worked, the parents noted that their son required Mannitol to bring down the ICP even if he had not required any intervention for elevated ICP for one or more days. The parents were then able to predict that when they saw that this nurse was on duty, even though he was very kind, compassionate, and competent, the ICP would go up and their son would require Mannitol.

To help develop self-awareness regarding one's own energy field and learn how others react to it, an individual may find it helpful to seek feedback from others and practice a variety of techniques for sensing and modulating it. Several exercises for centering and sensing personal energy fields are included in a mental health text by N. C. Frisch and L. E. Frisch (1998) and related tips and suggestions may be found in various texts on energy fields and healing modalities. The importance of focusing on energy fields when discussing Nursing practice in multicultural situations is that there is more to communication than the spoken word and nonverbal body language. Nurses can communicate a great deal to clients and colleagues when they do not speak the same language by being aware of and effectively utilizing their own energy fields. Likewise, they need to be aware of potential untoward effects from projecting uncaring, discounting, or demeaning attitudes towards others.

A particular challenge in a multicultural situation is that the nurse and client are both at risk for misunderstanding each other at some level, thus impeding the speed and likelihood that their energy will resonate well as their fields come together. Thus, nurses must take great care to be sensitive to their own as well as client variations in body language, verbal and emotional expression, cultural beliefs, attitudes, health practices, and need for privacy, control and affiliation. Some nurses are more insightful and intuitive. It is, therefore, of great value for nurses to do careful self-assessments on their own or in an educational setting. Discovery of one's own stereotypes and tendencies to discriminate against people of certain groups can enhance one's ability to provide culturally-competent and congruent care. Andrews and Boyle (2008) suggest that nurses do their own assessments before conducting them on others and provide a tool for this purpose in their text (Box 2-2, pp. 18-20).

Communication and Assessment

Becoming competent in cross cultural communication is also essential for compassionate, respectful clinical care and begins with the authentic desire to understand another's way of seeing the world and acting within it (Nance, 1995, p. 255). It includes the ability to express respect and caring through both verbal and nonverbal interactions, as well as to identify potential communication barriers, especially as related to culture.

There are some general guidelines to follow that may facilitate interactions between client and nurse if language is a problem and no interpreter is available. Many of these are adapted from Andrews and Boyle (2008). When greeting the client, it is wise to be polite and formal, using the complete or last name of the person. The nurse can point to himself or herself when stating his or her name. Handshakes, head nodding and smiles are helpful. It is really important to proceed calmly without seeming hurried, to speak in low, moderate tones using simple words and short, direct sentences, addressing one topic at a time.

Excessive wording, use of medical terms, acronyms, abbreviations, idioms and slang, and speaking loudly can create confusion for the client who is trying to understand and be understood. Nurses have a tendency to speak louder than may be necessary when people take time to decide how to respond. This often happens with older adults. Talking louder than needed could agitate the client who may perceive that the nurse is angry or demanding, and some people, (e.g., Navajo Indians), might consider it rude (Purnell, 2005). The use of pantomime and simple actions can help clarify the meaning of instructions. It is important to determine the reading ability of the client and to validate client understanding by having him or her repeat instructions, act out their meaning or demonstrate a procedure. Obviously, if printed information is given to the client, it would ideally be at the appropriate reading level and in the client's primary language.

For any given client or client group, nurses need to understand accepted use and meaning of direct eye-contact, spatial proximity, touch, silence, tone of voice, posture, facial expressions and gestures. They can use open-ended questions to elicit culturally-specific information (Jackson, 1993) essential to establishing a relationship and forming an accurate picture of the client situation as well as identifying major support and contact persons and how to reach them. It is also important for nurses to consider the seating arrangement and meeting space in which an assessment interview might be carried out. Clients of some cultures, for example Middle Eastern and Latin American, may want to be very close to the nurse, while others might want to keep a greater distance (Andrews & Boyle, 2008).

To make culturally-relevant assessments, nurses not only need to consider the cultural and ethnic affiliation of their clients, but also have some knowledge and understanding of their sense of timing, health beliefs, sense of modesty and privacy needs, as well as communication styles. In discussing a clinic visit of a Jamaican woman with a persistent cough and fever of several weeks duration, Brennan (1999) observes that one might want to move fairly quickly to the physical assessment; however, she notes that before doing so, an appropriate period of time should be spent expressing caring concern and establishing rapport. The occurrence of illness is anxiety-producing for most Jamaicans and as such, is frequently discussed and generally treated with folk remedies before help is sought from western healthcare practitioners. Jamaicans view the psychosocial or spiritual aspects of an illness as more important than the biological, and expect the practitioner to carefully address these areas before assessing various body systems.

Additionally, nurses must determine client needs and preferences regarding the presence of a family member, interpreter or translator. Further, it is important to find out if the client can read and sign consent forms and understand the implications of any procedures to be done.

Despite the U.S. legal requirement to obtain informed consent, it is contrary to Hmong tradition for individuals to make decisions for themselves. The Hmong culture requires the male head of the family, or clan, to make decisions for all family members. Understanding and respecting this world-view, can help the nurse establish a trusting relationship and instill a sense of perceived control with the client and family. Purnell (2005) observes that the Hmong have very little experience with and understanding of western medical practices and surgical procedures. Furthermore, most of them are unable to read in their own language, unwritten until the 1950s, much less in English. Thus, they have little trust in the healthcare system, and often feel as if they are being experimented on, especially if students care for them.

One of the authors had an experience with some Native American women who were unable to sign consent forms, even if they could read, because of their cultural norms. Most American Indian tribes are matrilineal, and family decisions are made by the appropriate female elder. Healthcare providers can address older clients as Grandmother or Grandfather to show respect (Purnell, 2005). In Mexican families, regardless of who makes the decisions, the husband or father is expected to be the spokesperson.

Part of creating a nurturing space for clients involves understanding what it will take for them to feel enough trust, respect and safety to be able to explain their problems or concerns. Perceiving they have some control during the initial encounter with the nurse, can go a long way in their being able to tell their story. Thus, it is essential for nurses to determine, as soon as possible, what the client understands and expects regarding direct eye-contact. Native American and Asian clients, for example, might consider direct eye-contact aggressive or impolite and avoid looking directly at the nurse. Further, Native Americans might maintain a downcast stare to indicate they are listening. Hispanic clients might turn their eyes downward to indicate respect for authority, age, economic status or other reasons, although they do expect direct eye-contact from their nurse (Andrews & Boyle, 2008).

Other issues of importance in creating and maintaining a nurturing space include learning about the client's understanding of silence, touch and space proximity. Nurses are usually encouraged to allow periods of silence to provide time for clients to think about their response. In some cultures, silence is an indicator of respect, whereas people from France, Spain and Russia might consider silence a sign of agreement. Some African Americans use silence in response to a question they consider inappropriate.

Many people have concerns about the appropriateness of various kinds of touch, particularly between males and females, perhaps more in some cultures, than others. With Arabs and Hispanics, for example, concerted effort must be made to ensure same-gender healthcare providers for clients. There are also some taboos regarding touch and examination of infants from different cultures, so it is advisable to ask the mother's permission and/or ask her to hold the child in her lap.

Some people have beliefs about illnesses or specific symptoms that may be unique to their culture, i.e., are culture-bound. *Pujos,* or grunting, for example, is perceived by Hispanics as an illness in which a baby exhibits grunting and a protruding umbilicus. These families attribute this condition to the baby being touched by a menstruating woman, or even the mother, if her menses returned less than two months post partum.

Another example related to touch in infants and children is *mal ojo*, or evil eye, which is common in many parts of the world. Evil eye is thought to be caused by someone looking at an infant or child without touching it, usually for a benign reason, but in some cases, the family might think there was intent to inflict harm. A nurse observing a child without touching it could be blamed for causing an illness that occurred soon afterwards. Evil eye can be prevented by just touching the infant while looking at him and perhaps remarking to the mother how cute or beautiful her baby is. The importance of this behavior should not be underestimated. If the infant becomes dehydrated from fever, nausea, and vomiting, the family might attribute the symptoms to evil eye. Careful teaching is required, especially as the family may not understand the importance of close monitoring and the need for fluid and electrolyte replacement, preferring instead to consult a traditional healer; for example, a *curandera* (female) or *curandero* (male) in Mexico, *a hilot* in the Phillipines (Andrews & Boyle, 2008; Purnell, 2005).

Sometimes, the family will accept something from both western and traditional systems, as well as whatever the grandmother suggests. A Filipino family, for example, may want traditional healing with herbs and massage, religious healing involving prayers or exorcism, and visits to shrines or to make sacrifices to appease spirits (Purnell, 2005). Knowing about these culture-bound afflictions and health practices helps the nurse model the client's world, to accept the situation as it is, i.e., the perceived cause and need for the *traditional healer,* and to determine with the client healthy ways to manage the illness (Role-Modeling). Establishing trust and instilling a sense of perceived control can help the client accept what the healthcare practitioner recommends.

There are numerous culture-bound syndromes and the intent here is not to discuss them in depth, but to bring awareness of them to the interview and assessment process. It is very important for nurses to be culturally sensitive and open to possibilities, so that clients sense caring intent and a safe, nurturing space, or field, in which to share information. Further, understanding the client's perception of the illness is important in order to avoid misdiagnosis and facilitate the client's getting well. One of the tenets of MRM theory is that people know at some level what caused their problem and what they need to resolve it. Thus, if the nurse understands that perspective, he or she will also seek to help the client obtain what is needed. Additionally, knowledge of how clients relate to the concept of time is important, because they may have a more relaxed notion of it than westerners do, showing up for appointments several hours earlier or later than scheduled.

Some healthcare facilities have a checklist, or section of an assessment tool, that facilitates gathering specific, culturally-based information from a client or family spokesperson on admission. Such data might include immigration status, spoken language, degree of acculturation and economic situation, among other things. However, even with a readily accessible questionnaire, it might be difficult to obtain much detailed information from a client admitted in any significant amount of pain or with difficulty breathing, seeing or hearing. Therefore, the interviewer might need to get the initial information from someone besides the client and elicit more data later. If a thorough assessment guide is desired, Andrews and Boyle (2008) provide one for individuals and families that addresses a variety of areas, including communication, cultural variations of disease incidence, nutrition, social networks, developmental considerations and health-related practices and beliefs (pp. 453-457). Another useful, but less comprehensive, questionnaire is provided by Luckmann (1999, pp. 195-197).

Using an interpreter

If there is an obvious language barrier, it is important to seek out an appropriate interpreter as soon as possible in order to begin relationship development and obtain basic admitting data. Many facilities have approved interpreters listed on the clinical units, available by phone or for on-site interpreting. Whether the client speaks little or no English, or can speak some English under normal situations, but has difficulty when experiencing anxiety and stress in a new environment or discussing sensitive issues, an interpreter familiar with the client's primary language should be requested. A trained medical interpreter has knowledge of health care, patient rights, and interpreting techniques, as well as cultural beliefs and practices. Thus, they may be able to offer advice regarding the appropriateness of any recommendations made (Andrews & Boyle, 2008). The situation can be challenging, however, with or without an interpreter.

Using an interpreter requires more time than when working with clients who speak the same language as the nurse. Thus, prioritizing what information is most important to obtain and what procedures must be accomplished right away is fairly critical to avoid fatigue in any of the participants. It is important to address the patient rather than the interpreter, maintaining eye-contact, as appropriate, for the patient. The nurse should use simple language and both nurse and client should speak no more than one or two sentences before allowing the interpreter to translate. It is helpful to let the client speak in his or her own language and then have the interpreter summarize what was said. It is important to watch for nonverbal cues from the client although Nailon (2006) noted that a skilled interpreter will write these down and give them to the nurse. Speaking privately with the interpreter may provide opportunity to learn about and clarify subtle emotional and cultural nuances. In this way, the interpreter can serve as a cultural broker to interpret not only language, but also culture.

In a phenomenological study of fifteen nurses and their use of interpreters caring for Latino patients in the emergency room, Nailon (2006) found that availability of interpreters, the ability of nurses to work with them, their engagement with their patients, and their accuracy in their interpretations either enhanced or hindered effective care. Nurses tended to spend less time with non-English-speaking Latino patients, taking shortcuts during assessments and relying too much on vital signs and observations rather than firsthand information from the patient. The study also showed that when interpreters were available, nurses were more apt to use them for discharge teaching than for assessments or when providing care.

It can be concluded from Nailon's (2006) study and others that education for both nurses and interpreters is important preparation for working together effectively to provide culturally-appropriate communication that is meaningful and accurate. To implement special programs for this purpose in healthcare facilities, however, there must be adequate funding and administrative support. Nurses may need assistance to learn how to develop grant proposals for funding and the appropriate sources to submit them to. In addressing the importance of such a program, it will be helpful to cite national guidelines, standards and evidence-based practice recommendations, such as those Nailon (2006) listed. The first set of standards in this country concerning professional medical interpreters was developed by the National Council on Interpreting in Health Care (2005). This document addresses issues such as accuracy, confidentiality, bias, role boundaries, respect, and advocacy. More recent efforts have focused on developing standards for a national certification process to ensure competency of healthcare interpreters as well as to increase health care access and quality for clients with limited English proficiency.

Reflective Practice

Nurses must recognize and acknowledge their own ethnocentric assumptions and biases that might interfere with accurate perception of client attitudes and behaviors. They also need to be sensitive to issues of cultural repression, oppression and dominance that stimulate feelings of fear and mistrust, effectively silencing a client and potentially interfering with appropriate care decisions, leading to unsafe behaviors or treatments. Berggren, Bergstrom and Edberg (2006) found in their study of twenty-two African women in Sweden that nurses, midwives and physicians were unsure how to deal with them in labor and delivery and in making family-planning decisions because they had been circumcised. The women felt that staff just stared at them, speaking among each other without involving them or listening to their suggestions, even in the presence of interpreters. Because of this, many of the women did not come to the prenatal clinic until late in their pregnancy, creating potential high-risk situations.

Even when a client comes to the clinic in a timely way, he or she may not be able to reveal the real reason for seeking health care. An example of this occurred between Steve, a nurse practitioner, and a client, Tillie during her first visit to the clinic. As Steve was talking with Tillie during the intake interview on an exceptionally busy day, she started becoming increasingly anxious because his large frame and abrupt, hurried manner of questioning brought up old feelings she had of being pushed around and "treated as dirt" by a former boss. Although she really wanted to get some treatment for an itchy rash, Tillie was unable to tell him what she needed and made up an excuse to leave the clinic without treatment.

Perhaps nothing Steve could have done would have changed the outcome, because Tillie might not have been comfortable sharing intimate information with a male nurse. Or, maybe because Tillie, an African-American who had worked under very bad conditions for several years in a chicken factory, was afraid that Steve, a white southerner, might berate her for behavior he would presume caused the rash. Most likely though, had Steve taken a moment initially to center and calm himself, re-balancing his energy with intention and focus, the entire interaction might have taken on a different energy, resulting in a more positive outcome. With focused intent, he could have set the stress of the busy clinic day aside for the moment, in order to be fully present with Tillie. She might then have felt calmer and more able to trust him with her personal information, even if that did include her preference for a female nurse or invoked racist fears. Without hearing the client's view of the situation, the nurse will never know for sure. Yet, thoughtful reflection could lead to alternative approaches attempted in future interactions. Since the interaction was not successful, it is valuable to consider other approaches that could have been taken.

Sometimes there is no option for another interviewer, so it becomes even more important to spend the time needed to establish a caring, trusting relationship, especially in a multicultural situation. We talk about the importance of the nurse accepting a client unconditionally, regardless of the circumstances. There is, however, no obligation on the part of the client to accept the nurse unconditionally. One of the authors of this chapter remembers all too well a situation that occurred many years ago in a southern university hospital, when an indignant female patient ended up leaving the unit before completing the admission process, after learning she would be cared for by a nurse of a different race than she was. Even though she raised a ruckus and demanded a different nurse, she was told the hospital policy and that she would have to accept the available staff. She refused and left as quickly as she could.

Fortunately, much progress has been made since that event occurred and the U.S. population has become far more diverse with greater acceptance and understanding of others with different backgrounds, beliefs and practices. Community, federal, and educational institutions have made great strides in recognizing and accommodating people with diverse needs. Cultural competence is a well-recognized standard of care for Nursing practice and healthcare agencies and has been addressed by a number of accrediting and credentialing organizations for some years now. Despite this progress, the problem of health disparities and access to care still exists and in some situations is increasing. Prejudice, racism, stereotyping, ethnocentrism and discrimination remain to some degree in all healthcare settings (Andrews & Boyle, 2008). Thoughtful reflection following any multicultural situation, whether undertaken as an individual or within a supportive, non-judgmental small group setting, is helpful in promoting and providing cultural competent care in future situations.

MAJOR MRM CONCEPTS AS THEY RELATE TO CULTURAL DIVERSITY

The Aims of Intervention

The Aims of Intervention as identified in the theory of Modeling and Role-Modeling (Erickson, H. 2006; Erickson, et al., 1983/2009) remain appropriate and applicable in any culture.

Establish Trust

The first, and perhaps most important, of the Aims of Intervention using Modeling and Role-Modeling Nursing theory is to build trust–a prerequisite to establishing rapport and health-promoting interactions with any client, regardless of ethnicity, culture, geographical location, or clinical setting. To build trust, nurses must take great care to observe their own body language as well as that of a client, using attentive listening postures and mirroring those of the client when appropriate. Visual observations of the client and the client's facial expressions and body postures are especially important when languages differ. It is also important for nurses to take plenty of time, to permit periods of silence (if culturally appropriate) and ask open-ended questions. The use of reflection, paraphrasing, validation and other therapeutic techniques of purposeful conversation will show caring intent.

Being empathetic and caring requires nurses to maintain a perspective of cultural relativism; i.e., to understand client behaviors within the context of the client's culture (Outlaw, 1994). If nurses keep their own feelings in abeyance and refrain from comments such as "I know what you mean" or "I know how you feel" they can avoid closing off further exploration of feelings and discussion of alternate possibilities as well as prevent explosive outbursts of pent up frustration and anger or fear. Retaining the stance of unknowing is, therefore, essential in getting to know the client and the meaning a situation has for that person. A social worker stated that when she worked as a counselor in a multicultural mental health center in Alaska, she always kept "a beginner's mind" and asked clients to tell their stories as a way of beginning to uncover what was going on and what it meant to them.

Promote Positive Orientation

Promoting hope for the future as well as promoting an individual's self-worth is important to include when role-modeling and intervening with any client. Reframing can help change the perception of a situation from hopeless to hopeful or from a threat to a challenge. Attention must be given to customs and beliefs when including reframing in culturally-sensitive care. For example, wailing is a customary demonstration of grief in many cultures. Attempting to reframe when an individual is demonstrating grief may be offensive to the individual and be interpreted as the nurse being disrespectful of the grieved person or situation. Reframing would be appropriate at another time. It is also important for the nurse to remember that in many cultures and religions, death is perceived as hope and a new beginning and not as an end or as hopelessness.

Promote Perceived Control

It is important for individuals to perceive that they have some control over their lives. Regardless of the cultural background of the individual, it is not enough that the nurse believes that each individual has control, but that the individual perceives that they have control. Control over one's own life may be direct or indirect as viewed by the nurse. In other words, an individual patient may perceive control by granting decision-making to another based on custom or belief. If client control is gained by delegation or deferring to another such as a spouse, parent, or elder, the nurse needs to include that person at such times when there will be teaching, gaining informed consent, and discharge planning, for example.

Supporting the individual's sense of being able to act autonomously promotes a sense of control and confidence in one's ability to provide self-care. This perception has been identified by Hertz (1997) as Perceived Enactment of Autonomy (PEA). Many nurses believe that self-care requires independent activity. However, choosing to rely on others also is a form of self-care and is especially pertinent in cultures that value decision-making by designated family members, for example, the eldest male or female. Promoting self-care actions that are congruent with an individual's cultural values can strengthen his or her perception of control. In fact, research studies with older adults from Taiwan (Hwang, Lin, Tung, & Hu, 2006), Japan (Matsui & Capezuti, 2008), and Germany (Personal communication, I. Wulff, December 8, 2008) validated the concept of PEA. Furthermore, social support was found to be a significant predictor of PEA in Taiwanese and Japanese individuals.

Affirm and Promote Strengths

In the face of illness or any stress, an individual may not be able to identify or mobilize his or her strengths or self-care resources. It is not uncommon, during illness, for a person to focus on perceived personal weaknesses or failures. Assisting the client to identify strengths and then promoting mobilization of those strengths as resources will aid in recovery and reestablishing equilibrium. Examples of cultural differences in self-care resources and personal strengths are presented throughout this chapter.

Set Mutual Goals that are Health-Directed

The ability to set mutual goals that are health-directed is the epitome of culturally competent care. Setting mutual goals implies that the nurse is focusing on the individual's innate drive to be as healthy as he or she can be. If goals are not mutual and the nurse's goals are different from the client's, the nurse has most likely not fully modeled the client's world or has not used that model in role-modeling. Inadequate data gathering or a lack of knowledge for analysis and interpretation of collected data can lead to goal-setting patterned after the nurse's model of the world rather than the client's. Caution must be taken when setting goals to include all subsystems that make up the holistic person and not limit the focus to only one subsystem such as the biophysical.

Self-Care

In any culture, individuals can often describe what they perceive to be their health problem, what caused it and what they perceive will make it better, worse, or have no effect. People also strive to be the best they can be, which includes maintaining the best personal health possible within their situation and resources. There are three aspects to self-care in the Modeling and Role-Modeling theory: Self-care Knowledge, Self-care Resources, and Self-care Action.

Self-Care Knowledge

The nurse always acknowledges the uniqueness and individuality of the client and appreciates that individuals, at some level, know what makes them ill and what will make them well. In an analysis of case studies reported by Erickson (1990), the following four themes found, that relate to the nature of self-care knowledge are shown in Table 11.1

Table 11.1 Themes found in Self-care Knowledge study

1. An individual's perception of factors associated with his or her personal health problems are rarely obvious to the healthcare provider.
2. The individual's perception of what is needed to help him or her can best be defined by that person.
3. One nursing role is to facilitate clients to articulate what *they* perceive to be associated with their problem and what can be done to help them feel better.
4. Another nursing role is to assist the clients to resolve their problems in ways that meet personal needs and are health- and growth-directed (p. 186).

These four themes are important for the nurse to remember when involved in providing culturally-competent care. Beliefs are often perceived to be far more credible than any "scientific fact" that the nurse or other healthcare provider can suggest. While doing family follow up through a genetics clinic in the late 1970s, one of the authors remembers visiting a family in north Georgia when trying to trace an autosomal dominant trait of a client seen in the clinic. The clinic client had two fingers fused together and family members denied any instances of syndactylism anywhere else in the family. After further discussion, one family member remembered an uncle who had a "gloved" hand where all of his fingers were fused together. The family also all agreed that the uncle's situation had no bearing on the current client since his gloved hand was quickly explained as having occurred because his mother was frightened by a large turtle during her pregnancy. Providing culturally-sensitive care includes that it is not always necessary to try to dispel a held belief with a "scientific fact." Self-care Knowledge is in the language and belief system of the client. Although the nurse might translate the data into medical language for the purpose of recording information, the client's language should also be recorded so that healthcare providers can talk with the client in his or her own language.

Self-Care Resources

All individuals have internal and external resources (strengths and support) that are important for their health and healing. The nurse assists individuals in recognizing and obtaining resources (internal and external). It is important for the nurse to assess internal resources which are characteristics resulting from appropriate need satisfaction and positive resolution of developmental tasks. External self-care resources can include perceptions, social support, types of resources used when ill and well, and transitional objects. The perception of adequate resources is itself a resource (Hertz & Baas, 2006). For many individuals a "non-Western medicine" healer is an important self-care resource. Supporting the involvement of the healer in care when there is no direct conflict in approach may well enhance the client's healing and general health. The use of objects seen as transitional objects or resources for self-care can often be accommodated when providing culturally-competent care. Encouraging the use of special blankets or clothing, providing a place for a special photograph, being respectful of religious objects are all ways of helping individuals recognize and obtain self-care resources.

Self-Care Actions

The nurse facilitates the individual's use of self-care resources. Several decades ago, a member of a large nomadic-type of family was hospitalized. It was important to the patient and the family that the entire family be present at the bedside and that they burn candles in the room. After a great deal of information was shared between the family and the nurse, the patient was moved to a larger room to accommodate the large number of family members (half of the members at a time). They agreed to use "flameless" battery-operated candles around the room since there was too great a fire hazard with live flame. Culturally-competent care may involve negotiation, but the culturally-sensitive nurse can often accommodate self-care resources such as objects, pictures, or people without major disruption to "standard practice." Facilitating the mobilization and use of self-care resources based on self-care knowledge can significantly impact the health and well-being of an individual and promote his or her sense of autonomy and control.

Affiliated-Individuation

The Modeling and Role-Modeling concept of affiliated-individuation describes the interactive process of connecting to another while retaining a sense of individuality. Affiliation and individuation are both inherent human needs; however, there are individual as well as cultural differences in the values attached to affiliation and individuation. In other words, in some cultures, there is greater value for individuals to be more affiliated, and in others, to be in balance is to be more individuated. Over time, as the nurse is able to satisfy some of the expectations and needs of the client, a sense of attachment can occur that helps the client to develop, regain and/or strengthen resources and health-promoting behaviors. The nurse must remain aware of his or her own needs for affiliation and individuation and avoid fostering mutual dependence while encouraging appropriate independence on the part of the client. If this does not happen and the client's needs continue unmet, the likelihood for continuing health problems and unhealthy, unsafe or risky behaviors is great.

Adaptive Potential

Stressors are unique for each individual, and circumstances that are not considered stressful in one culture may be considered stressful in another. Behavior indicating equilibrium, arousal, and impoverishment may also vary from one culture to another. Mourning behaviors in one culture may indicate equilibrium, while the same behaviors in another culture may indicate arousal or even impoverishment.

Facilitation

In the theory of Modeling and Role-Modeling, the nurse is seen as a facilitator and not as an effector. The nurse aids the individual to identify, mobilize, and develop his or her own strengths. There are occasions when the nurse must intervene by providing direct and total care for another individual, but even then, the nurse is aiding the patient to identify, mobilize and develop his or her own strengths.

Nurturance

In its literal sense, nurturance is to feed and encourage growth. So it is as a characteristic of the nurse. Nurturance also conveys the idea of warmth and affection. When considering nurturance in a culturally-sensitive way, the nurse must remain mindful of the differences in the appropriateness of demonstrations of care and affection. The use of touch and the amount of personal space required by individuals will differ among various cultures as well as between individuals of different genders, ages, or position. In many cultures, there is an overriding need to save face. It is helpful for the nurse to incorporate "saving face" for the client no matter what the cultural situation is since self-worth is important "food" for the growth of any individual. Facilitating physical, psychological, emotional and spiritual growth of another holistic individual involves an interactive interpersonal relationship.

Unconditional Acceptance

Cultural barriers can silence the voices of minority, disenfranchised and marginalized persons and inhibit their ability to assume control of their lives, including health care. This is why it is so essential that nurses clearly demonstrate unconditional acceptance of their clients. Many people of diverse cultural and religious backgrounds do not feel comfortable revealing their traditional beliefs and healthcare practices to nurses and other care providers, at least until a reasonably secure level of trust has been established. Even then, it is only by suspending judgment and remaining open to possibilities that nurses will be apt to uncover what a client may have been reluctant to share.

Nurse Manager Considerations

Just as clients may have their prejudices and racial biases, many staff members bring their negative cultural baggage to work and may find themselves yielding to peer pressure to reject others whose behavior, language or color are different from theirs (Andrews & Boyle, 2008). The desire to be affiliated with others as insiders, not outsiders, is very strong and can influence the behavior of nurses who haven't worked through their own issues well enough to avoid joining in to be part of the group. Standing up for what is right and advocating for others takes inner strength and determination as well as the ability to deal with conflict. That is why nurses need to do their personal-growth work, know their values and beliefs, learn what triggers they have and how to avoid or deal with them. This is especially true for the nurse manager who must be acutely aware of his or her own issues to avoid getting caught up in a brewing storm without realizing it.

Healthcare providers often use their own cultural frameworks to establish their norms and may view people of culturally diverse backgrounds as problematic. To better address the problems of language and other cultural needs of people from diverse backgrounds as well as those that experience unequal access to care, the Health and Human Services Office of Minority Health (2000) established standards for culturally and linguistically appropriate services. However, even with standards of care and increased education and experience with culturally diverse populations, nurses and other health care workers may have to cope with negative attitudes and behaviors where they work. This is where the importance of what nurses, and especially those in leadership positions as unit managers and supervisors, value and believe about relationships with others becomes critical.

Many people were raised in families with longstanding feelings of distrust, prejudice and bigotry toward one group or another for various reasons. Without experiences to change these attitudes and perceptions, nurse managers may find their employees making derogatory remarks such as racial, ethnic, age or gender-based slurs, showing favoritism, or depicting outright hostile behaviors, including violence. Sometimes a person may unintentionally make an offending remark not realizing the biases reflected in terms commonly heard in childhood. Another person, hearing the comment, may not realize the naïveté on the part of the speaker and take offense. To address these problems, the nurse manager might want to develop a plan to change the unit dynamics. Since the underlying attitudes and perceptions can run so deep that some staff might not even be aware of them, changing them will take time, strong commitment, and a willingness to deal with conflict.

Additionally, the common use of idioms, slang and proverbs not generally understood across cultures, can lead to misunderstandings at times when rapid communication is critical, possibly even compromising patient safety. Furthermore, cultural differences in role expectations, family obligations, and religious observances can create scheduling conflicts, absenteeism and unexpected requests for time off. How various cultural groups deal with conflicts such as these can create difficult interpersonal situations on a unit. Many Americans believe it is important to be assertive, even aggressive, and confront differences head on. However, many Asian and Native Americans emphasize harmony and avoidance of direct conflict. Nurses from China and Japan, for example, might use covert means, such as finding another staff person to mention a problem to, rather than go to their supervisor directly, so as to not be seen as aggressive and uncooperative.

Organizational Change

Although organizational change is generally most effective when all levels of management are involved, some approaches may involve individual assessments and a variety of educational media. Other approaches may incorporate group process, education, team-building and problem-solving. Andrews and Boyle (2008) suggest that no matter the approach used, staff will be more motivated to incorporate what they learn if they are rewarded for their efforts. Furthermore, they assert that a top down mandate for staff to embrace cultural diversity is rarely effective.

Communication is key throughout the process, regardless of approach. Ideally, individuals and groups will be willing to explore their values and how they influence their own behaviors. "Values underlie perceived needs, what is defined as a problem, how conflict is resolved, and expectations of behavior" (Andrews & Boyle, 2008, p. 307). When individual and organizational behaviors conflict misunderstandings and problems among staff members are to be expected. The nurse manager can view these conflicts as difficulties or as opportunities to enhance communication and promote cross-cultural understanding among staff from diverse backgrounds.

Using Modeling and Role-Modeling, the nurse manager would apply the same Principles of Nursing and associated Aims of Intervention (Brekke & Schultz, 2006, p. 63) to work with staff members as with any client, whether in a group or individual diversity awareness program. Getting individual members "on board" may present challenges for the nurse manager, and it might take some time to build enough trust and buy in from staff to commit to the process and assist in setting goals that are mutually compatible with the system as a whole. In addition, it is important to apply principles of change theory and leadership to ensure staff members at all levels are involved. The nurse manager can get as creative as desired within budget constraints to utilize appropriate media, facilitators, mediators, team building exercises, multicultural projects, etc. The more the staff feel included, heard and valued as contributing team members, the more likely successful outcomes will be achieved.

Throughout the process, the nurse manager needs to demonstrate unconditional acceptance of staff members, facilitate their process and nurture their efforts and growth toward the agreed upon system goals. "Saving face" is important in many cultures and is congruent with several of the Aims of Intervention identified in the MRM theory. Finding ways to promote the self-worth of staff members and helping them feel a sense of control in this process may be particularly challenging in cases where members may have been instigating or contributing to dysfunction on the unit. It will be well worth the effort involved, however, so that members feel safe in revealing their issues and being open to hear what others have to say. Affirming member strengths individually and as group members is important to their feelings of self-worth, satisfaction and contribution to overall goal achievement.

ISSUES FOR NURSE EDUCATORS IN A CULTURALLY-DIVERSE SOCIETY

Traditionally, when a faculty member is responsible for teaching "cultural issues" in an undergraduate Nursing program, the content consists of comparing generally accepted practices, customs, beliefs, foods, religion, etc., of the federally defined population categories of white, black, Hispanic, Asian/Pacific Islander, and American Indian/Alaska Native. There is also some time spent on comparing religious practices of the major religions of Catholic, select Protestant groups, Jewish, and perhaps, Buddhist and Islam, especially as the practices are related to health care. The information and empirical knowing is valuable and increases the students' general awareness and knowledge about practices that are different from their own with the intent that they gain some understanding of the uniqueness of various groups.

The empirical knowledge imparted through lectures comparing ethnic groups or religions is "shared knowledge" as explained in Chapter 3. This is knowledge common to all professional groups that provide care and is not "unique-to-nursing" knowledge. According to Capers (1992), "The manner in which cultural diversity is handled within any given curriculum depends on the values and beliefs in the nursing philosophy and conceptual or organizing framework" (p. 21). The theory of Modeling and Role-Modeling views individuals as holistic and believes that "nursing is a process between the nurse and client and requires an interpersonal and interactive nurse-client relationship" (Erickson, et al., 1983/2009, p. 43). An "interpersonal" and "interactive" relationship between two "holistic" individuals necessitates an appreciation that both individuals in the relationship have unique cultural components. The nurse, in the professional nurse-client relationship needs to be aware of his or her own cultural influences on beliefs, language, values, moral principles, health care practices, help-seeking practices, and affiliations as well as the cultural influences on the client's beliefs, values, health care practices, and help-seeking behaviors.

The nurse needs an understanding of the common beliefs and practices of specific ethnic and religious groups, but more importantly, needs to know the unique implication of ethnicity or religion to an individual client. A client may indicate a religious preference during an intake interview, but that statement of preference gives no indication of the extent to which that religion plays a part in the individual's life. Teaching Nursing students, at any level, to model the worlds of their clients implicitly teaches nurses to always consider the client's unique culture.

Faculty Preparation

The specific practice of every nurse is greatly influenced by his or her personal beliefs, philosophy and view of the world. It is important that Nursing faculty are clear about their own beliefs and how they influence their interactions with clients and students, so that they can enlighten students about the relationships between personal philosophy and Nursing practice. Faculty members need to recognize their own biases, preconceptions and assumptions about cultural issues and gain awareness of their reactions to people from cultural settings different from their own. In addition to being aware of their own beliefs and philosophy, teachers need to be aware of the culture of their student population. They also need to be aware of what they know and don't know about them as individuals and as a group. They also need to accept that they may never be able to identify all that they don't know.

The Expanded Ways-of-Knowing Matrix (Table 3.3. p. 67) in Chapter 3, shows the progression or hierarchy of ways-of-knowing, and indicates the stages that faculty use in learning about their students, just as their students will use to learn about their clients. The Matrix demonstrates that the pattern of "unknowing" (Munhall, 1993) is an important aspect of interacting with any student population after faculty members acknowledge their own personal beliefs and philosophy, reflect on how those influence personal practice, and accept that the learners will be the best source of information about their own world views. Munhall writes that "…'unknowing is a condition of openness and, 'Knowing', in contrast, leads to a form of confidence that has inherent in it, a state of closure" (p.125).

The student populations of today, whether undergraduate, graduate, agency in-service, workshop, or continuing education, tend to be culturally diverse. When teaching about cultural diversity to a group, shared knowledge about various ethnic groups, cultures and religions is important to include because, as already indicated, it helps nurses understand the parameters of behaviors and practices within cultural groups under usual circumstances. Some knowledge of intercultural communication, both verbal and nonverbal is useful prior to interacting with clients from diverse cultures. This common, shared knowledge is important to Nursing, but is *not* nursing science. Nursing science comes from knowledge gained from an "unknowing" attitude. Teaching about cultural differences is to teach students and practicing nurses to begin the nurse-client interaction with an acceptance that they don't know the subjective world of the client.

Although the student may be aware of the generally accepted knowledge about a specific cultural group, she doesn't know what meaning any specific aspect of the culture has for any one individual in that culture. This holds true even for individuals sharing the same cultural situations. For instance, a client may indicate a religious preference that is the same as the religious preference of the nurse. The nurse will still approach the client with an "unknowing" attitude, since it is not known what meaning the religion or the practices have for the client or if they are the same as the nurse's.

Students' Life Experiences

Life experiences and exposure to cultures different from one's own influence cultural competency in Nursing practice. Life experience is not necessarily related to age, in that many students in North America now spend part of their high school education outside of their primary culture. They may partake of educational exchange programs, religious mission work, or international sports competitions. A 19 year-old student may have more exposure to diverse cultures than an older student who has lived his or her whole life in a fairly homogeneous community.

The Nursing Code of Ethics (ANA 2001, p. 5), states that nurses "practice with compassion and respect for the inherent dignity, worth, and uniqueness of every individual…" (p. 4). Even students who are young in age and those who have had little life experience and exposure to different cultural situations accept the philosophy of accepting "the uniqueness of every individual." With limited exposure, however, students may encounter situations they never expected or thought about and have no pre-existing personal context in which to place the experience. An example of this can be seen in an experience of a young undergraduate Nursing student assigned to care for a young pregnant woman.

Through modeling the client's world, the student learned that the client had been artificially inseminated and that she and her partner were very excited about the prospect of becoming parents. Later in the day, when the client's partner visited, the student was startled, upon entering the client's room, to learn that her client and partner was a lesbian couple. The student had limited life experience and exposure to situations different from her own, but her personal distress was not that this couple was different from her own beliefs, but rather that her reaction was one of being startled rather than being accepting as she thought, and intellectually believed, she should be.

An important component of helping students appreciate the "uniqueness of every individual" is helping them understand their own uniqueness. Being startled because of a lack of personal context in which to place an experience is different from being startled because of preconceived bias or belief that a practice is inappropriate or taboo. Teaching students to approach the nurse-client interaction with an "unknowing" attitude and teaching them to model the client's world can help any student develop a context for the experience by gaining an understanding through the model of the client's world.

Teaching Students to Model the Client's World

Teaching students to model the world of their clients is to provide them with the best foundational skill for Nursing. To begin Nursing education by teaching skills such as bed-making, taking vital signs and giving bed baths puts the emphasis on the nurse and what the nurse *does*. Beginning education with modeling the client's world puts the emphasis on who the client *is* rather than on what the nurse *does*. Focusing on the client rather than the nurse is the basis of culturally-competent nursing. When we began teaching beginning undergraduate students about modeling the client's world before exposing them to their first nurse-client interaction, the results were incredible and exciting.

Post-conference discussions following the first-ever clinical experience of beginning students focused on who the clients were and what challenges they had. Historically, the post-conference following the first day in the clinical setting would focus on what each of the students saw (dressings, wounds, equipment, etc.), what they did (helped walk, feed, bathe, change a bed, etc.), and how awkward or uncomfortable or incompetent they might have felt in a new situation. With a short amount of instruction about understanding the client's world so that nursing practice can occur within the context of that world, the post-conference topics were about "how difficult it must be to be in the hospital when the client spoke and understood so little English"; and "how hard it must be to be ill, homeless, have a wife and child to provide for and worry about losing his job because of being ill"; and "my client told me that no one had ever listened to her before and she really appreciated being able to tell me how she felt."

When beginning students focus on modeling the client's world, they are focused on the client and feel confident in what they are doing. They demonstrate the intent to understand the client, and the client perceives the nonverbal behavior of really wanting to understand, just as they can clearly notice when the focus of a student (or nurse) is on themselves and what they are doing.

There is an entire chapter covering facilitation of the Modeling and Role-Modeling processes (Chapter 7). This section will briefly identify the introductory information that is helpful for facilitating beginning undergraduate students to model their client's world during their first nurse-client interaction adopting an "unknowing" attitude and assuming that all nurse-client situations are culturally diverse.

Communication Techniques and Building Trust

The most important concept to teach students about communication is verbal and nonverbal congruence. It is most helpful for students to gain the awareness that when verbal and non-verbal communication (behaviors) is incongruent, the listener or "receiver" will most often believe the non-verbal. This knowledge will best facilitate fostering *intent, client focus,* and an attitude of *unknowing* and true *concern* for the client. Focusing on the verbal techniques, although they are useful, important and more concrete, encourages students to focus on the use of the technique and thereby focus on themselves and what they are doing rather than focusing on their clients and who they are. Understanding the power of non-verbal communication and a genuine desire to understand the client within his or her world allows the students to engage in any multi-cultural situation, even if there is a language barrier.

With intent and true focus on the client, the student is open to learning a great deal about the client without needing to use a pre-printed list of assessment questions. One student in particular demonstrated this lesson very well when assigned to a hospitalized client who had a life-style and culture very different from the student's and very different from any other staff member in the agency. The student wanted to model the client's world, but was asking questions from his own cultural experience. The student was frustrated because the client gave one-word answers to his questions and didn't seem to have any trust in the student (or any other staff member for that matter).

After talking with the student about unconditional acceptance, intention, and truly wanting to develop a model of the client's world, the student said that he wanted to go back to talk with the client. The student's awareness was exceptional. He explained to his classmates that by asking the client questions such as, "What type of work do you do?" (He was jobless); "Where do you live?" (He was homeless) and referring to his "wife" (They were not married), the student was explaining to the client just how different their worlds were.

By answering in one-word answers, the student related that he finally realized that the client was "trying to model *MY* world instead of me modeling his." During his second interaction with the same client, the student used more open-ended questions, showed genuine interest in the client's world, his needs, and concerns. They developed a trusting relationship and a week later, when the client came back to the hospital for a clinic visit, he remembered that the student would be on the medical-surgical unit that day and came to find him. This was the student's second week as a student nurse and only the second day of engaging in any nurse-client relationships. The client wanted to discuss the treatment regimen the clinic prescribed for him and wanted to know what the student thought about the drugs that were prescribed. The client said that the student was the only healthcare worker he felt comfortable with!

Sympathy and Empathy

Helping students differentiate between these two concepts is also useful in facilitating modeling the client's world and becoming culturally competent. Attempting to understand how another person is experiencing a situation by thinking how that situation would be for you within your own cultural context is *sympathy*. Attempting to understand how another person is experiencing a situation by thinking how that situation is being perceived and met within that person's cultural context and model of the world is *empathy*. If a client relates that she is pregnant or that her mother has recently passed away, the student might consider either of those situations based on a previous personal situation, and utilizing a sympathetic response, indicate that they “know just how you feel.” Of course, what the Nursing student is really saying is “I know how I felt in a similar situation” and puts the focus on his or her own experience rather than the client’s.

If the student has no previous personal experience in these situations, he or she might think about what it would be like for them if they found themselves experiencing an unexpected pregnancy or sudden loss of a parent. A sympathetic response might sound something like “I can’t imagine what that would be like” or “I don’t know what I would do in that situation.” Again, the sympathetic response puts the focus on the student nurse and his or her world rather than the client and the client’s world. The professional empathetic response presents an open and unknowing attitude with the intent of understanding the situation from the cultural context and within the world of the client.

An empathetic response could be reflective such as “You’re pregnant?” or “You recently lost your mother?” putting the focus on the client and inviting her to explain the situation within her own cultural context. Differentiating sympathy and empathy is especially important for the younger student who often thinks that because they have such limited life experience, they have no idea what any healthcare situation would be like, and therefore, have nothing to offer. Of course, they may have an advantage because they have no personal experience to share and take the focus away from the client!

Unconditional Acceptance

According to the Modeling and Role-Modeling theory, “Being accepted as a unique, worthwhile, important individual–with no strings attached–is imperative if the individual is to be facilitated in developing his or her own potential” (Erickson, et al., 1983/2009, p. 49). Unconditional acceptance implies acceptance of the individual and his or her potential to grow and develop.

It does not imply that there is no room for growth, and it does not imply acceptance of all the person’s behaviors. Unconditional acceptance comes from the genuine belief that every individual proceeds through each day doing the very best he or she can do given their current ability to utilize internal and external resources. Although beginning students may not understand a specific cultural practice or may believe that some practices are not healthy, they can still be guided in accepting any individual with all of their potential, their needs, need assets and need deficits, their healthy and not-so-healthy developmental residuals, and their striving to be the best that they can be.

CULTURAL RELEVANCE OF THE MRM THEORY

So far in this chapter, we have identified important issues that should be focused on to ensure that culturally-sensitive and competent nursing care is provided to clients. The key concepts and propositions from MRM theory along with other literature served as the basis for this discussion. We also discussed application of MRM theory in management and education. In this section, we will discuss application of MRM theory to guide education, practice, and administration from a systems or "big picture" perspective. The focus will be on determining cultural congruence and relevance when MRM theory is to serve as the guiding framework for nursing practice throughout a healthcare system, in an educational program, or in any other setting where the theory is to be utilized.

Prior to implementing a particular theoretical perspective in a healthcare system or in an educational program, the first step is to determine if the theoretical perspective is culturally congruent. A conceptual model will be presented to guide the process of determining cultural relevance from a systems perspective. Based on our experiences as consultants to healthcare systems and educational programs within and outside the U. S., we believe that this model can be used by other consultants, educators, and administrators in their settings.

Overview of Conceptual Model for Application of MRM Theory

The story at the beginning of this chapter illustrates some of the issues to consider when planning to use a theory in a practice or educational setting that differs from the culture in which the theory originated or when planning to utilize a theory to guide nursing practice throughout a system or setting. Our purpose for consulting with the school in Taiwan was to teach nurse educators about MRM theory and its application in their educational setting. To accomplish this goal, we developed an approach based on MRM theory combined with some aspects of cultural theories (Leininger, 1991, 1996, 2007; Purnell, 2005). The process and approach that we originally developed and applied in Taiwan has been refined and is represented by the Framework for Cultural Relevance of Theory Utilization (Figure 11.1).

When applying MRM theory in a new setting or system, the theory's underlying values, assumptions, foundational theories, and propositions provide the backdrop for evaluating cultural congruence. In Figure 11.1, those aspects of the theory are incorporated within "Modeling and Role-Modeling Theory" and are placed in the background at the top of the-+ circle.

As illustrated in the figure, we modeled the worlds of our nurse educator clients from several perspectives. Key characteristics of the individuals who would be applying the theory needed to be identified. Those individuals are identified as the target population. In addition, key characteristics of the environment in which the theory would be applied were assessed and understood.

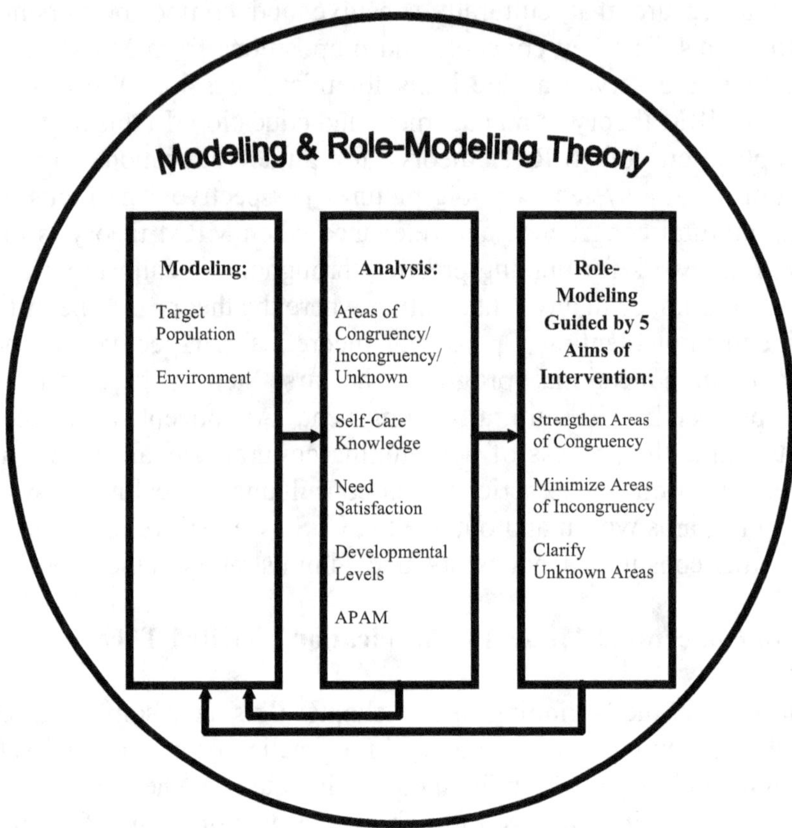

Figure 11.1 Framework for Cultural Relevance of Theory Utilization

Target Population Characteristics.

Specific target population characteristics that should be assessed include concepts integral to MRM theory such as self-care knowledge, need satisfaction, developmental levels, and adaptive potential. In addition, areas typically delineated in a cultural assessment should be assessed (Leininger, 1991, 1996, 2007; Purnell, 2005). These areas include beliefs and values regarding health, life and death as well as religious beliefs and values. Common family structures and roles, typical living arrangements and norms of behavior in everyday life must be considered. Language and communication patterns along with typical social networks must also be assessed. The importance placed on education and use of technology should be understood. Finally, information about typical health practices including beliefs about different types of health care and healers should be gathered.

The environment includes individuals receiving nursing care, norms and standards of nursing practice within the school and local clinical practice settings, along with the regulations guiding the scope and legal aspects of nursing practice. For individuals receiving nursing care, specific areas of assessment are similar to those assessed in the target population. The norms and standards of practice at the level of the setting are important to understand; they will determine the degree of acceptance of new nursing behaviors when the theory is implemented. Obviously, the regulatory aspects are important to understand because they, too, will determine if implementation of nursing practice guided by a specific theory would be legally acceptable.

After these areas are assessed, judgments can be made regarding the congruence between target population and environmental characteristics and theory characteristics. In essence, these judgments represent an aspect of modeling, gaining an understanding of the client's perspective and view of the world. Areas of congruence, incongruence, and uncertainty are identified and depicted in the model. Subsequently, the Aims of Intervention in MRM theory are used to guide role-modeling to provide interventions that will strengthen or build upon the areas of congruence, minimize areas of incongruence, and clarify unknown areas.

A Fluid Process

Although this model depicts the process of ensuring cultural relevance as progressing in a step-by-step manner, the actual process is more fluid. For example, it is not necessary to complete *a comprehensive* assessment of the target population and environmental characteristics in order to make initial judgments about cultural congruence and then to plan and implement interventions that will enhance areas of congruence, eliminate areas of incongruence, and clarify unclear areas. Furthermore, the target population's perceptions and views might be altered after role-modeled interventions are implemented. In other words, the target population and environment might respond and change in some way during the process of ensuring cultural relevance. Therefore, the person applying this model is simultaneously gaining deeper understanding of the target population and environment while analyzing, planning, and implementing role-modeled approaches that influence the target population and environment.

Applying the Model for Cultural Relevance in Theory Utilization

In this section, we will provide an example of how the model was applied during our consultation in Taiwan. Although the basic elements were actually applied during our experience, the model has been refined over the years.

The process of determining cultural relevance of MRM theory prior to using it in Taiwan began prior to our traveling to the country. First, we began modeling the world of the target population of nurse educators and their environment by learning as much as possible about the country and the values, beliefs, and behavioral norms of individuals residing in the country. We read numerous travel and scholarly publications and communicated with the individuals who would serve as our interpreters and translators. Since there were two of us consulting, we were fortunate to be able to share our own perceptions with each other and to cross-validate our baseline understanding about the country and the values, beliefs, and norms of the persons living there.

After arriving in Taiwan, we used all our senses to directly observe how values, beliefs and norms of behavior were actually carried out in the country. Because neither of us was fluent in Mandarin Chinese, the primary language spoken and written in Taiwan, it was important to rely on our senses to gather information. Discussing our individual observations with each other intermittently throughout each day, aided us in modeling the world of the target population of nurse educators and the environment at the school.

In the end, a major limitation for us was our lack of fluency in the language. We relied heavily on our interpreters for communications with faculty and students at the school. Although many individuals at the school spoke or understood some English, we were never quite certain if our messages were understood the way we intended or if the messages we received from faculty and students were what they intended.

This is one of the problems with using translators and interpreters. Also, we learned that often words in English could not be translated into Mandarin and words in Mandarin did not translate into English. Idioms and phrases that held common meaning in our native land, had no meaning in Taiwan. This became obvious when we were driving on a highway along the ocean at sunset with silver reflecting behind each cloud. One of us commented that "every cloud does have a silver lining," a phrase commonly used and usually understood in the U. S. This phrase had no meaning for our colleagues from Taiwan. An hour later, we were still trying to explain the phrase to those colleagues. Words just could not explain the meaning.

Nonetheless, over the year when we consulted at the school, we did gain a deeper understanding of the culture in which the theory would be applied and were, therefore, successful in modeling the world of the target population and environment. This understanding was partly due to our using multiple methods for data gathering and our validation process with each other. Despite the fact that it took a full year to feel like we gained an in-depth understanding, we began teaching MRM theory within the first two weeks of our arrival in Taiwan!

Faculty at the school seemed to be accustomed to large group meetings. Faculty meetings often included as many as 50 persons; both of us were accustomed to faculty meetings comprised of a maximum of 20 persons. We were also accustomed to sitting in meetings where each faculty member had their own desk or expansive space. In the faculty meetings we observed, faculty often sat around long tables and in close proximity to one another. Since this was the norm for faculty meetings, we taught the basic premises of MRM theory in that same type of setting.

We took turns leading these classes. That afforded us the opportunity to present materials while having the other person observe the responses to the teaching. This approach to teaching further enhanced our ability to model the world of our target population and the environment in which they taught.

We also observed that in faculty meetings as well as when faculty were teaching in the classroom, the usual instructional method was for the leader or teacher to talk or lecture to persons in the class. We adopted this approach, but experimented with active learning approaches such as role-playing or case analyses, too. We found that those approaches were successful when faculty participants told us they liked them or when they participated with smiles on their faces. At other times, we obviously were not successful since faculty appeared confused rather than actively engaged in the activity. We were not certain whether it was the activity or the content being taught that failed to engage the learners. Obviously, we were not always accurate in role-modeling interventions with this target population. In those instances, we returned to the process of modeling prior to the next teaching session.

It should be noted that we did not follow a checklist or use a formal tool for documenting the data we gathered in trying to understand the target population and environment. Instead, our approach was to determine what others wanted us to do; in other words, to learn what the problem was. Then, we asked what they wanted to learn as a way to identify their needs. This was followed by asking how they thought they would best learn the material; in other words, we tried to find out what they thought would meet their learning needs. Assessing these areas, informed us about the faculty's perceived situation, expectations, resources, and goals. These are all important components of modeling and not only represented primarily aspects of self-care knowledge, but also provided clues about need satisfaction, developmental levels, and adaptive potential.

After gathering assessment information, we could analyze whether or not the values, beliefs, and behavioral norms that we identified were compatible to the values, beliefs, and approaches in MRM theory. When we identified areas of agreement between MRM theory and the cultural values, beliefs, and norms, we reported those back to the group and then emphasized those aspects during our teaching sessions. For example, we learned that faculty taught Erikson's developmental stages to their students. We were able to point out during a teaching session that this content area about which they were already knowledgeable was foundational to applying MRM theory with clients.

For areas where there seemed to be a lack of agreement between MRM theory and the cultural factors, we addressed those areas in teaching sessions and tried to minimize the disagreement. Although faculty members were not familiar with the concept of affiliated-individuation and it was not a highly valued concept, we were able to analyze and discuss the aspects of affiliation and individuation separately. Then, after faculty indicated the value of each, we could address the balance between meeting needs for affiliation and individuation, simultaneously.

Sometimes we lacked sufficient information to make a judgment about cultural congruence. In those instances, we purposefully attempted to gather additional information from various sources. For instance, we read publications or talked to a variety of faculty members. This happened several times in relation to environmental characteristics. For example, we were not certain what government or private or professional body legally regulated Nursing practice in Taiwan and what those Nursing practice regulations entailed. We tried to gather this information from multiple sources, but they were unable to clearly answer our questions about professional Nursing regulation. Nonetheless, as the teaching sessions unfolded, we did learn that there was compatibility between legal norms for Nursing practice and MRM theory-guided practice.

Overall, there were more areas of agreement than disagreement. Also, there were relatively few areas that were unknown. Therefore, our task of teaching MRM theory to this population of nurse educators was made easier. We could build on already existing areas of congruence between MRM theory and the culture at the school.

Thus far, the discussion in this illustration has focused primarily on the processes of modeling and analysis. We also designed methods for teaching MRM theory to the faculty. We incorporated the Aims of Intervention, as delineated in MRM theory, to guide these role-modeled teaching approaches. For example, we endeavored to build trust, promote control, and promote a positive orientation among the nurse educators with whom we were consulting. We did this by providing resources as requested by faculty, ensuring that we were well-prepared for teaching sessions, requesting input from faculty regarding topics for discussion, requesting feedback at the end of each session, and recognizing areas of increased understanding. An example of our responsiveness to requests follows.

Quite often, when we arrived at the teaching session the faculty attending the session would request that we not use an interpreter. So, despite our having prepared a lengthy script for the interpreter, and having been prepared to use an interpreter which takes twice the length of time as not using an interpreter, we would respond to their request. This aided us in building trust with the faculty at this school. *We listened to them.*

As previously mentioned, after our teaching sessions were implemented, we always evaluated our teaching strategies through a debriefing session with each other. We found that sometimes the role-modeled approaches we chose were successful while at other times, they were not. When those approaches were unsuccessful, we purposefully resumed the processes of modeling, analysis and role-modeling.

At the end of the consultation experience in Taiwan, we concluded that our approach and model for promoting cultural relevance in utilizing MRM theory at this school was a valid one. Our consultation ended with a two-day invitational conference for educators, managers, and clinicians from throughout Taiwan. At this conference, we presented MRM theory to that national group of educators. We also showcased the expertise of faculty from the school where we consulted. Several of them presented cases where they had applied MRM theory. Indeed, we found that faculty members were well-prepared to use MRM theory in their program, and that MRM theory did have cultural relevance for them!

SUMMARY

In this chapter, we examined cultural issues involved in applying MRM theory. An overview of considerations for nurses practicing in a culturally-diverse society was presented. Then, we highlighted the cultural aspects of applying MRM theory concepts before addressing specific issues for nurse managers and nurse educators. We ended by presenting a model to guide determination of cultural relevance for theory application in educational or healthcare systems.

As we reflect back on this content, it occurs to us that the recommendations we made for application of MRM theory in multicultural situations really addresses application of MRM theory in all nurse-client interactions. Whenever nurse and client interact, each brings a unique perspective and cultural background into the relationship. Therefore, all nurse-client relationships entail a multicultural situation. Furthermore, we conclude that using MRM theory is an effective pathway to ensuring culturally-competent nursing care for all clients.

CHAPTER 12

EVIDENCE-BASED NURSING PRACTICE, HOLISTIC CARE AND ADVANCED PRACTICE NURSING

Linda Baas and Lynn Smith

A journalist sat on his hospital bed listening to the physician lay out the course of treatment for chemotherapy, surgery, and radiation to treat a malignancy. "I think that you should...and at that point I will schedule you for...I'm willing to go so far to see what works here...." At which point the journalist said to his doctor, "When are you going to realize that this is not about you?"

OVERVIEW

Evidence-based practice (EBP), the ubiquitous moniker for provision of the *most current and competent healthcare possible*, is commonly thought of as advanced practice nursing based on research findings. Practice based on evidence speaks to the empirical way of knowing in Nursing that was described by Carper (1978), and discussed in Chapter 3 of this book. Our goal in this chapter is to demonstrate that evidence-based care is important, but is not currently applied by most advanced practice nurses (APN) *within the context of the discipline of Nursing*.

We will discuss the importance of the *context* for advanced practice nursing as we review historical events that led to the rise of evidence-based care. We will include the benefits, forces driving the movement, underlying philosophy and ethical principles, and then critique the APN's reliance on the current model of EBP, often applied in an atheoretical or paradigm-less manner. Finally, we offer a model that incorporates a holistic nursing framework. This chapter ends with examples of how the advance practice nurse can apply EBP within the discipline of Nursing to work toward nurse and client's mutually-agreed-upon goals.

EVIDENCE-BASED PRACTICE

Nursing's Problem with Evidence-Based Practice

The Conduct for Research Utilization Project (CURN Project) (Horsley, Crane, Crabtree, & Wood, 1983), projected research utilization into the Nursing practice arena, setting groundwork for the EBP movement in Nursing. In 1992, the Evidence-Based Medicine Working Group published, "*Evidence-based medicine: A new approach to teaching practice of medicine*" (Guyatt, Cairns, Churchill et al., 1992). Instantaneously, evidence-based medicine (EBM) became the golden standard for medical care. Nursing followed almost immediately with a call for research-based protocols of care soon identified as Evidence-Based Nursing (EBN). The rest is history.

Today, Magnet hospital designation by ANA depends upon a nursing service that demonstrates EBP. All baccalaureate and graduate Nursing students taught the basics of EBP, learn how to search and review the literature to determine the best plan of care for groups of patients. This approach is reinforced for the advance practice nurses (APNs) who are taught how to perform an extensive and in-depth literature search and review, and are expected to become leaders in EBP.

APNs include nurse practitioners, clinical nurse specialists, nurse midwives, and nurse anesthetists. All four categories perform their practice with much more autonomy and different responsibility than staff nurses. APNs are able to practice independently, guide clients in their health care and sickness management in multiple settings, and interact with other professional groups as peers.

Although the legal boundaries of the various professional groups are established by state practice acts, there is considerable overlap in roles and responsibilities between the APN and the physicians. This is because much of the APNs' educational process focuses on technical skills, advanced assessment, and diagnosis and treatment of disease—courses deemed necessary by Nursing faculty if the APN students are to become experts in evidence-based practice.

Another trend, parallel to the EBP movement, is the tendency for educators to discount the importance of Nursing theories as the base for advanced practice nursing. As faculty focus on the *advanced knowledge needed for EBP,* they argue that Nursing philosophy and theory are no longer relevant for advanced practice nursing. Today, many programs have replaced such course work with content on health promotion or adult education theories. As a result, their APN graduates have never been exposed to, or have lost sight of other ways-of-knowing important to Nursing. All too often the APNs use EBP as the sole way of practice. As a result, atheoretical practice is becoming institutionalized.

A concerted effort is needed to revisit where we are in our orientation to advanced practice nursing and to reevaluate our practice models. We aim to demonstrate the importance of applying EBP within a Nursing framework. We also think that advanced practice nursing would be strengthened if it is based in a Nursing theory. We propose that practice models of care should demonstrate clearly and emphatically that Nursing theory guides practice, and that certification for APNs should include Nursing theory application in testing situations.

Later in this chapter, we will discuss the current EBP model based primarily on empirical knowledge related to the medical model of care. We also propose an alternative holistic practice model that incorporates multiple types of knowledge. We will discuss the implications for practice, and the alterations required to create a change from the current model to a more holistic one for advanced practice nursing.

First, we will discuss a few select forces that reinforce the current status quo.

Multiple Forces at Work

In Chapter 1, H. Erickson described Nursing as a part of a multidimensional suprasystem that constitutes the healthcare system. She discussed various characteristics of systems including the power bases, the actions and counteractions of driving and restraining forces, and other factors that affect outcomes. We think that it is important to consider some of these forces and their influence on our current situation before we propose alternatives. Without a full understanding of these movements and how they relate with one another, it is difficult to appreciate the importance of change or even the potential effect of change.

With this in mind, we offer a brief discussion of several forces at work in today's healthcare system. We'll start with the events happening in other areas of the healthcare suprasystem and then discuss the APN movement. We hasten to point out that the advanced practice movement in nursing did not occur in isolation of others, but probably *because of* other movements across the healthcare suprasystem.

Some of the forces we see today started in the early part of the last century and evolved at an exponential rate over the last fifty years. As the professional groups evolved, the need for social accountability increased, and with it, professional groups responded. New models were created, mandating other groups to change as well. Over time, the various forces have evolved and history is blurred, depending on how it is perceived and reported. Today, it is sometimes difficult to discern where one movement started and another ended. Nevertheless, we can be certain that they are interconnected—one professional group affecting another by way of power bases. Changes in one have the potential to affect change in another. Key forces include the society's push for financial accountability, the professional groups' aim for practice accountability, educational shift, and consumerism.

Financial Accountability

Healthcare costs provide a significant force that impacts healthcare services. The costs have been rising for the past 30 or more years, and continue to rise at an alarming rate, exceeding the cost increase of any other developed country. Despite these expenditures, the health of the American people continues to decline. The real needs of the clients are not addressed in current guidelines. As a result, we have witnessed approaches from Medicare/Medicaid, private insurers, government, industry, and public health groups calling for fiscally responsible health care.

Medicare and Medicaid fund only approved procedures performed by approved providers in medicine or APNs. Institutions that provide services must be accredited by the JCAHO (the Joint Commission on Accreditation of Healthcare Organizations). When a new procedure or diagnostic test is developed, it undergoes a review by Medicare to determine if it is of sufficient benefit to be incorporated into practice. This review is based on the evidence to date. If approved by Medicare, it is likely to be approved for reimbursement by Medicaid, and eventually, private insurers adopt the same practice. With rising health care costs, the evidence must be strong to necessitate a practice change, especially when the cost or the number of people likely to be affected by the change is great. APNs practicing in these systems are again receiving reinforcement for practice that is driven solely by medical outcomes instead of ones that reward nursing.

Private insurers have instituted a number of initiatives over the past two decades to reduce costs. Few pay for preventive services despite the potential benefits. This is, in part, due to the relatively short period of time that any insurer covers an individual. It may also be related to the fact that we have yet to identify what unhealthy behaviors we want to prevent. Healthcare insurers are awarded contracts with employers or industry based on costs, and everyone is striving to reduce these. Fee for service, fee for group care, primary provider organization, the medical home, and many other catchy phrases surface every few years as new approaches to provide cost effective care are attempted.

Practice Accountability

Standards of Care. The national movement to be concerned with *outcomes* rather than *process* is another movement that has affected how Nursing roles are defined. While we can trace this movement back further, our current situation started around the same time as the movement for graduate education of nurses; it started as agencies responded to society's demand for *standards of care or practice accountability*.

Professor Avedis Donabedian's (1966) rash of publications launched in the 1960s introduced a framework for classifying three types of standards, *structure, process* and *outcomes*. *Structure standards* provided the rules for what should exist. As applied to hospitals, these rules include the guidelines for the unit structure, the equipment, and staffing. *Process standards* defined the way people perform the work. The process standards provide the "how to" of the work to be done. The *outcome standards* defined the results of having structure and process standards in effect. *Outcome standards* are the most difficult type of standard to achieve. His work, instrumental in instituting quality improvement in healthcare throughout the western world, was foundational for the development of standards used by what is now the Joint Commission on Accreditation of Healthcare Organizations (JCAHO).

Donabedian's framework for setting standards is designed to be used across disciplines, assuming that the way the standards would be implemented would vary depending on the profession. That is, standards were intended to be developed, mindful of the professional group that would use them, and shaped by the philosophical orientation of the profession. If this happens, nursing standards should be shaped to guide and assess the *well-being of the person*.

Initially, various professional organizations issued statements of standards for practice, which were structure- and process-oriented. Hospital reviews were based primarily on structure and process standards for several years. Later, the standards became less focused on the profession and more on the recipient or consumer of the care provided. And when this happened, there was a shift from *professionally-related* structure and process standards to outcome standards.

Stipulating Outcome Measures. Since the medical profession had already defined its focus of care, and *had the major power bases* in the healthcare system, they were ready and able to stipulate the nature of the outcome measures that evolved. That is, they were able to stipulate outcome measures consistent with the medical orientation to healthcare. Outcomes consistent with other professional orientations were overlooked or considered irrelevant, in spite of their history with relations among structure, process and outcome standards.

Certainly one of the earliest healthcare providers who published in the area of outcomes was Florence Nightingale, honored by nurses for her efforts in the Crimean War to provide direct care to the wounded, and to improve conditions in the military hospital. But Nightingale was not just a wonderful nurse; she was also a great researcher and statistician. During the Crimean War, Nightingale developed the Coxcomb method for tracking outcome data for the wounded (Dossey, 2000).

In her later years, Nightingale became a respected consultant to the British Empire as they worked to improve the community health of their countries and colonies. A basic consideration in their plan was to use the best evidence to improve the health of many. They concluded that the only way the health of the community could be evaluated was through outcome measurement.

Although Nightingale was recognized by the American Statistical Association as one of the top statisticians of her time, after her death, outcome measurement became a worthy cause without a champion. As a result, outcomes were of little interest to the physicians and nurses providing patient care for a number of years. The more pressing issues for both professions was forming organizations to promote standards, improving education of nurses and physicians, and establishing professional licensure to protect the public.

Nevertheless, in 1916, Dr. Ernest Codman proposed that all hospitals be required to track every patient to determine whether treatment was effective. If ineffective, hospital personnel were told that they should try to identify the causes and aim to eliminate them in the future. Since the physicians and surgeons of the time were most interested in survival, Codman identified *mortality and morbidity* as the significant outcomes to track (Codman, 1916).

JACHO. In 1913, at the urging of Dr. Codman and others, the American College of Surgeons was founded. Soon thereafter, a set of hospital standards, contained on a single page, was developed. Inspection of hospitals commenced in 1918; only 89 of 692 hospitals met the requirements. By the 1950s the American College of Surgeons, the American College of Physicians, the Canadian Medical Association, and the American Hospital Association had joined together to form the Joint Commission on Accreditation of Hospitals (JCAH) (later renamed Joint Commission on Accreditation of Hospitals Organizations [JCAHO]), which has served as a hospital review commission ever since. Initially, the standards set to guide hospital care of patients included structure and process standards, but over the past two decades, JCAHO has emphasized outcomes standards (JCAHO, 2009).

While institutional review by JCAHO may be voluntary, reimbursement by various government and private insurers necessitates review and demonstration of meeting these standards. In 1965, the US Congress passed the Social Security Amendments which linked reimbursement for Medicare and Medicaid to meeting JACHO standards. Private insurers soon followed suit; the link between standards and financial reward has become firmly cemented. Now the "Core Measures" of hospital performance are published as a *Report Card* for the public to review and evaluate.

Educational Shift

A shift in education, with a focus on evidence-based practice is a natural result of these movements. When the organizational emphasis shifts to outcomes that reflect how well disease and conditions are managed or controlled, then schools tend to prepare their practitioners to be able to achieve these goals. Starting in the early 1990s, Guyatt and Rennie (1993) published the first of a series of twenty-five EBP related articles to appear in the JAMA. Later, these articles were published in a book that quickly gained popularity with medicine as well as Nursing and other healthcare professions (Guyatt & Rennie, 2002).

This publication gave rise to numerous organizations issuing practice guidelines based on the framework provided by Guyatt and Rennie. For example, in the area of cardiology there are standards issued by: the American Heart Association, American College of Cardiology, Heart Failure Society of America, European Society of Cardiology, and many more groups. Sometimes, the standards from one prestigious group conflict with another.

Nursing has also prepared a few guidelines that mirror the method used by medicine. For example, The University of Iowa Nursing Interventions Research Center has been a leader in developing nursing protocols that are evidence-based. Many of these protocols are in the area of gerontology and cover topics such as "Management of relocation in cognitively intact older adults" (Hertz, Rossetti, Koren, & Robertson, 2005) and "Detection of depression in cognitively intact older adults" (Pivens, 2005).

Unfortunately, the number of nursing EBP protocols that have a true Nursing basis is far fewer than medical protocols. Perhaps, this is because Nursing has not yet agreed on the theory, values, and philosophy underlying professional practice, so they have accepted the standards of other professions.

Consumerism

AARP. About the same time that EBP was being advanced as the prototype *of best clinical practice,* consumers became more aware of their potential power in determining the nature of the health care they received. The rise of the American Association of Retired Persons provides an exemplar of consumers involved in healthcare. This organization provides a strong lobbying force at the federal, state, and local levels. They stay informed on trends in health care and outcomes. The AARP has led the drive for reform in healthcare and improved access while remaining cognizant of the cost to providers.

HIV and AIDS. Another example of a strong consumer force from two decades ago was in the area of HIV/AIDS research, pharmaceuticals, and healthcare. Early activists in this movement pushed to have many medications moved through research and approval by the FDA in an expedited fashion. Now AIDS has taken its place with other chronic health conditions in the United States; however, access to drugs at an affordable price remains a concern in many developing countries. Activists continue to push to improve outcomes for those who bear this diagnosis and the stigma that often accompanies it.

The Report Card. Still another consumerism-related force that has had a recent impact on the stability of the healthcare system is the Health Care Report Card, mentioned above. Consumers can now search the web and look at the outcomes report of their local hospital; they will soon have access to outcomes of provider groups. Their findings influence the decisions they make regarding which provider to select for personal care needs. The results of these report cards also influence insurers and industry when faced with which health care plan to make available to employees, and who will be the providers on the plan.

The problem with these report cards is that they track medical outcomes and medical practice. They do not track nursing care. This may be because there is an assumption that nursing care exists to facilitate medical care; all else is irrelevant. In reality, people come to hospitals because they need intensive nursing so they can recover from their sickness or condition, or so they can mobilize sufficient resources needed to manage their disease process.

Conflicting Views. Most scientists accept the adage that benefits must outweigh the risks. For instance, you do not want too many false positives from a test that would require more invasive and risky testing in order to rule out a diagnosis. Likewise, too many false negatives will result in a larger number of people with the disease who are not diagnosed by the test. This orientation is valid for those whose perspective is disease management and/or control.

However, consumerism, alive and well today, can overpower science, and not all consumers are focused on disease management or control. Some perceive that prevention is more important. For example, there are times when *the evidence* indicates that a particular test is not beneficial for screening certain groups of the population, but consumers perceive otherwise. When this happens, there is a great cry of "Rationing Health Care." Often, the attempt to initiate a guideline deemed *rational* by those who interpreted the scientific findings is overruled by the public.

A good example is the 2009 Screening Mammography Guideline that increased the starting age to 50 years instead of 40 years. There was a vocal group voicing outrage and blocking any attempt at limiting this testing for women in their forties. One reason for this is that the interpreters fail to consider the data that describes the individual or group differences that are important in healthcare, data that might explain much of the outcome variance. Nevertheless, most people realize that healthcare resources are finite, as are the moneys available to pay for healthcare.

Ethical Considerations

We might ask then, why is the system so closed? How can we philosophically justify the current status quo? Some might say that EBP is really paternalism with the professionals determining what is best for the individual. Others would argue that EBP comes from the roots of two positive ethical perspectives, Justice and Beneficence. When considering health care from the justice perspective, all people are entitled to the best care available, and that would be what is supported by scientific evidence. Beneficence is based on the belief that it is best to do the most good for the greatest number of people. When viewed from these latter perspectives, the paternalism criticism is negated.

What is missing in this debate is that the issue is not about scientific evidence for practice, but about the original intent or philosophical perspective of the profession. When considering Nursing, the philosophical bases must be Justice and Beneficence as *paternalism* is not a basis for the profession. Instead, Justice and Beneficence would be thought of as providing, to all people, care that will enhance their quality of life, facilitate their well-being, and help them find meaning and meaningful relationships in their lives. Advanced practice nurses have the potential to fulfill this role.

Advanced Practice Nursing

The Early Days. The role of the Clinical Nurse Specialist (CNS), started in the 1960s and devised to be an expert in nursing care and systems change, emerged as healthcare systems were pressured to develop strategies important to structure and process standards. Soon after, the Nurse Practitioner was articulated secondary to an anticipated shortage of physicians in primary and episodic care of individuals and the shift toward outcome standards. Although the early CNS's role was designed to help other nurses provide high quality care through education and mentoring, by the 1970s some CNSs provided direct care to specialized groups of patients and to individuals, but almost always within the confines of a hospital system. On the other hand, NPs had branched out into the community, working with physicians and in some cases, independently. In some schools of Nursing the CNS and NPs were educated together, separated only for specific role definition seminars and clinical experiences. Others separated post-graduation for seminars that would prepare them for licensure or certification.

In the 1990's. While nurse anesthetists have practiced for many decades, their growth in numbers intensified in the 1990s and coincided with the move from hospital schools to graduate nursing education. The most recent movement to add nurse anesthetists and to increase the number of nurse practitioners as healthcare providers grew directly from the need to fill roles in the 1990s when physician shortages were projected again, *and* the healthcare system was confronted with growing patient needs due to the aging population. Due to multiple forces at large at the time, both the nurse anesthetist and the nurse practitioner of the 1990s followed the medical model and focused on diseases and conditions, rather than adapting their roles within the context of Nursing. Midwives had a more unique role in that they were a hybrid of the inadequate number of obstetricians and the lay midwife movement. Nurse midwives were educated in a model of care that blended the unique perspectives of the person-centered, lay model, and the empirical model of medicine.

During this phase, debate raged in Nursing regarding the *essence of advanced practice nursing.* By the mid 1990s, The American Nurses Association (ANA) had developed the *Scope and Standards of Advanced Practice Registered Nursing* (1995), and the American Association of Colleges of Nursing (AACN) had produced *The Essentials of Master's Education for Advanced Practice Nursing* (1996). The National Association of Clinical Nurse Specialists responded, producing their own document, *Statement on Clinical Nurse Specialist Practice and Education* (1998). Shortly thereafter, it was decided that all four roles, the CNS, NP, nurse midwife, and nurse anesthetist, would be considered Advanced Practice Nurses. About one third of the states now recognize CNSs as direct care providers with prescriptive authority, assuming they have the course work required. Although the roles of advanced practice nurses have evolved in different ways, all APNs are now expected to be the *standard-bearers* for Advanced Practice Nursing in an evolving healthcare environment.

Today. Nearly all nurses seeking any of the four APN roles are taught that *research findings provide the primary bases* for their practice, and that their practice should be *outcomes-oriented* rather than be concerned with the processes of care and caring. They are taught how to develop guidelines using a series of steps. First, they do an intense search of the literature; requirements for the studies to be included in the review are clearly specified. Most often the criteria stipulate that the studies have undergone a peer review process, and meet specific inclusion criteria related to the topic of interest in the review.

Next, a panel of experts reviews the research, extracting details of the studies for further comparison and analysis, and then rates the studies in terms of the strength of the evidence. As indicated in Table 12.1, descriptive research (i.e. case studies) is considered the weakest form, and multiple meta-analyses provide the strongest form of evidence. Finally, guideline statements are prepared, based on the type and strength of research.

Table 12.1 Hierarchy of Strength of Evidence and Types of Research.

EVIDENTIAL STRENGTH	TYPE OF RESEARCH
Weakest	Case studies
	Focus groups
	Descriptive studies
	Quasi-experimental studies
	Randomized, controlled trials
Strongest	Meta analysis

Even though APNs are educated within Nursing schools and colleges, much of their educational process emphasizes technical skills and advanced assessments needed to diagnose and treat disease or conditions, and their outcomes *of concern* are those that assess how well they have managed or controlled these problems. As a result, their literature searches tend to focus on research related to diseases, disease management, or conditions.

Because of the emphasis on diagnosis and treatment of conditions, sickness, and/or disease, many advance practice nurses have not been taught how to put empirical knowledge within a nursing practice framework or how to integrate it with other ways-of-knowing. Instead, the overlap of the roles and responsibilities of many APNs and physicians is so great that there is a blurring of role distinction. This state of affairs exists even though legal boundaries are determined by the state practice acts for nursing and medicine.

This is probably a greater problem for the NP and Nurse anesthetist, and less of a problem with CNS practice due to their role within nursing services. However, the education of new CNS nurses is moving in the same direction as that of other APNs with less emphasis on nursing theory and more on pathophysiology, pharmacology, adult education, and lifestyle behaviors. The problem arises when APNs are taught EBP from a medical model perspective, with a focus on disease and conditions—a focus consistent with outcomes that assess management or control of a disease of condition, rather than outcomes that assess quality of life.

We are not arguing against outcome measures or science, but aim to emphasize that the *outcomes measured* depend upon the nurses' orientation to the *phenomena important in the process,* and so does the type of knowledge needed for practice.

When nurses are taught to think about phenomena that are linked primarily to disease, conditions, and sickness, their outcomes of concern are consistent with this orientation. On the other hand, when they are taught to think about the *person who has a disease, condition or sickness,* the outcomes of concern will be broader; they will also include other dimensions of the human being, or as indicated in earlier chapters, other ways-of-knowing.

FINDING A BALANCE

As indicated above, there are multiple forces that merge to shape the nature of healthcare. Some have stronger power bases than others, yet there is constant exchange—and opportunities for change. In the most part, the intent behind most of these forces is *to do good.* The problem is how one defines *good* and what is perceived as important *to do.* One thing that we know for certain is that evidence-based practice is fully entrenched in the healthcare system. What we, as nurses, have to decide is how we want to balance the use of science with other ways-of-knowing common to Nursing. The following section discusses evidence-based practice as it relates to Nursing today.

Evidence-Based Practice and Types of Knowledge

The National Institute of Health (NIH)

NIH is currently promoting and supporting translational research, originally described as bench-to-bedside research. Translational Research is described by the Center for Clinical and Translational Sciences as:

> *Translational research includes two areas of translation. One is the process of applying discoveries generated during research in the laboratory, and in preclinical studies, to the development of trials and studies in humans. The second area of translation concerns research aimed at enhancing the adoption of best practices in the community.* (NIH, Feb 24, 2010)

T1 Translational research occurs as the bench (or basic) scientists identify *something new* that can serve as a marker of variance in a specified outcome, and then use randomized, controlled studies to test its effectiveness. The *new* factor might be a previously unidentified gene, a new drug, a behavior or sets of behaviors, new protocol, etc.

T2 translational research is the phase where the new "factor" is applied to a larger population, in a clinical setting, to further evaluate its effectiveness. A newer version of translational research, T3, evaluates changes in real practice arena (Westfall, Mold, & Fagnan, 2007)

NINR. Currently, the National Institute for Nursing Research (NINR) has a call for a two-year initiative to develop strategies for dissemination of interventions into the community. Two principal investigators with an established relationship are required: one that represents the research institution and one that represents the community might be considered. A list of potential studies is shown below in Table 12.2.

Translation research identified important by NINR (Table 12.2) offers Nursing an opportunity to capture the best way to apply evidence-based interventions and guidelines, so that patient preferences and other ways of "knowing" can be applied to the care of the individual.

Table 12.2 Call for Proposals identified by NINR as Important Translational Projects for Nursing.

1	Evaluate strategies that promote interdisciplinary research collaboration between investigators and members of vulnerable/underserved communities.
2	Utilize strategies that enhance community-based networks and infrastructure to translate research in collaboration with vulnerable and underserved populations.
3	Identify technologies and environments that enhance and support the effective dissemination of research findings.
4	Develop strategies that encourage investigators to integrate community and cultural factors in the dissemination of biobehavioral and clinical research findings.
5	Evaluate strategies that promote consumer access and interpretation of health information based on research findings.
6	Identify methods for assisting populations and communities in the adoption of results of biobehavioral and clinical research.

Clinical Application. Over the years it has been found that despite the best education, evidence-based protocols are not applied consistently. This may be because the defined protocol is not perceived by the APNs as relevant to their practice.

Carper's Ways-of-Knowing identified empirical knowledge as one of the ways-of-knowing. The other ways included: esthetical, ethical, and personal ways-of-knowing. In Chapter 3 of this book, H. Erickson and M. Erickson combine the ways-of-knowing with the Metaparadigm of Nursing (health, environment, person, and nursing). While bench research can be powerful, and when applied properly, demonstrate positive outcomes, it is not the only aspect to consider in patient care. Because empirical knowledge used by many APNs is usually focused on biophysical phenomena, often it does not address well-being or quality of life. In order to use evidence-based knowledge within a nursing framework, you must combine empirical knowledge with knowledge derived from other ways-of-knowing. Within that context, nurses are then able to practice person-centered caring, either from a Totality or Simultaneity paradigm.

This view is consistent with the work of Guyatt and Rennie (2002), who repeatedly argued that patient preference must be included in the plan of care. Nevertheless, many who influenced the creation and mainstreaming of the current version of EBP in the healthcare system did not make that distinction. We believe that nurses must use basic science—it is a part—and weave it with the art and ethics, and personal knowledge to plan the best mutually-devised and agreed-upon plan of care. We think this is the kind of knowledge that Nursing needs to develop in a T3 model of translational research.

> Many forces have come together to devise and promote evidence-based care. Nursing benefits from using EBP as the foundation for the empiric way-of-knowing in professional practice, but only when applied within the nursing framework in an effort to provide holistic care. The key is to use all types of knowing within nursing.

TWO MODELS OF PRACTICE

There is an anonymous, old saying, "An elephant selling for a quarter is only a good deal if you both have a quarter, and need an elephant." What should be done when medical protocols and patient preferences, or the nurse's personal philosophy, conflict? How can the nurse provide holistic care in the face of evidence-based practice?

The challenge for holistic nurses, who practice within the healthcare system is to weave together two models of care that represent two different worldviews. While the objective of both models is the safe, effective care of the client and their family, the current model of EBP and the proposed alternative model that incorporates holistic care approach that objective very differently. We will identify them as Model 1 and Model 2.

Current-Status Practice. Model 1.

The current, predominate model of care is shown below in Figure 12.1. In this model, EBP (as currently operationalized) is the center platform from which protocols and order sets are derived. Contributing factors include financial resources, hospital peer-review systems, Risk as defined by the tort system, and the patient and family.

The goal of this model is positive patient outcomes, *defined as survival, and hospital report cards, including morbidity and mortality statistics, and overall achievement of benchmarks for low incidence of complications, such as falls, infections, and medication errors*; not to mention amputation of the wrong limb!

Under this particular model, healthcare institutions secure their own survival based on reimbursement from third party payers and the continued use of institution facilities by the community. Physicians who are recruited to practice in these institutions must also meet the current EBP criteria. And their practices must show good outcomes, for e.g., keeping patients out of the hospital, throughput of patients in the hospital, and positive physical outcomes without excessive use of tests.

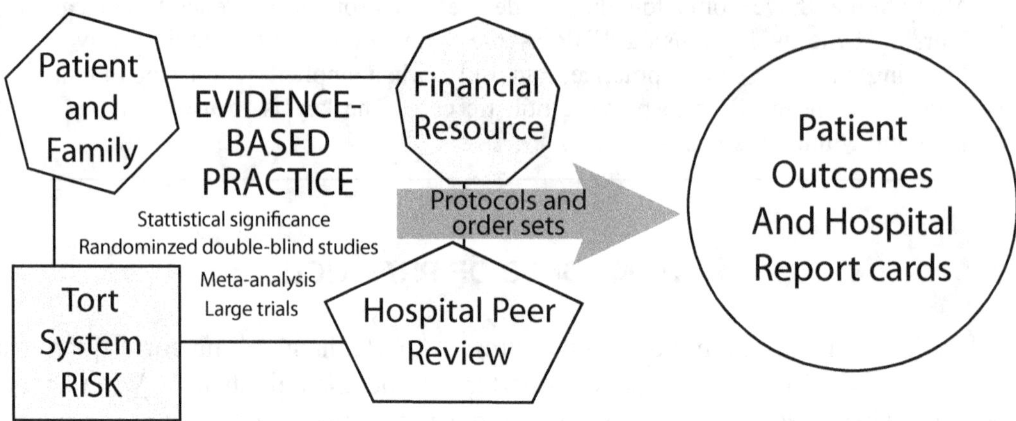

Figure 12.1 Evidence-based practice, focus on physical problems. Adapted and reprinted with permission from L. Smith, (2010), unpublished manuscript.

The patient and family have little input in this model. Consultants and practitioners manage the body system of their specialty; patient and family are told what is happening in their kidneys, their heart, or their liver, but rarely are they involved in discussions in regard to their overall quality of life given the synergy of the disease processes from which they suffer. Procedures are scheduled at the hospital and at the physician's convenience, and reports are discussed in a paternalistic manner that assures the patient that the physician has brought the best science available to bear in the care of the patient. The following, provides an example of a case under this model.

> *Mary is a thirty-five-year-old with a history of hypertension and diabetes. She has been medically managed with glipizide, lisinopril, and hydrochlorothiazide. Her primary healthcare provider now wants her to start on simvastatin, even though her cholesterol has been within a reasonable range. Mary refuses this treatment, even though she recognizes that it is now routine treatment for those with her health problems. According to the NCEP Guidelines, a person with diabetes mellitus is now considered to have the equivalent of clinical cardiovascular disease, and should have an LDL goal of 100, and even 70 if there are strong risk factors for heart disease.*

An Alternative Practice. Model 2.

Model 2, shown in Figure 12.2, places great emphasis on the science that guides practice, but proposes that empirical, basic science is not the primary focus of nurses who seek to understand the world in which their clients live. The client's goals and the resources available or potentially available to the client, and the person's readiness to accept information and make a change are central to the holistic practitioner's approach.

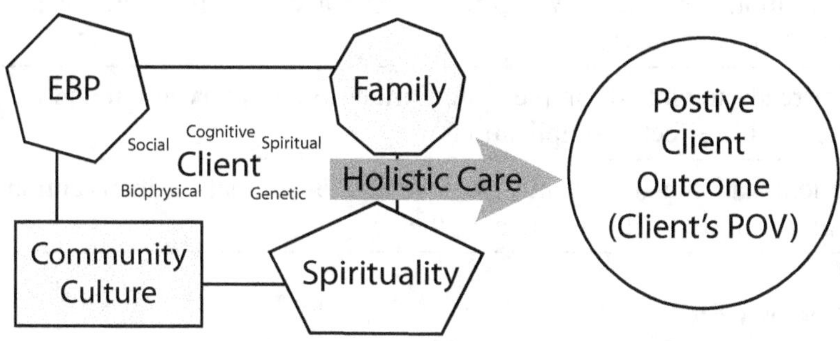

Figure 12.2 Evidence-based practice, focus on clients point of view. Adapted and reprinted with permission from L. Smith, (2010), unpublished manuscript.

Anecdotal evidence drawn from similar situations, deep, active listening to the client's story, and an advocacy that seeks to make the client's goal primary, are the essential tools of holistic care. In essence, this is research that is highly qualitative in nature, and yet, uses quantitative measures, when appropriate.

The practitioner's aim in Model 2 is to create an environment that is conducive to facilitate the client's growth and healing, with positive outcomes from the client's point of view (POV). The ultimate goal is to use the best science available that meets the client's cultural, financial, spiritual, mental, and physical needs. This work requires a partnership between the healthcare provider and the client. One framework that supports this partnership is Modeling and Role-Modeling. This framework considers not only what has been statistically accepted scientifically, but how the choices of best-practice fit into the client's world, relate to the availability of their internal and external resources, and have the potential to meet their needs, starting with physiological and safety and security needs.

Factors that Confound the Use of Model 2

Above, we quoted the anonymous statement, *"An elephant selling for a quarter is only a good deal if you both have a quarter, and need an elephant."* APNs need a model of care, but it is only useful if their clients perceive that it will benefit them. Otherwise, they are practicing without consideration of their client's preferences, one of the keystones of evidence-based practice (DiCenso, Guyatt & Ciliska, 2005). We propose four rhetorical questions that must be considered in order to begin to weave EBP into a holistic care framework as suggested in Model 2. These are shown in Table 12.3 and discussed below.

Table 12.3 Rhetorical questions for APNs using a Nursing Model for EBP.

Does the intervention that is being introduced fit with the client's goals, ethics, religious and personal beliefs?
Is the intervention sustainable within the client's access to resources away from the prescribing healthcare provider?
Is the client ready to embark on the commitment to the intervention and the possible consequences (side effects, complications)?
Has the client had the opportunity to investigate alternative interventions, weigh questions and concerns with significant others?

Is There a Fit?

Nurses need to ask themselves if the intervention they are considering fits with their client's world-view, including their ethnic, religious, and personal beliefs. This challenge is seen often in people who are scheduled for surgery, but because of religious or personal reasons refuse to accept blood administration. It is also commonly encountered in the pregnant mother who refuses amniocentesis to detect birth defects, and who, because of her personal beliefs will not abort the fetus regardless of the findings. Others include those who are making autonomous, end-of-life decisions even though medicine has not yet run out of options. This group has chosen to forego "exceptional" treatments.

In each of these cases, the EBP gives guidelines for safe, ethical choices. The client, however, working in affiliation with his or her community, church, family and friends, makes individual, autonomous decisions to decline further treatment.

The nurse is charged with the responsibility to assist the client to gather the resources needed for this self-care action, and to provide the context in which the decision can be made from a platform of *self care-knowledge, not of despair*.

Is it Sustainable?

Many factors influence a client's access to healthcare resources. Finances, geography, and family support are just a few of these factors. One of the newer protocols being adopted for diabetic clients is Intensive Blood Glucose Management. This protocol provides for long-acting basal insulin, followed by precisely regulated prandial doses of short-acting insulin. This regimen is supplemented by additional doses of short-acting insulin, titrated to the preprandial blood glucose level. Research studies indicate that this method of tight blood glucose control considerably reduces complications from diabetes.

These complications are substantial and include hypertension, kidney disease, blindness, acute coronary disease, and stroke. However, the complexity of the intervention may be beyond the ability of a single mother with small children and a limited budget. Model 2 makes APNs accountable to search for other options, sources of resources, and help the client balance the burden and benefit of intervention.

Is the Client Ready?

A scenario, played out over and over again in the past 40 years in women with breast cancer, illustrates this issue. The option of a lumpectomy preserved body image to a great extent, but many times left the client with the nagging fear of return of the malignancy. The option of mastectomy violated body image for many women, and with it, self-esteem.

And yet, physicians in the past were certain that the only way to secure remission and cure was to "cut it all out." Newer debates on the safety and efficacy of Hormone Replacement Therapy carry the same burdens. Men with prostate cancer face a similar dilemma. With a slow-growing cancer, EBP indicates no clear superiority of radical surgery, radiation, hormone therapy, or simply doing nothing. All options have widely variable burdens and benefits.

It is often difficult for practitioners using a medical model or Model 1 to accept that they simply do not know the "right way" to go, or the "best" decision to make, even when working one-on-one with each client. In comparison, practitioners who use Model 2, share what is currently known including possible complications and risks, and then ask the client, "How can I help you make your decision?"

Those using Model 2 support the client's choice of intervention and its largely predictable consequences, recognizing that this support reinforces the individual's self-care resources, helping them withstand unforeseen complications and supports remissions. It also eradicates the parentalism that is so embedded in the healthcare system.

Organ transplants provide another example that illustrates this consideration. Certainly the potential benefits of receiving a transplant are great, but the burdens are heavy. The cost of immunosuppressive drugs, the need for frequent, long-term surveillance, and the mental and spiritual experience of receiving an organ from a donor, either live or cadaver, are not small issues for the client to consider. When these issues are brought out and made clear and the client supported and encouraged throughout the decision-making process, the client's personal needs can be met.

What About Alternatives?

There is no greater gift to the client than time and support in which to make important decisions. The healthcare provider who limits the choice of interventions to the statistically-beneficial FDA-approved list that matches the practitioner's values does the client incalculable harm by practicing parentalism.

If the client feels forced to make choices based on statistics in the face of personal knowledge of other outcomes, the dissonance that may occur can produce added stress and stress responses to a person already under duress. The old adage that a mortality rate of 1% is great only for the 99%, applies to this situation. Openness to questions, investigation of alternatives, and time in which to digest information and reflect on one's goals is an essential element of holistic care.

EBP provides good statistics in regard to physical outcomes, but the responsibility falls on the holistic caregiver to facilitate the client's stretching beyond those boundaries, and becoming aware of the total impact of their decision on their mind, body, and spirit. There are benefits to time of solitude in this deliberation and reflection, but ultimately, the client lives in a community with significant others, and their input is of great value, as well.

Bottom Line

Holistic Care is client-centered. The beginning of all activity resides with the client's physical, social, cognitive, and spiritual being. Family plays a large part in the determination of self-care action and the resources from which it is derived. The community and culture in which a client lives has great influence over choices and decisions made, as well. In this model, EBP is simply a tool with which the nurse provides information and choices to the client, all based on the client's needs. While disease management and control are important, the overall goal of Model 2 is more appropriately defined as eudemonistic health as discussed in Chapter 4. The *outcome measures* of eudemonistic health include a sense of well-being and perceived quality of life reported by the clients. The following story provides an example of care offered using Model 2, care aimed at helping clients find meaning in their life journeys.

> *A newborn preemie with a severe birth defect is taken by helicopter from the county hospital where she was born to the tertiary care center with a Level III nursery. The NICU has just adopted a protocol for treatment of premature infants including ECMO with sedation and paralytic agents. The parents ask about the child's prognosis, and are told that it is poor. They are told that even if the lung function improves, the baby would be severely impaired both mentally and physically due to the genetic birth defect. Mom and Dad spoke with pastoral care who called*

their own pastor and facilitated the trip to the hospital for him. Baby's grandparents joined in the discussion. After requesting a second opinion regarding the child's prognosis, which did not differ from the first, the family declined the extraordinary treatment. In addition to being competent with the technology and pharmacology involved, the nurse was able to focus on comforting the family, and help them prepare for the loss. The baby died in the NICU 12 days later, in her mother's arms. The parents sent a card to the NICU staff thanking everyone for the care of their daughter.

The foundations of holistic caring must be taught from the beginning of the curriculum in schools of Nursing. When classes are divided up into systems, and psychiatric nursing is isolated from the physical diseases in the medical surgical course, faculty set the stage for novice nurses to fragment their thinking and build knowledge on a medical model.

"Why did I do that?" is a good question to teach critical thinking in nursing. The answer to the question is two-fold. There is usually a scientific answer, based on empirical knowledge, as to why a certain intervention might be used. For the nurse, however, there are always other types of knowledge that are important. When we use Modeling and Role-Modeling, data assessment always begins with the clients' view of the world, their goals and needs. The practitioners' interventions aim to empower the client to mobilize their own resources and meet mutually-set goals. Another case below provides an example.

A seventy-seven-year-old Vietnamese man was admitted to the hospital with pneumonia and COPD. He became weaker and weaker, and although his pneumonia resolved, he refused to eat hospital food, or drink the supplements that were provided. His family requested permission to bring in a rice steamer so that they could cook his food. A case conference was held with family, nurse, physician, nutritionist, and maintenance department staff. Permission was granted, and the family cooked and fed the client rice with small pieces of fish and vegetables. The patient ate well, gained strength, and recovered to return home with his family.

SUMMARY

Evidence-based practice (EBP) is an entrenched model of care. Advanced practice nurses are educated to use EBP. Currently, EBP is primarily based on a medical model focused on disease management and control. Rigorous studies on appropriate populations have determined statistical best-practice for disease management. Medications and other interventions have been shown to improve survival. Because the goal of holistic healthcare providers is to assure outcomes that fulfill the client's multiple types of needs, it is important to find ways to approach and interact with the science available.

This chapter offered a discussion of the current status of EBP in advanced practice nursing and some of the factors that have influenced its emergence and continuance. It also offered an alternative model of advanced practice care that holistic nurses might consider. Bottom line for the holistic nurse are the beliefs that *only the client can decide whether survival alone is the goal; only the client can define the end points and outcomes that are meaningful in their own journey of healing.*

SECTION 3

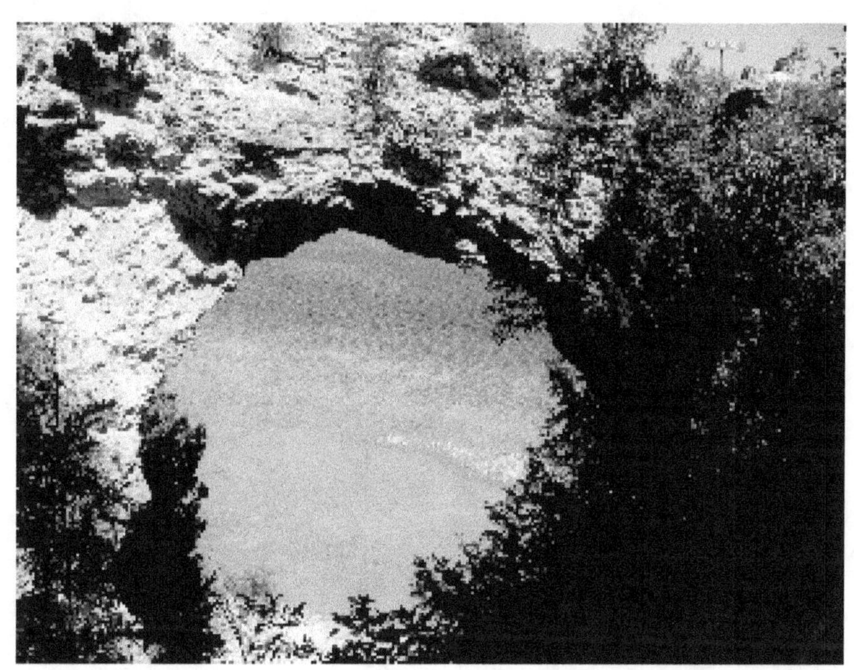

SECTION III

CONTINUING THE JOURNEY: FINDING MEANING

What can we do as educators to facilitate nurses to become integrated holistic professionals?

In the previous section, we discussed a number of issues relevant to mentoring competent, ethical, altruistic holistic nurses in both the academic and clinical setting. This section goes beyond these issues and addresses a factor often overlooked by educators. Specifically, it concerns *what we can do as educators to facilitate nurses to become integrated holistic professionals, each on a personal journey, seeking meaning in their life experiences?* While the preceding section addressed issues related to the acquisition and use of knowledge, the importance of facilitating nurses to become *integrated as human beings* was only mentioned sporadically. This section addresses this issue more directly.

The first chapter discusses the importance of the individual's experience as a source of knowledge. It addresses both positive and negative experiences, noting that the latter can result in unresolved loss and associated behaviors. The authors suggest that there are two options currently known to help nurses learn how to integrate their clinical experiences into their repertoire of knowledge. These include reflective practice and story-telling. They recommend that educators incorporate story-telling as a technique to facilitate students to learn to value reflective practice.

The second chapter involves a discussion of reflective practice as a *way-of-being*. The author argues the importance of self-reflection as a way of learning about self and self as professional. Models that facilitate self-reflection are offered for consideration. The last chapter provides the reader an inside-view of one nurse's life-journey, uncovered through self-reflection. It describes the stages she experienced, including the years of just living to becoming aware, and being enlightened and challenged to finding meaning in her experiences and discovering her life purpose. She concludes with a discussion of the process, including mentors who have facilitated her process and persons in power who have impeded it. She concludes with a few words of wisdom for those who wish to mentor others like herself.

CHAPTER 13

THE NURSE'S EXPERIENCE: SOURCE OF KNOWLEDGE

Da'Lynn Kay Clayton and Margaret E. Erickson

We need to remember that there are times that people need more help with spiritual healing and growth than they do with physical healing. They need help contextualizing their life experiences. Erickson, H., 2005, cited in Clayton, D., Erickson, H., & Rogers, S. 2006.

...experience and thought-or empirical knowledge and speculation...these two methods supplemented each other, and they alone, under the direction of reason, lead to the attainment of truth. Ernst Heinrich Haeckel, (1905), *The wonders of Life*, Chapter I *(cited in Seldes, G. (Ed) The Great Thoughts)*

OVERVIEW

Nurses who work with individuals and families in all circumstances and walks of life are privileged to share some of the most important times in their lives. They are with clients as they bring new lives into the world, as well as when they transition from this world. Being with people during important life experiences can be both amazing and awe-inspiring. These experiences can also be challenging; some are even traumatic. In any case, being with people at pivotal times in their lives can be transformative experiences for both clients and nurses.

Some nurses are able to find an audience to listen to their stories, either verbally or in writing, when experiences are awe-inspiring or challenging. But when they are traumatic in nature, nurses are less eager, and/or able to share their stories. This could mean that this latter group of nurses has more difficulty resolving losses related to these traumas. According to Modeling and Role-Modeling, unresolved loss can result in morbid grief (Erickson, et al., 1983/2009, p. 69, pp.121-22, p. 154, p. 230; Erickson, M., 2006, p. 225, pp. 233-34). Unfortunately, although both groups of nurses would benefit from being able to process their stories, discuss what happened, how they felt, and explore what they can learn from the experience, this usually does not occur. This chapter addresses these issues.

Nursing has not fully addressed the potential for nurses to have spirit-altering situations in the course of their daily work.

NURSING'S UNTAPPED POTENTIAL

Positive Experiences

When nurses have experiences with clients that help them gain new insight, they are often eager to share their newly-found knowledge with others. They want to talk or write about their experiences, describe what happened, and how it affected them. They also want to share their new ways-of-being and transformation, initiated by such nurse-client experiences.

Knowledge Dissemination

Currently, the primary venue for knowledge exchange is through professional publications. Although little is traditionally printed, when it is, it is usually about the nurse's inspirational or challenging experiences. But this venue only accommodates the few nurses who are willing to write or talk about their experiences, *and* are able to find a publisher interested in their work. What about the others whose stories are untold? Their experiences are also wonderful opportunities for nurses to learn from one another, and to advance knowledge about the nurse-client relationship and what it involves. Finally, what about the traumatic situations nurses experience as they provide nursing care? These, too, merit attention.

Traumatic Experiences

Nurse-Client Relations

Terrible things happen to people. They have life-altering accidents, fires, acts of violence, and other experiences that affect them profoundly. Many result in their needing nursing care. What is it like for the nurse caring for a child whose parents and siblings were killed while they were traveling to a relative's house for the holidays, or caring for a severely wounded soldier who is the only survivor of his unit? Nurses regularly have these experiences with clients. They are there to care for battered spirits and bodies, share their experiences, comfort them and their loved ones, and try to help them regain some semblance of dignity and hope. Sometimes, this is at a great personal expense to the nurse.

Nurse-Colleague Relations

Nurses also have traumatic experiences with colleagues. How do they process experiences that occur as they see clients harmed by other professionals? Sometimes this happens *even* when providers seem to be operating within professional standards of care. For example, one nurse reported observing infants and toddlers who were held down by professional colleagues for two hours while they were trying to start an intravenous solution drip; toddlers whose burned skin was washed with a wet cloth for 20 minutes without any analgesic; and infant circumcisions without analgesic. Although we know these conditions exist, such stories are rarely talked about, much less processed by nurses. As educators, we need to consider the cumulative effect of these unprocessed negative experiences on nurses.

Gunther and Thomas (2006) asked 46 registered nurses (RNs) representing diverse clinical specialties to tell them about a time they provided nursing care to a patient. Nurses described extraordinary events, some are tragic events and some are not. Yet, they all caught them unprepared, leaving them to ponder the event—wondering whether the outcome could have been altered, if they had done something different. They were also left feeling that they were either alone and different, or had no input from colleagues.

Literature Support

Constructs discussed in the literature (Bush, 2009; Corley, 2002) such as *stress*, *burnout*, *moral distress, compassion fatigue*, *vicarious trauma*, and *secondary trauma,* are some of the effects experienced by nurses. Table 13.1 includes definitions, samples and research findings for each of these. Both *vicarious trauma* and *secondary traumatic stress* are predicated on the assumption that healthcare providers with preexisting unresolved traumas will be more likely to develop symptoms.

Many experiences nurses have in an otherwise normal workday are challenging at best; many are traumatic. It is important for nurses to have an opportunity to process these experiences. Professionals like police, firefighters, and first responders have programs available to assist them when there has been a critical incident. These incidents are professionally recognized experiences that can cause psychological harm if not properly treated. Nursing, on the other hand, has few on-site professional resources.

Aycock and Boyle (2009) looked at compassion fatigue among oncology nurses nationally and the resources available to assist them. Sixty percent reported using "employee assistance programs," but the number of sessions and fees vary among institutions, while 51% used pastoral care. Forty-five percent of the nurses reported no educational offerings on workplace-related coping. Although 22 % reported having access, only 3% reported mandatory off-site retreats to promote renewal

Table 13.1 Conceptual definitions, samples, and findings

Concept and Definition	Concept Identification and Usage	Sample Groups of Nurses Studied	Findings
Burn out: a psychological response to work related stress that consists of emotional exhaustion (a depletion of work-related emotional resources), depersonalization (pulling away from those associated with the job), and reduced perceptions of personal accomplishment (a belief that one is not as good at the job as he or she was (Maslach, 1982); Halbenleben, Wakefield, Wakefield, & Cooper, 2008, p. 561)	(1974) Freudenberger a psychiatrist working with health care providers (1976) Maslach, social psychologist (Maslach & Schaufeli, 1993)	Oncology nurses (McElroy, 1982); Nursing administrators (Harris, 1984); Critical care nurses (Cronin-Stubbins & Rooks, 1985); Hospital staff nurses (Ceslowitz, 1989); Acute mental health nurses (Jenkins & Elliott, 2004)	Work conditions such as role ambiguity, workload, age, hardiness, active coping and social support effect burnout more than patient conditions (Duquette, Kerouac, Sandhu, & Beaudet, 1994)
Moral Distress: "…the painful feelings and/or the psychological disequilibrium that occurs when nurses are conscious of the morally appropriate action a situation requires, but cannot carry out that action because of institutionalized obstacles: lack of time, lack of supervisory support, exercise of medical power, institutional policy, or legal limits" (Corley, 2002, pp. 636-637).	(1984) Jameton defined term in nursing ethics	Examined in clinical nurses, RN, & diverse specialties	Effects on job satisfaction and staff turnover, but not the nurses' psychological responses and how they are managed (Corley, 2002).

Table 13.1 Conceptual definitions, samples, and findings (continued)

Concept and Definition	Concept Identification and Usage	Sample Groups of Nurses Studied	Findings
Compassion fatigue: viewed as a broader concept of burnout. While burnout focused on workplace issues, compassion fatigue encompassed workplace issues that result in a nurse being too tired to care for self (Joinson, 1992). Cognitive restructuring caused by listening to traumatic client experiences (McCann & Pearlman);	Used by US government relation to immigration (1981); news media homeless problem (1990); Joinson applied to nurses (1992)	Palliative caregivers (Mulder, 2000) Pediatric intensive care nurses (Meadors & Lamson, 2008) Oncology nurses (Aycock & Boyle (2009)	Secondary traumatic stress can occur in people helping those with PTSD (Figley, 1995). Both are predicated on healthcare providers having preexisting, unresolved traumas.
Vicarious Trauma: Therapists' reactions to their clients' traumas; therapist's unique responses to client material as shaped by both characteristics of the situation and the therapist's unique psychological needs and cognitive schemas (McCann & Pearlman, 1990, p. 136).	(1990) Psychological term identified by McCann & Pearlman	Mental health professionals (Devilly, Wright & Varker, 2009)	
Secondary Traumatic Stress: Incorporates concepts of *compassion fatigue* and *vicarious trauma*, and also includes symptoms of post traumatic stress disorder (PTSD) (Bush, 2009).	(1995) Psychology term identified by Figley	Hospital trauma teams (Laposa & Alden, 2003); Emergency nurses (Dominguez-Gomez & Rutledge, 2009)	

Student Nurses

Our experience informs us that these experiences are also a part of *Nursing students' lives.* Student nurses have challenging experiences that are awe-inspiring. They frequently write about these in their clinical papers and in courses such as the one described in Chapter 9.

On the other hand, many of them also have very traumatic experiences during their Nursing education. Few discuss these experiences in a manner sufficient to resolve the related losses and learn from the experience. Instead, they graduate with the attitude that nurses should be tough and ignore the distress and pain they experience as they care for some of their clients; many conclude that to do otherwise is unprofessional.

Through the years, as nurse educators, several of us have had the opportunity to teach the *Synthesis* course described in Chapter 9. We have had Nursing students who experienced a life-changing trauma which they have been unable to explore and analyze with a mentor; in some cases, they have been further traumatized by faculty responses to their experience. Occasionally, students deduce that they might not be "cut out" for Nursing, and think about finding jobs that will require minimal interaction with people, or leave the profession all together.

Potential Problems

Nurses are people first

Nurses, as human beings, need to find meaning in their life experiences. However, most faculty, mentors, charge nurses, supervisors and others responsible for facilitating learning in younger nurses, focus on *teaching* content, skills, and strategies related to empirical, esthetic or ethical knowing (see Chapter 3). Few focus on facilitating these novice nurses to expand their understanding of alternate ways-of-knowing, i.e. personal, unknowing, and reflexivity. This limits their understanding of both their positive and negative nursing experiences, and creates two problems for Nursing.

Loss of Opportunity. First, almost all nurses have wonderful inspiring and challenging experiences that could inform nurses about the essence of the nurse-client relationship if these experiences were evaluated and reported. They could also help nurses learn about themselves as humans and gain greater understanding of the nature of people as clients.

Loss of Self. Second, traumas, often inflicting feelings of loss, can result in morbid grief if unresolved and prolonged (Erickson, et al., 1983/2009, p. 69, 89, 93, 230; Erickson, M., 2006, pp. 228-237). Morbid grief interferes with growth, health and well-being. As indicated in the literature mentioned above and reported in Table 13.1, it predisposes nurses to compassion fatigue and secondary traumatic stress. We would propose that this means that these nurses would learn to detach from the humanity of their clients to protect themselves. They would also learn to treat clients as objects or conditions rather than humans with needs. Furthermore, they would have difficulty learning about their own humanity, their own life purpose and reason for being (Erickson, H., 2006a, pp. 5-32).

Solutions

Reflective Practice

Christopher Johns' work (Chapter 14) on reflective practice is a wonderful option for nurses who wish to advance their own understanding of self and self-in-relations-with-others. Many nurses have found that this approach has helped them to more fully fulfill their potential. This approach is particularly useful for practicing nurses who have limited access to faculty. As indicated in Chapter 5, reflexivity, as a way-of-knowing, could be built into Nursing programs as part of the curriculum. If this happens, nurses would graduate from school with a very powerful life-time technique that would help them learn how to think (Bruner, 1965/1971).

Story Telling

Another option, the *synthesis process*, described in our earlier work (Chapter 9), can also be used to help nurses *reflect on and analyze* experiences that "stick with them." Faculty members who have used the Synthesis process have discovered that many students enter their senior year with unresolved loss due to traumatic nursing experiences. Sometimes, these experiences are described in the students' case stories; sometimes, in one or two poignant lines. Other times, they emerge as the students report their cases to one another. And there are times when they are never mentioned. Instead, the student has difficulty aggregating the data and finding similarities among their cases. When this happens, the "real issue" will emerge when faculty ask the student to tell the rest of the story, listen intently, affirm the student's experience, and reinforce the importance of sharing the experience. The first step involves getting students/nurses to share their story.

SHARING THE EXPERIENCE

Through the years, we have read many stories written by Nursing students and nurses. These can easily be classified. While all of them were challenging for the students, some of them were also distressing. The difference in the outcome of those that were challenging and stressful versus those that were distressful was significant. Theoretically, people who have the resources needed to contend with the stressors are better able to cope. Generally, when people reflected on experiences and reported them as challenging or stressful, they were able to cope with the events. In comparison, events remembered as distressing indicate difficulty mobilizing the resources needed to cope. When students have the resources needed to cope, they are more likely to learn and *grow*. On the contrary, when they are unable to mobilize resources (internally and/or externally) what they learn will not necessarily help them grow. Instead, these experiences might impede their growth.

In either case, we think that it is beneficial for students to tell their stories. In the first case, they are able to reflect, think about what transpired and integrate it into their knowing. In the latter case, they need to be able to debrief, to find meaning, and to be able to reframe the experience. These processes help them let go of the loss related to the event, learn and grow.

> Bottom line: all students need to be facilitated in telling their stories, to share both awe-inspiring experiences and those that are difficult to resolve. The faculty's role is not to be the psychiatric consultant, but to facilitate the student in disclosure and processing.

Facilitating Disclosure

Story Prompting

Story-prompting involves creating opportunities for genuine expression of a person's story. If mentors want nurses to share significant and meaningful stories, it is important that they value story-prompting techniques. They have to believe that facilitating people to tell their stories is a valuable way to gain insight into and understanding of their experiences. Teaching Nursing students how to write their stories, reflect on them, and use what they have learned to articulate their practice, is an important aspect of Nursing education.

Encouraging nurses to share stories they are proud of is more easily done than encouraging nurses/students to share the painful stories; telling painful or chaotic stories, can be difficult (Frank, 1995). Painful and chaotic stories may not have the expected story sequence or ending, and they frequently show evidence of not being able to control life. To tell these stories, a nurse or student must be willing to revisit the experience(s). Many nurses have disclosed that they cried as they reflected on or wrote about such painful stories. A nurse or student may need to be prompted and facilitated to go further or deeper into the story. Initially, they may only be able to tell it in part as it is just too painful to "remember" in its entirety, or they may be hesitant to disclose the most painful aspects of the story for fear of being judged. Techniques used to facilitate clients to tell their stories (H. Erickson, 2006b, pp. 309-317) can be used to help any vulnerable person to disclose their personal knowing.

Story Receptivity

Once the story has been prompted, the challenge for the reader is to be receptive to the story. As nurse educators, we have been impressed with the number of extremely painful situations Nursing students had experienced before graduation. Hearing such stories can be challenging. The educator needs to be comfortable praising others for insight and excellent care. They also need to be comfortable with the process of reading very difficult situations and dealing with the anxiety or pain it can stir within self.

Listening to these painful stories can be difficult. Frank (1995) found listeners typically want to steer storytellers away from their feelings. Yet, the story-teller must be allowed to express their feelings. Story receptivity is essential to facilitate healing for the nurse—the storyteller. Story-receptivity involves rapport, unconditional acceptance, and nurturance (Erickson et al., 1983/2009).

According to Sandelowski (1991), the relationship between the teller and listener is generally asymmetrical and this is certainly the case with a student and teacher. Therefore, it is important that rapport is developed and maintained by the teacher respecting the student's story as the experience evolves by initiating at least a written dialogue. Unconditional acceptance of the storyteller, accepting people as they are, their stories, and the nursing care given is also essential to this process.

When the story is an experience in which the nurse is proud or was personally challenged, it is important to validate the nurse's experience with comments written in the margins, such as 'that must have been hard for you,' 'how difficult,' 'oh my!' 'good for you,' 'excellent nursing care,' 'so glad you know this,' 'insightful.' At the end of the story, we write a note thanking the student for sharing this story with us. With an extremely difficult story, the nurse educator can meet with the student to further process the experience and facilitate healing.

Students' Stories

The challenging and harrowing experiences undergraduate students have been exposed to are impressive. If we had not purposefully designed a course which required students to write their stories and faculty to listen as they reflect on their experiences, it would be impossible for us to fully appreciate the depth of their unresolved grief, the fragmentation of their understanding, and the lack of meaning attached to the experiences.

Traumatic experiences, left unresolved, have state-dependent memories, also known as stored memories that are associated with them (Brekke & Schultz, 2006, p. 62; Hertz & Baas, 2006, p 107; Walker & Erickson, 2006, pp. 75-77). The individual relives the feelings whenever they are reminded of the original experience consciously or unconsciously, and are unable to create healthy, cognitive schema with a logical order. It is only after they tell the stories that they begin to *remember* the beginning, middle and end of the experiences, integrating feelings with thoughts and sensory information. Until they do this, they cannot objectively understand what happened, make meaning of the experiences, or have positive learning outcomes from them. Unresolved losses may precipitate irrational or unexpected behaviors, sometimes not even understood by the student.

Take as an example the story about Doreen in Chapter 5. Ann was not upset about Doreen's mother, but the loss of her own grandmother and her inability to show her grief at the time. If Doreen had responded to her differently, reprimanded her for unprofessional behavior or enhancing her (Doreen's) own grief, Ann would probably have learned to *bury* her grief, only to have it resurface at another time in an unexpected way.

CASE EXAMPLES

We draw from our experience to provide the reader with examples of student stories which can be used to develop knowledge. When invited to write about a case that "just comes to mind," they tell stories that come from various settings and at different times in their lives. They share stories that come from traditional and untraditional clinical experiences as well as from summer work internships. We offer the following stories because we want the stories that are challenging and stressful as well as those which are traumatic and distressing. It should be noted that the stories that follow represent the full range of experiences. When students are able to cope, they often have wonderful "*a-ha*" experiences as an outcome; our goal is to help more students have the "*a-ha*" experience in any case. We believe that life has its pitfalls; we just need to learn how to make meaning of them, to grow and continue on the journey.

The first story was told by a student practicing in a traditional clinical setting. The second student story came from a nontraditional, third-world clinical experience.[1] The third student story comes from a summer work internship experience. Each of these was told by contemporary students. The last story

---

[1] Since many students in our Nursing program go to third world countries, it is imperative to have our students write about their experience, to validate them and to facilitate their healing process.

describes a nurse's experience when she was a student, some 30 plus years ago; one that she remembers vividly today, and reported with a sense of sadness. Clearly, she was traumatized by the experience. Perhaps sharing it with readers today will help her find meaning in the experience.

Each of these stories illustrates a type of challenge that Nursing students experience every time they enter the clinical arena. You will note from the students' postscript that they learned about Nursing as a profession and themselves as human beings by telling their stories. The stories range in the degree of humanity and compassion shown by the healthcare providers.

We hope that you, the reader, may discover that reading the life experiences of young nurses will help you remember similar stories, perhaps yours or those of your students. We know that if they remind you of *forgotten experiences*, it is time for you to reflect on them, to learn and find meaning in your current life situation. We also hope that these stories will help us all remember the importance of our own life experiences as professional nurses, as a source of knowing and a way to uncover the essence of nursing.

Kelli's First Day at the State Mental Hospital

> *In my second semester of Nursing school, I met the most challenging client I have worked with thus far. It was the first week of my psychiatric rotation at the State Hospital. The charge nurse selected a client for me. Before heading out to the floor to meet my client, I was extremely nervous. I was instructed not to look at the diagnosis or the client's chart before meeting him because my teacher wanted me to go into the experience with a clean slate. I did not even know how old he was!*
>
> *Upon meeting my client, I was surprised at how young he was, 18 years of age. I learned he loved origami and paper, he liked to talk to people, and he had several brothers and sisters. One more thing I learned, the hard way, was that he did not like talking about his parents. When I brought up his home life, he told me to stop making fun of him and he was going to hurt me if I did not go away. He became very loud and yelled at me to go away. At this point, I stepped back from the table that we were sitting at and slowly walked to the nurse's station. However, I could still hear him yelling that he was mad, that he did not like me, and that I better stay away from him.*
>
> *I was very shaken. I did not know what to do or how to feel. I felt upset that I had hurt him so badly, but I was also confused because I was not sure what his trigger was. I did not know what I was going to do for the rest of the shift because he said he did not want to speak with me again.*

I decided to look through the chart. I gleaned that this client had been severely abused physically, emotionally, and sexually throughout his childhood by his parents, who also abused drugs. He was one of six children, and the only one in the family who was treated in this manner. His parents thought he was "retarded." They would buy him presents for his birthday and before he could open them, they would take them away and give them to the other children. They would feed him scraps from the table after everyone else had already finished eating. They threw things at him, burned him, hit him, and verbally attacked him with unkind words. The abuse began at a very young age, and his grandmother was the only person who was kind to him although she never took action to remove him from the home.

As a result, this client began to act out. He would not go to school because people would make fun of him. He would act violently towards animals and he began to use drugs and alcohol. Eventually, he ran away from home and lived on the streets. These actions resulted in legal trouble and his being admitted to the State Hospital.

There were many challenges in working with this client. One challenge was comprehending the immense hurt in his past, and the fact that this would affect him for the rest of his life. It was hard for me to accept that he had such a hard life ahead of him and so many things to overcome. Another challenge came from the fact that not reading his chart before interacting with him made it hard for me to equate the boy on the chart with the boy I met. It was hard for me to put the whole picture together. Looking back on the experience, I was glad that I did not read the chart before our interactions because this gave me a clearer view of him upon our first meeting. Not reading the chart before our first interaction helped me to not see the darkness of his past and to not pass judgment when we interacted. This allowed my first impression of him to be clear.

I saw a pleasant boy, with slight mental retardation, who loved to talk and make origami. I was able to treat him like any other person. I think this was healthy for him and for me. However, it did make it difficult when reading the chart because I did not want to believe what I read. Another challenge was the struggle with understanding "Why?" When going through the chart and reading the horrible life that this boy had suffered through, I began to cry and struggled to comprehend why God would let this happen to someone. I also struggled with how another human being could cause so much pain and so much hurt. I wanted to find a way to make it all better, to make it all go away, but there was nothing I could do for him. I felt like I could not do anything, which is difficult for a

Nursing student. In all my other rotations, I felt that I at least helped out in a small sense with someone's physical or emotional needs, but in this case I felt lost. I did not know how God was going to use me. I was upset that there was not an answer for how I was supposed to help this boy. Another challenge was leaving at the end of the day and not knowing what would happen to this client.

After reading the chart, it became obvious why the client reacted as he did and I did not blame him for his behavior. However, I did not know how I was going to recover from our first interaction. I was scared to be near him because I thought he was going to hurt me. I knew that he did not want to speak with me again, so I gave him space. After about 30 minutes of sitting in the women's lounge and talking with a few other clients, the behavioral therapist came to get me saying that someone wanted to talk to me. I was confused, but when I arrived at the nurse's desk I saw my client there looking down at the ground. I kept about five feet between us and I allowed him to initiate the conversation. He told me that he thought I was making fun of him and that I thought he was "retarded." He said he should not have yelled at me and scared me. Then he apologized.

After his apology, I apologized to him for talking about things that he did not want to talk about. I told him that it was my fault that he was angry and that I would not "make fun of him" again; I also told him that he could trust me and that I did not want to hurt him.

The next thing he did took me by surprise. He took a few steps forward and offered me the origami that he was making for his grandmother. From that moment on, I was able to sit down and talk with him about his feelings. He even taught me some origami. Throughout the rest of the shift, I paid close attention to both the nonverbal and verbal communication. This allowed me to gauge how I needed to respond to him and what he needed from me. I also took cues from the client on what he wanted to talk about; I let him take the lead in communication, so I knew where he felt safe and where he wanted to go with me. I allowed him to open up to me in his own time, which created a trusting relationship between us. I also used a gentle tone and made sure not to enter his personal space during our interactions.

We were able to create a strong bond. This was evidenced by the fact that week after week of my psychiatric rotation, whenever I was at the canteen, this client found me and sat with me. He even asked me if I wanted to go to the Valentine's Day dance with him.

Faculty Note

Most of the time, we do not see the clinical experience from the perspective of the student. We are only aware of what we see as we make rounds and talk with the student, or read in their paperwork. When students *write* their stories, educators have the opportunity to talk with students about what they have experienced, to clarify things that might not be clear, and to assist them to process the experience so it can be integrated into their knowing. When stories are shared, students' strengths are also illuminated, i.e., the students' awareness and use of presence, communication skills and techniques when interacting with their client. Educators can then affirm these insights, reinforcing their students' strengths—a strategy which helps them to learn new skills, and integrate what they have learned into a new way of thinking.

Lessons Learned by Kelli

I learned many important lessons from working with this client, lessons that will remain with me throughout my Nursing career. I did not know, at that time, how important communication is to developing a positive relationship with a client. Before this, I thought that the emphasis was always on the physical needs of the client and the fact that I needed to meet these needs in the best way possible. After working with this client, I realized that healing begins with the heart and from developing relationships with other people. I learned that sometimes when you feel like there is nothing you can do to help someone, you could listen. You can be there for them and show them that someone in this world cares about them; you can also show them that God loves them and cares about them too, even when it seems like they are all alone.

I also learned that everyone has a past; a past that has developed them into the person they are today. For this reason, it is never appropriate to judge a person based on their actions or attitudes. People do things for a reason, and at times I may not understand or agree with the way they act or feel, but I should not pass judgment. Often times, they are acting in a way they think is appropriate and who am I to think that my ways are better? We all have a past and we all have hurts; events in our lives have shaped us into the people we are today. From this experience, I also learned that it is sometimes hard to walk away from the hospital and leave your worries and concerns for a certain client with God. However, this is necessary in order to maintain health and wellness. Even though it is hard to leave at the end of the day, it is important to know that just being there and showing God's love is enough to start the healing process.

Faculty Note

Kelli learned many important lessons as she reflected on this experience. Initially, she focused on his physical needs; however, by reflecting on her practice, she learned about the importance of caring for the whole person. She began to understand the importance of presence, active listening, heart-to-heart connections and holistic nursing care. She learned that all behavior had meaning, and it was important to look for the meaning behind a person's behavior rather than judging the behavior. I was impressed by the professional behavior she displayed as a second semester Nursing student.

Whitney's African Experience

> *This past summer, I traveled to Tanzania, Africa, with the College of Nursing and worked at the Chimala Mission Hospital. To this day, I am still haunted by the images of the young and old I saw die because of AIDS. In Africa, we were able to do several things we would not have been allowed to do here in the states. We assisted in surgeries and delivered babies. One of the most difficult, yet rewarding things I did was to perform neonatal resuscitation.*
>
> *During my third week, a doctor said there was a woman who needed an emergency cesarean section because she was hemorrhaging. She was at thirty weeks gestation and had not had complications until now. He said, "If we do not do this cesarean section now, we will lose the mom and the baby." He asked me and the other Nursing students to assist in surgery.*
>
> *As we prepared the woman for surgery, I tried to comfort her. I was only able to speak a small amount of Swahili, and she did not know any English. I believe I can communicate well with my patients without using any words at all. I sensed the mother was nervous, because she continued to look around the room at everything that was going on around her. As we transported her to the operating room, I made eye-contact and smiled at her. She smiled back at me and reached out to hold my hand. In Tanzania, holding hands is a friendly gesture made between members of the same sex.*
>
> *During the surgery, another student and I were responsible for recording the babies APGAR, cleaning the baby, and performing neonatal resuscitation, if necessary. There was a nurse midwife in the operating room assisting us. I had been told this midwife was hard to work with because she did not want us touching the babies. I thanked her for letting us be in the operating room. I wanted to cooperate with her. She*

continued her work and did not respond. I made sure that our baby station was set up with the needed equipment (suction, bulb syringe, stethoscope, oxygen, and an ambu bag).

When the baby was delivered, I heard the doctor say, "Good luck, Whitney!" As I looked over, I saw the baby was not moving much and was very cyanotic. I felt my heart begin to race as the midwife carried the baby over to the table. As the midwife laid the newborn on the table, I said a quick prayer to God asking that this child live, if it was God's will. I felt a rush of adrenaline and began to focus solely on the baby. I noticed that she was still not making any noise. As I listened to her heart rate, the nurse midwife told me to stop. She then pushed me away from the baby saying, "Stop! The baby is premature!" I knew the baby was still living. I replied, "I think we can still help her." The midwife did not know much English.

We had already delivered a couple of premature babies and had learned that the Tanzanians, usually, do not fight to keep them alive. They also believe if the baby does live through the birthing process, she might not be able to suck and, thus, would starve to death. The hospital did not have an incubator to care for an extremely premature newborn.

Her APGAR for the first minute was a 3. I knew we needed to start resuscitation if this baby was to live. I lifted the baby into my arms and began chest compressions while the other student used the ambu bag. The midwife continued to tell us to stop what we were doing, slapping at us. "The baby is premature," she said. "Yes," I agreed, "but I think we can help her if you will let us try." I continued to try to work around the midwife to resuscitate the newborn. I began talking to the newborn, asking her to cry for me. The midwife then looked at us, wrapped the baby up and told the doctor that the APGAR was zero/zero. Then she took the baby and ran out of the operating room! I just remember thinking about the baby, knowing that I would regret not doing anything for her when I knew I may be able to help her. I made eye-contact with the surgical nurse and stood in shock for a second. I then looked at the other student and said, "Let's go!" We followed the midwife into the ward with our surgical gowns and masks still on.

In the ward, the midwife unwrapped the baby to clean her. Other nurses were standing around her. As we walked up, the midwife looked at us, then looked at the other nurses and began speaking in Swahili. The other nurses began laughing. I had built a strong relationship with one of the nurses who spoke English well. I asked her why the midwife would not let us resuscitate the newborn. She said she did not know. She encouraged us to try working with the baby, so we began resuscitation once again.

While we were working, the midwife continued to speak in Swahili and the nurses continued laughing and looking at us. Even though my main focus was on trying to help the baby, it was so discouraging to hear these women laughing at us. I remember having tears roll down my face as I continued giving chest compressions.

After about thirty minutes, the baby's heart rate had risen, she was pink in color and her respirations were within normal limits. We gave oxygen to the baby. I was going to place her under a heat lamp so she could stay warm, but I did not want to leave her. So we decided to take turns holding her.

When I was holding the newborn, I felt a strong bond. I continued talking to her, telling her she had done a great job. I was still in shock with all that happened, but I felt a sense of peace knowing the newborn was still alive and in my arms. As I sat holding the newborn, I reflected on how fragile the gift of life could be. If I had not followed the nurse out of the operating room, the baby in my arms may not have been alive. I also realized that, at 30 weeks, there was a long road to recovery.

When the mother came out of surgery, I went over to see her. Though she was still highly sedated, I was able to tell her that she had a beautiful baby girl. I held her hand for a moment. I continued checking in on the mother and baby throughout the day. The mother continued to recover, but the baby was not getting better.

The next morning I learned the baby had not made it through the night. Words seem inadequate to describe the sorrow I experienced. I felt like my heart had been ripped in two pieces and my whole body went numb. To this day, it still brings tears to my eyes to remember this moment. I knew that the newborn was not making improvements and in the back of my mind I knew that this could happen, but I could not help asking myself, "What if I would have been here? Maybe I could have saved her again." I went out to see the mother, held her hand and told her "Pole sana" which in English means, "I am very sorry." She thanked me for all that I had done for her.

That night, I sat down and wrote in my journal about the experiences of my day. I reflected back. When I was holding the newborn under the lamp, I said a prayer of thanksgiving to God. That moment is fixed in my mind, with the realization that life truly is such an amazing gift! I had formed a special bond with this baby and I know that our education, along with God's blessing, allowed the newborn to live long enough to meet her mother. The mother at least had the opportunity to hold her and for that I will be forever thankful.

Faculty Note

Whitney's feelings of excitement, fear, awe, discouragement, and encouragement are interwoven throughout her story. Her feelings of unresolved loss are also apparent. This is an important, yet difficult experience for Whitney. This student began to share this experience with the instructor as soon as she turned in this assignment, giving me an opportunity to validate her experience, and to see where she was in the process of incorporating this into her world.

Lessons Learned by Whitney

Two lessons emerge from this reflection. First, the same type of communication errors could easily occur in America, and extra efforts will be needed when trying to communicate effectively during emergency situations. Second, we must always be aware of the resources we have available to us because saving a person to go through near-death episodes over and over again is not necessarily the optimal choice. Was the midwife actually right in this situation?

Faculty Note

How wonderful that Whitney could look at this experience from the context of the American and African cultures and resources, given the difference in perspectives. Through the writing of her story and the processing of the experience she was able to work through her feelings of loss. She now speaks of this experience with a smile.

Ashley's Most Challenging Nursing Experience

While working on a pediatric Neuro/Trauma Intensive Care Unit (ICU) this summer, we received a call. There had been a car accident with one fatality (the mother) and two children. The two children were in transit to the hospital. Later, we learned only the eight-month-old girl had survived. Her four-year-old brother died in transit.

When the child arrived on our floor, we were told the father was being escorted to the hospital by the police who had gone to bring him to the hospital. The trauma team, neuro-surgery team, my preceptor, and other nurses came to help. For the most part, my job was to retrieve any supplies they needed. Occasionally, I would be asked to move the patient or attach some sort of equipment. With this child they still were not sure what internal injuries there were, so the team was being extra careful. The client was intubated and receiving sedation.

I was asked to clean the blood off her to find any cuts. It was very evident that all the blood on her was not hers as there were no lacerations besides one to the head and ankle. It was amazing to see the team work assessing everything so carefully while waiting on the results of the scans and x-rays. Tests eventually revealed she had a small skull fracture and both legs were fractured.

When the father came in, all the doctors left the room so he could be with his child. My preceptor and I were in the room to assess the client every fifteen minutes. The chaplain was in and out of the room getting things organized for the father, but left him alone when he was on the phone. We gave him the nurse's chair to sit by the crib as he cried.

This was a man who had lost two of the most important people in his life and was stuck in a room with people he did not know. My heart went out to him, so I simply stood next to him without saying a word placing my hand on his back, silently lifting up prayers for him. I thought using silence was appropriate. Eventually, his parents arrived where I witnessed the most heart-wrenching sight as a grown man cried in the arms of his parents. Multiple times the family questioned us about the progress of their little girl. We reassured them that physically she was going to be fine, but it would take time to heal her injuries.

This was my first experience with death while working in a hospital. This was a difficult situation for me. But what made it even more difficult was when I turned to see the next two faces to walk into the room, my preacher and his wife. I had this sinking feeling in the pit of my stomach, the one you feel when you receive bad news praying to God it does not involve your loved one. I had become very close to my preacher and his wife the previous summer while serving as a church youth intern.

This difficult situation had become very personal to me. The father of the client was my preacher's wife's cousin. They were very shocked to see me. We exchanged hugs and I formally introduced myself to the father.

When someone you know and trust is taking care of a loved one, burdens suddenly become somewhat lighter. Through this conversation with the family, I could see this happening amongst the pounds that were thrown on them in one afternoon.

The client's family was so thankful to me for the emotional support even though there was not much I could offer to help their little girl. I will never forget the fear I could see in her eyes as I began my assessment. This fear of being in a strange place and looking around, not seeing anything familiar besides the faces of her family. After a few minutes of talking to her and telling her what I was doing, she would calm down.

Each day I worked, I visited this family even when they were not under my care. I was assigned to care for this little girl on the day of the funerals for the mother and brother. Even then, I could see the slow healing process of the family. The family told me how thankful they were of the care and kindness I had shown them.

There was an instance where I had come in to find the little girl's hair in cute pigtails. As I began my first assessment of the day, the father stood next to me smiling and said, "I have no clue who did the pigtails; it must have been the night nurse while I was sleeping. I don't even know how to do that." By the tone of his hopeless voice I felt that he needed some encouragement for the future, so I replied in a soft, kind voice, "Yeah, that's okay. You will."

Over time, the father slowly opened up to me and I saw his thinking change from, "I cannot believe that has happened" to "How do I move forward and raise a little girl without her mother?"

Faculty Note

Ashley had finished two semesters of Nursing school before this experience. Although she had not yet had her pediatric and family theory courses, she was able to be professional and effective in a complex emotional situation.

Lessons Learned by Ashley

I learned to open my eyes and look closely at situations God puts in front of me. To always know God has a plan and I may never know the reason why I've been placed in certain situations. To find my role in each challenge I am placed before. I learned firsthand what it means to simply 'be there' for the client and family. We are not only taking care of the client, but the family also. I now realize I was there to be a familiar face to them and bring comfort in the midst of chaos.

Faculty Note

This situation would challenge many experienced nurses. Ashley has learned some very important life lessons. She learned about herself, how important it is to be "present" with others, and that she is responsible for caring for her client as well as the family. She also learned about her ability to assume her role in challenging situations. Specifically, she learned the importance of providing support to help facilitate clients' healing on their life journeys.

Mrs. Edwards, A Story From the Past

Mrs. Edwards, a small, slender 78-year-old woman was admitted to the unit at 6:30 p.m. with abdominal pain and oral bleeding related to a diagnosis of metastatic liver cancer. In an agitated whisper she stated, "I don't want to be here. I have so much to do to get ready for Thanksgiving." Then with sparkling eyes, she said, "My kids are coming home and I am so excited to see my grandchildren." As she talked, she clasped and unclasped her hands. Her husband, meanwhile, was intermittently at the bedside holding her hand or pacing about the room. With a furrowed brow he asked the nurse, "How long do you think we will be here this time?" The nurse stated that she wasn't sure. The doctor would be in to see her soon, and maybe they would know more then.

I asked why she had come into the hospital she said, "I have been having some abdominal pain and a little bleeding from my bottom and there has been some blood on the tissues when I wipe my mouth. I thought they might be able to give me something for the pain and send me home. Can I please have something for the pain now?" At that time, the doctor walked into the room, closely followed by a couple of medical students and an intern. The doctors all stood at the end of the bed looking at the charts. None of them approached the patient or her husband. "Good evening Mrs. Edwards. I am Dr. Doolittle. We are going to draw some blood, and do some tests to see what is causing the bleeding. You'll be NPO until we run the tests." She asked, "Will I be able to go home soon?" He replied, still not looking at her, "I won't know anything until I get some results back." Mrs. Edwards huddled in the bed as the doctor talked to his chart and she seemed to shrink and get smaller as he told her what the plans were. When she asked for something for the pain he replied, "I will order something for it." With backs turned to the Edwards', the doctors discussed her "case" and her plans. Then, the entourage left with the noise of rustling papers and flapping coats, without another word to the Edwards.

Mrs. Edwards received pain medication. An hour later, she still complained of pain. She received additional medication with some relief obtained. I checked on her every 20 minutes doing mouth care, offering ice chips, giving a massage, changing her bed linens or adjusting blankets and pillows. Sometimes, I just sat for a few minutes to hold her hand as Mrs. Edwards talked about her grandchildren and Mr. Edwards took a break. He refused to leave his wife alone. "She needs someone here with her." Mrs. Edwards rarely asked for anything, but smiled gently and always thanked me for "being there and checking to see if I am alright." When the shift was done, she asked me if I would come and see her again.

The next day, I was assigned to care for Mrs. Edwards (per their request). Mrs. Edwards was having a lot of pain and spitting up a lot more bright red blood, an upper GI was to be performed in the room, but so far Mrs. Edwards had refused to have it done. Upon entering the room Mrs. Edwards sat up in bed, leaned forward and said, "I am so glad you are here. You are such a dear and we were afraid you weren't working tonight. The doctor said I have to have a test done, but I told them I wouldn't do it unless you could sit by me and hold my hand."

The doctor arrived for the procedure. He was followed by several medical students and interns. They were discussing the procedure amongst themselves and what they might find or see. No one addressed the client or her husband. They sprayed her mouth with an anesthetic spray and told her it would numb it so it wasn't so bad. She asked, "Can we wait a few minutes? I'm not ready." The doctor said, "Oh no. You're fine. The spray works right away." Mrs. Edwards listened with wide eyes. She then frantically patted the bed where she wanted me to sit beside her. She clutched my hand as they began to tell her how they would proceed. When they inserted the scope down her throat, she pulled her body into the bed away from the violation of the painful insertion of the scope. Blood began to come out of her mouth because of the forced insertion of the scope. She was gagging. As I was holding her hand, several of the doctors' hands reached down to restrain her, pushing her fragile body into the bed, so the procedure would be easier for the doctor to do. After they finished, the doctor said, "We're sorry, but there isn't anything we can do. We will give you some blood and an IV to make you stronger before we send you home." She cried quietly.

I asked her if she would like to get cleaned up before I brought her husband back in. I helped her cleanup, gently washing her mouth and offering to change her sheets which were soaked with sweat and blood. I helped her with oral care, got her some soup and Jello, and gave her a back massage. After she was more comfortable, I asked if she was ready to have her husband come back in. When Mr. Edwards returned to the room, he went to her bedside and asked if she was alright. He took her hand and in quiet broken tones said, "I know it was really hard for you." His eyes were full of tears. She smiled gently and said, "I am a little better now." I also asked if she would like something to help her sleep. I stayed and quietly visited with them until she fell into a fitful sleep.

Four days later, I returned to the unit. Mrs. Edwards never got home for Thanksgiving. She died two days after the procedure.

Authors' Note

This case was reported by a nurse approximately 30 years after the experience. It is not unlike those reported by students who work as nursing assistants, technicians, or have extended clinical experiences. However, the level of care this student was able to offer is amazing. Many students find it very difficult to know how to help a client in extreme pain, but this student intuitively knew what to do.

This situation is complex, and like others, it involves unintended, inhumane care by healthcare providers. Some of them may have been operating within the existing standards of care, but had forgotten that the person they were privileged to be with was a human being with needs.

No one but the student heard *and understood the meaning of the client's words* when she said she wanted and needed to go home for Thanksgiving, and that she was not ready for the doctors to begin the procedure.

In Modeling and Role-Modeling, we call the client's knowing *Self-care Knowledge*. When a nurse responds appropriately to client expressions of self-care knowledge, it often makes a significant difference in client responses and outcomes.

Finally, it is important for us to report that after this nurse shared her story and had an opportunity to reflect on the experience, she had some important insight. Now, she knows that she provided the best possible care she was able to, given the circumstances. As a result of this insight, she argues that educators need to recognize that students need to learn how to be more assertive, skills they can use to support their clients in getting their needs met.

She also states that most nurses will have challenging experiences in the course of their practice. Therefore, it is imperative that nurse leaders develop better ways to support their colleagues, be aware of the potential for nurses being traumatized by their experiences, and develop models of debriefing or follow-up which will help them process their experiences.

This case also raised the issue of another problem in Nursing: nurses being traumatized by observing or being involved in unethical care. Stories that describe such care are not new to our profession. Sometimes, they are stories about situations where people are actually mistreated; in other situations, people are not actually mistreated, but are treated without compassion. As a result, both the client and the nurse suffer. In reality, the incidence of cases where lack of regard for the client's humanity occurs falls at various points along a continuum of inhumane care. In all cases, they violate Nursing's Code of Ethics (ANA, 2004); we as nurses need to take a more proactive position against such care.

Interestingly, Chapter 1, originally written in 1985, was based on the recognition of this same problem. Yet, here we are in 2010, raising the issue again. It is imperative that nurses explore and discuss these cases. We need to learn how to process what happened and understand the impact on the nurse and the client. When we do this, we will be able to ask important professional questions necessary to bring about a safer, more compassionate healthcare system.

SUMMARY

When the nurse educator prompts students to share nursing stories, students reflect on their experiences and explore their feelings. If nurse educators are receptive to these stories, they affirm that they value and respect student experiences. Student stories come from traditional clinical experiences, nontraditional clinical experiences, and internships. Their experiences range in the type of challenge and degree of stress experienced; some are traumatized by the nature of inhumane care observed. We described a model used to facilitate students to share their stories and process their learning. Interactive dialogues with the faculty help the student process and find meaning in the experience, and help them learn and grow on their life journey. We contend that facilitating nurses share their stories and process their experience as an important source of knowledge, important to the advancement of Nursing.

CHAPTER 14

REFLECTION AS A WAY-OF-BEING IN PRACTICE

Christopher Johns

There are very few human beings who receive the truth, complete and staggering, by instant illumination. Most of them acquire it fragment by fragment, on a small scale, by successive developments, cellularly, like laborious mosaic.

OVERVIEW

Reflective practice, derived from Schön's (1983) work, provided a background for the development of the Model for Structured Reflection (MSR) as a way to facilitate those who wish to pursue *being in practice.* This chapter describes the importance of this work, and how it relates to *knowing in practice.*

REFLECTIVE PRACTICE

Being-in-Practice

In this contribution, *I want to open, for you, a path to reflection as a way-of-being in practice.* I emphasise *being* rather than *knowing*, simply to suggest that an ontological concern with *being* has a more fundamental focus than an epistemological concern with *knowing*.

Ways-of-Knowing have been delineated in Nursing practice, notably the work of Barbara Carper (1978) as revealed and expanded in contributions to this book. Yet ways-of-knowing reflect a largely epistemological concern to impose a conceptual reality on knowing and knowledge. The fundamental, yet flawed premise is that *if we know something, we can control it.* Such a premise reflects a persistent, yet, perverse positivist legacy on Nursing. If we don't know something, we live with uncertainty.

Schön (1983) has illuminated that much of clinical practice is complex and indeterminate without easy solutions to the problems that face practitioners. He likened this to the swampy lowlands. He differentiated the swampy lowlands with the high hard ground of technical rationality.

Embodied Knowing

Survival in the swampy lowlands requires a certain *sort of craft* guided by knowing-in-practice, or everyday wisdom that knows, but often cannot quite tell how it knows. *It is an embodied knowing.* Schön suggested that this *knowing-in-practice* is the primary disciplinary concern, not technical rationality, simply because it has no answers to the issues that face practitioners day by day.

Given this appreciation, it is pertinent to inquire why Nursing curricula continue to be theory-driven rather than practice-driven, particularly since Nursing is a practice profession.

> I would argue that access to knowing-in-practice is achieved through reflective practice.

Knowing-in-Practice

Access to knowing-in-practice is achieved through reflective practice. Let me explain. Can you imagine a group of us sitting around a campfire? The flames are dancing; the smoke spiralling toward the sky. I am telling a story of my practice. Each of you relates to my story and tells your own story in return. In the telling, *we* lift *this knowing* onto the surface where *we* explore the contradictions or tension between what *we* seek to realise in our practice, our vision or values so to speak, and the way *we* actually practice. In doing so, *we* identify those factors both embodied within ourselves, and embedded within the practice environment, that constrain this realization. Reminding ourselves of our integrity, *we* act to shift those forces, so our visions can be realised as a lived reality through subsequent (reflected-on) experiences.

Being Mindful

Reflective practice is essentially learning through experience, moving forward, gaining insights, realising a vision of desirable practice as a lived reality. Vision is a statement of our beliefs and values about Nursing that gives purpose and direction to practice. It sets up intentionality–that by mindfully holding my vision I am more likely to realise it. *Learning through experience* is always within the moment, either the clinical moment itself, (if I am mindful enough) or after the event. When it is after the event, it happens as I experience a "looking back" which is often triggered by a sense of unease (Boyd & Fales, 1983); it is as if the emotion lifts the event into consciousness.

When I return to practice, I pay more attention to those things I have reflected on—it is as if seeds have been planted in my head to germinate at appropriate moments in practice. In this way, I become increasingly mindful of self-within-practice.

Being mindful is the quintessential nature of reflective practice. *It is the ability to be aware of self,* within the unfolding moment, without judgment. It is as if I am a witness to self, mindful of how I am thinking, feeling and responding. For example, I imagine the First Nations chief sitting within a circle of wise men, outside the ceremonial tipi, contemplating a decision that must be made. Their wisdom is deeply intuitive and compassionate. It comes from a deep appreciation of the *way things are* and a *commitment for doing good* that transcends self-interest and self-concern. Characteristics of being mindful are shown in Table 14.1.

Table 14.1 Characteristics of *being mindful.*

To *be mindful* is to *be:*
• A witness to myself without judgment; • Intentional of realising my vision; • Open to the possibility of the best way to be and respond within the moment; • Non-attached to any particular idea about what should be done; • Aware of any distraction that might pull me into self-concern—what I describe, adopting the Buddhist term Apramada—meaning the guardian at the gate of the senses (Sangharakshita, 1998).

> Being mindful integrates all knowing. It transcends the rational mind. It is stripping away layers of ego to reveal the true human core of being.

Coherence: A Unified Whole

I do not know things as ideas or parts, but as a whole. I know this 'whole' is in constant flux, as I engage the situation, moving through time and space. I also sense that the outcome is never predictable, that we move through uncertainty yet with intent, and that intent shapes the apparent chaotic space we move into, a strange attractor around which order moves (Wheatley, 1999).

The Rhythm of Relating

Through reflection *I tune into the rhythm of relating*, as if a synchronous dance, movements that seem both well-rehearsed and spontaneous, as if the body and mind are in unison. And yet, where a pause or breakdown in the rhythm manifests, the body adjusts, confident, like a silver stream finding its way around apparent obstacles, but in reality no more than the complexities of the situation revealing themselves.

In terms of Carper's Ways-of-Knowing, this dance might be described as *aesthetic knowing*–the way embodied knowing is reflected in the performance. Such knowing is always transient, *known within the moment*, difficult to express in words simply because it is so complex. It integrates all other 'ways of knowing.' As such, aesthetics is not a separate way-of-knowing.

> As I reflect on my practice, I wonder how I know things. I sense that knowing is coherence.

Aesthetics as Craft

Perhaps a more useful word than aesthetics is *craft.* The craftsman takes his raw materials with him to his work. He has an idea about the outcome, but he knows that the outcome is shaped by the local circumstances. He prepares himself, he ensures that he is in good condition and ready for the job. He wants to give it full attention. He makes himself fully present to the rhythm of the moment and to the forces that shape the rhythm. In the present, *he holds the moment between what has passed and what has yet to come*. The craftsman draws on knowledge to inform his art. *He acts for the best, in terms of a moral responsibility to do his best. Indeed, anything less, he sacrifices integrity.* He respects the wood for it is his material to work with. In this way *I am a craftsman; the person is my wood.* I am shaping practice and being shaped by practice. *It is resonance with the material*. As Barbara Hepworth, a sculptress, says, "One must be entirely sensitive to the structure of the material that one is handling. One must yield to it in tiny details of execution, perhaps the handling of the surface or grain, and one must master it as a whole (http://www.brainyquote.com).

> I sometimes feel that as a therapist my hands sculpt the person I work with, like shaping clay—I am shaping the person to become as they must. It is being fully present, paying attention, listening deeply, empathic resonance, tuning into the wavelength of the being of the person as the prelude to responding.

Things I Know, But Not for Certain

Of course there are things I know, *but not for certain* (Johns, 2009a) and these become food for reflection both within the situation—a mindful working-out-the-rhythm, and later for deeper contemplation. You too, can become a reflective practitioner. For instance, you can consider some basic questions shown in Table 14.2. Think about these questions. Take some time to write your answers. The last two questions are significant to consider because reflection is not easy.

Table 14.2 Self-reflection questions.

- What is the *vision* you hold as a nurse?
- Do you live this vision as a reality in everyday practice?
- What constrains you from realizing your vision?
- Are you satisfied with not living your vision and living a contradictory life?
- Are you being truthful to yourself in answering these questions?

> It requires commitment and integrity to face up to one's reality and *to become one's vision.* Skilful guidance may be necessary to help us see ourselves and beyond our own horizons, to become who we need to be.

A Narrative Example

Let me share a brief narrative of my own as an example.[1] I work as a volunteer complementary therapist within the in-patient unit one day a week. Richard was admitted to the hospice some days previously. He is dying with cancer of the lung. Ed, his son, also dying, has also been admitted to the hospice. Hettie is Richard's wife; Sophie is his daughter.

Friday 27th February.

Richard panics as sputum plugs his airway. With the help of nebulisers, he eventually shifts it. Hettie watches helplessly. Her suffering spills out as tears. How difficult it is for a spouse to watch someone you love slowly disintegrate toward death. Richard is exhausted.

---

[1] This narrative was first published in 'Engaging reflection in practice' (Johns 2006). It has been developed for this publication. I have interspersed my journal notes with my commentary to enrich your experience.

It is also difficult for me to watch him. I do not offer a treatment. I witness his distress without pity. I know he is comforted because we know each other. The resonance is simply in my presence, in my compassion that lifts the energy and comforts him and Hettie at this time.

My appreciation of presence is inspired by Joseph Rael (1993). He writes:

There is an energy that comes to all of us from the sacred place, the vibrations of an ancient past, wisdom we would come to find one day. Once the scared place is discovered, we begin to open to the wisdom. It descends upon us just as it did when the beings from the spirit world brought spirit to the people (p.29). *It starts to lift us to a higher place and when it happens to us, it also happens to other people who are also being lifted to the next level and something dramatic happens in our lives* (pp. 88-89).

These words *take me to the very core of healing*. Rael says it in words that *I know*. *You* also know this. Ask yourself, what lifts you at work and what drains you? You know being together with some people lifts you and with others it drains you. We need to know these things to help us be more present with our patients and colleagues.

Begin with yourself; be open to this ancient wisdom.

Monday, 1st March.

Richard and Hettie are behind closed doors with Daphne, the social worker. Time hangs in the air. Later, I collide with Hettie in the small kitchen. She is making tea. Her eyes are strained from crying, but she is also laughing. "That was good to get all that into the open."

Walls of silence broken down. How difficult for people who have spent a lifetime together to talk about dying, death, and loss. Hettie is keen to have a foot massage. Richard declines. He says he wants Hettie to have one. A familiar pattern.

I blend lavender, geranium and bergamot essential oils into the reflexology base cream massage. These oils have the ability to ease stress and fatigue. Hettie loves the smell "I love lavender... I use it at home to help me sleep."

She settles in the recliner, a blanket wraps her into a cocoon, and against the background noise of Richard's nebuliser she quickly falls asleep as I work her feet. Richard reads the paper. He becomes very relaxed during the treatment. His breathing and chest pain have eased, so much, that he now has no need to ask for oromorph. It seems to work both ways–if I treat the patient, I too become very relaxed and vice versa. It is as if Hettie's energy field spreads through the whole room intermingling with other energy fields. As I center energy and massage the physical foot of another, so I massage this wider energy field and help ease the tension. It is profound wisdom. The room becomes still, a sacred place.

Monday, 15th March.

Richard hangs tenaciously onto life. The staff felt he was dying last Friday and then Saturday, then Sunday, but still he hangs on. He moves his head in some deep recognition to my greeting, but then slips back into his oblivion. I stay with him, using Therapeutic Touch to move the heat out of his chest and body until he is cooler and breathes more easily.

Hettie and Sophie arrive. They are pleased but a little surprised to see me as I have not been at the hospice for the past 14 days. I feel guilty, mindful of my neglect. I sense I could have made more of an effort, but had gotten caught up in University work. Although the lack of continuity highlights the need for the hospice to employ therapists to ensure continuity rather than rely on volunteers, I also realise my responsibility to continue to support this family or at least to have informed them I would not be here for so many days.

What is the nature of my responsibility if I choose to be a volunteer? Given the situation again I would have prioritised differently, and yet do I assume I am significant in their lives? Perhaps I am dependent on being needed?

Hettie and Sophie have stayed at Richard's bedside for two days until they were exhausted and frustrated with the waiting and had to retreat to find respite and sleep, both of which have been elusive. Ed has also deteriorated even though he has been visiting and sitting with Richard. Ed's despair is sharpened by his own impending death, the whole family wilting in the face of this double tragedy.

Sophie has pain radiating up the right side of her neck. She accepts my offer to help. I mix marjoram, lavender and pettigrain in apricot kernal carrier oil. It is a delightful aroma. The oils will help with stress and ease her taut neck and shoulder muscles. She sits on a chair. I work the right side of neck and along her trapezius muscle. A large knot is the source of her pain radiating up into her neck. "Ouch," as I slowly untie the knot. Two lesser knots on the left trapezius are similarly loosened. She continues to speak with Kirsty, one of the staff nurses without pause in her constant talk, just like her father! Slowly her talk lessens as she relaxes into the massage.

Afterwards, the pain has eased. She can move her head from side to side again as though the stress has melted away. Her waiting will be easier now.

I say goodbye to Richard and wish him well on his journey for I shall not see him alive again. I give Hettie a hug and my phone number if she or Sophie need my help in the future. I feel sad for I have dwelt within this family and felt their suffering. It is difficult to move away. Part of me wants to sit with them as they journey this last stage. But I sense I would intrude. I must know when to retreat. But how does one know these things? Is it simply intuitive? A sense of being in tune?

Thursday, 18th March.

A blustery March day. Richard's name is missing from the name board. He died at 20:00 on Tuesday. Later, at home, I write a poem in memoriam, as I often do, a moment of closure. Poems capture meaning like no other form of writing. It is cathartic, enabling me to work through my grief for Richard.

Clay

The hard fecund earth beckons
I sense her vibration draw closer
I hear the thin wail of ancestors
Drift across the solemn distance
between this place and that
I hear the lisp of unspoken words
I hear the call of black birds as they
sail on silver currents
Maybe a raven's croak amidst the din
And gathering gloom of earthly life.

I am clay fashioned by spirit to be human
Strings of carbon linked in complex chains
evolved into the body wrapped in spirit;
How many lives passed and those yet to come?

Soon I will be clay again
Returned to the earth
Upon which tender feet will trip in play and dance
To nourish the harvest
So the wheat stands tall and fruitful

I hold the moist clay in my hands,
These hands that heal and ease suffering
And shape the giving clay into a head
Scoop sockets for eyes and lumps for ears;
The senses already formed
And perhaps a mouth so the breath
can flow amongst all the breaths that flow
Moment by moment across the distance
Pause now to sense the space
Turning the earth.

Tuesday, 6th April.

Another blustery cold day—one moment blue sky and the next a hailstone blizzard. Seems to me ideal hospice weather with its turbulent emotions and moments of deep peace, often shifting moment by moment.

Ed wants to get home, but his condition has worsened. He is having antibiotics for a chest infection. It's his birthday tomorrow. Tania, his wife, seems calm on the surface. Indeed she wants no fuss made of her. She copes in this way. Ed is restless, so he surprises me when I offer a foot massage, by saying 'up to me'. He knows how much his mother and father had benefited. During the therapy, his mother-in-law and son, Alex, arrive. Alex simply gazes at me quietly—most unlike his normal boisterous behaviour. Perhaps, he senses, even at his very young age, the significance of healing vibration. Tania's mother is intrigued with what I do. She enthuses about the smell of the aroma-stone I have set up with benzoin, thyme, lavender and marjoram. It is a beautiful mix. I've chosen benzoin to help ease Ed's dry cough, the thyme to help fight the chest infection, the marjoram to help ease his chest and anxiety, and lavender for every possible reason. Benzoin will also help Ed open his heart and mind as he approaches his inevitable death. Holding this intent, these qualities of oils manifest themselves. You might ask how I know this and the rationale for the claims–yet somehow I do know, although not for certain. It is the nature of intentionality to plant the ideas.

Ed thanks me. The foot massage has helped him to relax. Later, I see Hettie. She is tense, her tears on the surface. She finds it almost unbearable to visit because of Richard. She refuses to pass the door to the room in which he died. She rejects my offer of some therapy–that she is too wound up to relax enough to accept the treatment. I wish I could ease her suffering, but I know I can't at this moment. I can accept that. The quality of poise is to be fully present, to acknowledge her suffering, but not absorb it. She suffers and grieves, as she must do–losing her husband and now, helpless, as her son drifts toward death. Such pain and tragedy.

This brief narrative is part of a larger continuous narrative commenced in September 2000, and continuing today. It reflects my commitment as a practitioner to take responsibility for ensuring I am most effective in my practice. My patients deserve nothing less from me.

What I originally wrote in my reflective journal is transformed into a narrative that plots my reflexive journey of becoming more adept at easing suffering. In doing so, I throw light on the nature of suffering and ways in which it might be eased, opening a narrative space for others to consider in terms of themselves and their own practices. This is why I teach through story and narrative.

MODEL FOR STRUCTURED REFLECTION [MSR]

I developed and use the Model for Structured Reflection (MSR) to guide my work (Johns, 2009b, p. 23). Table 14.3, The MSR, comprises a number of sequentially designed cues to explore the depth and breadth of the experience. The first edition was constructed in 1990 through analyzing patterns of inquiry into experience. The intention of the MSR is to enable you to gain insights that will change your practice. Consider each of the cues in relation to my narrative above.

Table 14.3 The Model for Structured Reflection, Edition 15. Adapted with permission, Johns, C. Published in Johns, C. (2010), *Becoming a reflective practitioner*. 4th Ed. Blackwell Publishing: Oxford, In press.

Reflective cue	Link with Carper's Ways-of-Knowing/ reflexivity
Bring the mind home.	personal
Focus on a description of an experience that seems significant in some way [story/ video etc]	aesthetic
What particular issues seem significant to pay attention to?	aesthetic
How were others feeling and why did they feel that way? [empathic response]	aesthetic
How was I feeling & what made me feel that way? [sympathetic resonance]	personal
What was I trying to achieve & did I respond effectively?	aesthetic
What were the consequences of my actions on the patient, others and myself?	aesthetic
What factors influence the way I was/ am feeling, thinking and responding to this situation?	personal
What knowledge did or might have informed me?	empirical
To what extent did I act for the best & in tune with my values?	ethical
How does this situation connect with previous experiences?	reflexivity
How might I reframe the situation and respond more effectively given this situation again?	reflexivity
What would be the consequences of alternative actions for the patient, others and myself?	reflexivity
What factors might constrain me responding in new ways?	Personal/ reflexivity
How do I NOW feel about this experience?	personal
Am I more able to support myself and others better as a consequence?	personal
What insights do I draw from this experience? Am I more able to realise desirable practice?	Framing Perspectives and Being available template

The MSR Cues

The first cue is to *Bring the mind home*. By this, I mean bringing oneself fully present to the reflective moment. I do this by using my breath in much the same way as centering self for Therapeutic touch or meditation. In doing so, we learn to use this technique within practice itself, enabling us to be more present to ourselves and to others within the moment.

The second cue is to *write a description of an experience that seems significant in some way*. Through journaling, we learn to pay attention, so when we return to practice we are more aware of those things we have reflected-on. In doing so, we open all our senses.

The third cue is to tease out *what is significant within the experience*. One story is a microcosm of the whole; it is just a question of what we pull out (i.e., the foreground) from the whole (i.e., the background), to pay attention to, yet never losing sight of the whole. *This is holistic learning*, acknowledging that everything is related and cannot be viewed as separate without losing meaning.

The fourth cue challenges you to consider *how others were feeling and why they felt that way*. I mean *really* felt! The cue challenges the way I might make quick assumptions of others' feelings. It helps practitioners develop what I describe as *empathic inquiry.*

The fifth cue is the other side of the coin–inviting me to *reflect on my own feelings and why I felt that way*. It acknowledges that much of what we perceive is emotionally-driven and that such feelings may interfere with therapeutic work. This cue begins to take us deeper into self and understand what makes us tick. It leads to what I describe as *sympathetic resonance* that, together with *empathic inquiry*, is fundamental to accurately connect with the experience of the other without distortion.

The sixth cue, "*What was I trying to achieve and did I respond effectively?*" gets to the core of my practice. It assumes that all action is purposeful towards desired and effective ends. How would you know if you were effective? What criteria do you use to make such judgment?

The seventh cue challenges me to consider the consequences of my actions, both short-term and longer term consequences, especially those consequences that are hidden beneath the surface of the experience. Through this cue we develop practical wisdom or phronesis (Hansen, 2008). In Native American lore (Jones & Jones, 1996) people considered the consequences of their decisions for seven generations hence. From this perspective, we can sense the necessary far-reaching consideration of consequences.

The eighth cue, "*What factors influence the way I was/am feeling, thinking and responding to this situation?*" challenges me to go deeper into knowing self. Of course, *who I am* is my primary therapeutic tool, and hence, I need to know this 'tool' to use it effectively. Multiple factors influence me, such as expectations from self and others, limited knowing, comfort with certain responses, entanglement, pity, stress, prejudice, resources—the list is extensive (Johns 2009b). This is a difficult cue that usually requires guidance simply because we primarily view ourselves as normative. These influences are also difficult to change as *who I am* has been shaped by learned patterns of relating that tend to be reinforced within everyday practice.

The ninth cue, "*What knowledge did or might have informed me?*" opens the door for me to explore what is termed *evidence-based practice*—the idea of best practice in terms of known efficacy. As I have previously noted, using Schön's argument, there is little evidence to support much of clinical practice, for example, the therapeutic potential of essential oils. However, whatever evidence is available I can meaningfully draw on in relation to the specific situation. Perhaps, it is only through reflection that theory can be meaningfully assimilated into practice.

The tenth cue, "*To what extent did I act for the best and in tune with my values?*" challenges me to consider the ethical basis of my actions and to review my values in terms of their impact on practice. Do we respect autonomy or act with integrity? Words we might easily use to describe our values, such as *compassion* and *presence,* are now held up for scrutiny for their meaning as *something lived* rather than as concepts. To help with this cue I have developed ethical mapping (Johns 2009b).

The eleventh cue, "*How does this situation connect with previous experiences?*" acknowledges that the way we perceive situations, make clinical judgment and respond is governed by what we have done before. We are creatures of habit. It is how we make sense of the world. Unfortunately, these habits become largely unreflective leading to habitual unexamined practice. Thinking we know, we do not inquire. Worse, we become attached to these habits and defensive when challenged—not the recipe for best practice. Every situation within the human-to-human encounter is unique. It has never been experienced before. *As such you must be open to the possibility of the moment without being attached to ways of knowing or doing. It is the basic holistic stance.*

The next three cues anticipate future practice. The first, "*Given the situation again, how might I respond differently?*" is an act of imagination and research and opens the learning space. Of course, how you actually respond is not determined; yet, the cue plants seeds of possibility that might just germinate when faced with new situations (Margolis, 1993). The MSR continues with two supplementary cues, "*How do I now feel about this experience?*" and, "*Am I more able to support myself and others better as a consequence?*"

Reflection is cathartic and healing, enabling difficult feelings and stress to be worked out. Nurses often work in clinical environments that are not supportive; the cues help us to focus and consider how the care environment can become more supportive. I have moved along a reflective spiral, commencing from what is significant on the surface to drawing out *tentative* insights. *Insights change us as people*. They are not conceptual and as such are only recognized through reflection on subsequent experiences.

> Hence, my use of the word tentative; insights are always evolving within the reflexive spiral of being and becoming an effective holistic practitioner.

Reflexivity

As I designed the MSR, I recognized the way each cue opened into each of Carper's Ways-of-Knowing. As such, I adopted Carper's Ways-of-Knowing as a way to comprehensively frame insights (Johns, 1995). In addition, I identified *reflexivity* as another way of knowing—an *anticipatory embodied knowing* nurtured by contemplating potential new ways-of-being in practice, juxtaposed with previous ways of responding, made more explicit through reflection. I emphasize *embodied* because it is more than thinking about how the practitioner will respond in future, similar situations. The practitioner is changed through reflection by gaining insights, even though such insights may not be explicit. We are more than we can tell. Perhaps, another way of describing reflexivity *is being* the breath of life that turns knowledge into knowing as a dynamic, uncertain, ever shifting whole pattern of being shaped around what's unfolding.

> Through reflection on subsequent experiences, insights (or reflexive-knowing) are revealed within the *reflexive spiral of being and becoming*, guided by the intent to realize one's vision of desirable practice.

Moving Beyond Carper

If I grasp at the truth of being, then how can such knowing be captured with frameworks? Carper proved to be too abstract as a meaningful way to capture the essence of *holistic knowing-in-practice*. Holistic knowing, by its very nature, cannot be reduced into such patterns. Practitioners needed something more tangible and practical, more related to their everyday clinical practice. Hence, in the 12th edition of the MSR, I moved *from* framing learning within Carper to using the *Framing Perspectives* and the *Being Available* template.

Framing Perspectives

The Framing Perspectives (Table 14.4), an approach to framing insights and learning, span the breadth of potential knowing. Each is written as a question, such as, *How does this experience enabled me…?* The framing perspectives are, hopefully, self-explanatory. These are more thoroughly discussed and described in Johns, 2009a.

Table 14. 4 Framing perspectives.

Framing perspective	***How has this experience enabled me to:***
➢ Philosophical framing	Confront and clarify my beliefs and values that constitute desirable practice?
➢ Role framing	Clarify my role, boundaries, and authority within my role, and my power relationships with others?
➢ Theoretical framing	Access, critique and meaningfully assimilate relevant theory / research findings with my personal knowing?
➢ Reality perspective framing	Understand the barrier of reality whilst helping me to become empowered to act in more congruent ways?
➢ Problem framing	Focus problem identification and resolution within the experience?
➢ Temporal framing	Draw patterns with past experiences whilst anticipating how I might respond in similar situations in new ways?
➢ Parallel process framing	Make connections between learning processes within my supervision process and my clinical practice?
➢ Developmental framing	Frame my realising of desirable practice within appropriate theoretical frameworks?

As I thought about these questions, I realized that I had no adequate response for the last one, the Developmental Framing Perspective which asks, "How has this experience enabled me to frame my realizing of desirable practice within appropriate theoretical frameworks?" (Johns 2009a, p.78). In my view, no appropriate theoretical framework existed for framing holistic practice; no adequate, tangible models existed. Hence, I constructed my own. I extrapolated it from an analysis of experiences shared by practitioners, who seeking to realize holistic practice, used guided reflection[2]. I call it the Being Available Template (Johns, 2004; Johns & Freshwater, 2007, p.164) .

> A comprehensive approach to frame learning through reflection is offered by *Framing perspectives*. These are a set of lenses that represent the breadth of learning necessary for becoming an effective practitioner.

[2] This was the focus of my PhD studies working with practitioners who espoused holistic values in guided reflection between 1989-1993.

To be a congruent representation of holistic practice, it was essential that the template was not a collection of themes or parts, but something whole in itself. The 'Being Available Template' that was not reducible I called this the Core Therapeutic, expressed as:

> *The practitioner being available to enable the other to find meaning in their health-illness experience and make decisions about their health, and to assist the person as necessary to meet their health goals* (Johns, 2009b, p. 108) .

At its root then, *holistic practice is a working with relationship, centered on guiding others to find meaning.* The extent the practitioner *can* be available seems to be determined along six inter-related qualities, shown in Table 14.5. Whilst each of these qualities might be considered a way-of-knowing in itself, they are only partially sensed within the whole of the experience. They are only known within the unfolding moment in relationship with each other[3].

Table 14.5 Practitioner qualities that facilitate *Being Available.*

1. Intention to realise a vision;
2. Concern for the person/compassion;
3. Knowing the person;
4. The aesthetic response [the ability to make good clinical judgment and respond with skilled appropriate action towards meeting the person's health needs];
5. Poise [or equanimity];
6. Creating an environment where being available can be realised.

Qualities such as *compassion* and *poise* complement each other. Compassion is having room in your heart for the other's suffering, without conditions. Compassion is not so much for the individual, but a *way-of-being* towards the world. As such, it may leave the practitioner vulnerable to the other's suffering, and hence, require a sense of poise, being mindful of one's own and the other's suffering, so one can be fully present to the other without one's own concerns getting in the way. The Being Available template is discussed more fully in Jarrett & Johns, 2007, p. 164; pp. 177-178.

---

[3] For a detailed exposition of the Being Available Template, see 'Becoming a reflective practitioner' (Johns, C. 2009b).

The Burford Model

The quality of *knowing the person* is linked to vision. So if my vision is to ease the person's suffering, I must ask, what is suffering? Not an easy question as suffering is deeply complex. To guide practitioners to know the person, I constructed the Burford[4] model reflective cues, shown in Table 14.6.

Table 14.6 The Burford Model of Reflective Cues.

1. Who is this person?
2. What meaning does this health-illness experience have for the person?
3. How is this person feeling?
4. How has this event affected the person's usual life patterns and roles?
5. How do I feel about this person?
6. How can I help this person?
7. What is important to make this person's stay within the healthcare setting comfortable?
8. What support does this person have in life?
9. How does this person view the future for self and others?

These cues are internalized and become a natural reflective way-of-being in practice. In this way, they are constantly at work as caring unfolds, leading to a narrative approach to clinical practice. Again space does not permit a deeper exploration of these cues.[5] Of course, the beauty of these cues is that they reflect the way practitioners actually think, except perhaps, the cue, "*How do I feel about this person*?" However, as suggested above, this cue is the link to compassion and poise, qualities that are vital for holistic practice.

Finally, a rare quality, *creating an environment whereby the practitioner can be available,* requires assertion, strong self-worth, political nous, campaigning for resources, collaboration, positive conflict skills and the suchlike.

> *Narratives of self-inquiry offer a new approach to nursing scholarship that enables nurses and other health care practitioners to both understand and realize their therapeutic destiny* (Johns 2010, in press).

---

[4] Named after the Burford Community Hospital, England, where the cues were first developed.

[5] For a detailed exposition for the Burford model, see John, C. (2009b).

SUMMARY

The need to conceptualize knowledge is primary in a modernist world as the basis for dong research and teaching. If we don't know, then how can we practice it and teach it? Schemes such as Carper's ways-of-knowing emerged in 1978 in response to this agenda. Reflective practice fundamentally shifts the relationship between practice and theory. It gives primacy to experience, and then forces us to consider how theory might inform practice. It raises questions such as, *"What is the nature of knowing-in-practice?"* And, "*Are such ways really ways-of-being*?" This shifts our focus from an epistemological concern with knowledge to an ontological concern with being, demanding more sensitive and holistic ways to frame patterns of knowing-in-practice.

At the fundamental level, practice or experience can be systematically explored using a model or reflection as a guide. The MSR is the gateway to a hermeneutic spiral of being and becoming who you need to become, a dialogue between the whole and its parts, towards deepening understanding and gaining insights. More appropriate reflective ways of framing insights using the Framing Perspectives and the Being Available Template are proposed as being more sensitive to the nature of being a reflective and holistic practitioner than the use of Carper's Ways-of-Knowing. To be a holistic practitioner is to be a reflective practitioner. Indeed, being mindful is the hallmark of holistic practice—that deep sensitivity to the relationship between self and other based on wisdom and compassion.

Becoming a reflective practitioner requires commitment, curiosity and openness to self and others. It is a discipline, and it takes time and hard work. It is not instant illumination, but embodied fragment by fragment through successive reflections on experience and becoming mindful. Yet, reflection is also playful and imaginative, opening the right brain to its mystery, joy and ways-of-being. Imagine your life and then become it.

CHAPTER 15

EMBRACING THE JOURNEY

Christi A. Holland

Life is a journey. One that is neither linear nor circular in nature – rather one that is a spiral, ever achieving greater heights, with each new discovery, lesson and joy that is found along the way. Yes, life is a journey, but I didn't know it for the first forty-some years of my existence!

OVERVIEW

I offer my life-journey here to remind the reader that while we're all here together, each of us is on our own journey. Each of us has to find our own way, make meaning of his or her experiences, and each has to make choices at each turn in the pathway. This is not something that others can do for us, but it is something that others can help us achieve. Or they can impede our process, depending on how they choose to interact with us, here on this earthly plane.

This is my story. In telling it, I trust it will be of benefit. Perhaps, it will shed some light on your own journey and illuminate your path toward discovery.

Be open, flow with the story, and allow yourself to tap into your own inner knowing, to be activated to a greater and richer level.

BECOMING ENLIGHTENED

Just Living

So, there I was, living my life, moving along on the acceptable trajectory of education, family, career; eating, sleeping, working—just living—being "in the moment" of earthly tasks, oblivious to the fact that there might be a plan for me–a purpose for my existence—that perhaps, I was already on a journey of which I was totally unaware.

I grew up in a very strict, religious blended family, thought I would be a surgeon, but received a scholarship and went to school to be a nurse, got married to a minister, had a beautiful daughter. I did not thrive in the paradigm I found myself in, so I finished my BSN while getting a divorce, then completed my MSN, all while doing the single parent thing. Ultimately, I got married again, developed, built and implemented a heart center that I ran for a bit, went back to school to become a nurse practitioner, worked at that a few years, and once again began looking around for the next "new" thing to do with my career.

My career-path usually took a jog every four or five years, moving from one thing to another, looking for something different and unique. Most often, I would create the role myself, probably to fill a need or to explore a different facet of nursing practice. I had no conceptual understanding, at that time, that I was on a journey or following a plan set out for me.

Then came the first inkling that perhaps there was something more to this thing we call *life*.

A Discovery

We moved to Austin and shortly thereafter I attended a festival/event at Laguna Gloria–one that exhibited the art of many local merchants. I have since discovered that it was there that I had the first glimmer that I was actually being led on a journey....events were being orchestrated by a Higher power in concert with my Spirit to weave my path into the presence of those who would be instrumental in awakening my Soul to its purpose...enlightening my Spirit to fulfill its passion. I didn't realize it then–the clarity came later.

I was drawn to the booth of a local metal sculptor who invited me to visit his gallery. I did, and I met some amazing folks over the course of the next few months. Then, on a Sunday afternoon, I received a call from a person at the gallery, whom I really did not know, who invited me to take a course they were offering called "The Artist's Way" (a book by Julia Cameron, 1993). Now, you may have a little smile of understanding here if you are familiar with this course, but for those of you, who aren't, never fear...neither was I! So I thought, why not? It sounded fun, and off I went.

The first chapter in her book is about synchronicity; I didn't know what it was; it certainly hadn't *happened* to me (that I was aware of!). And then, during the first week, things began to occur—things others might call coincidence, but were now just too obvious to cast aside. It was as though I was suddenly *aware* that perhaps something was afoot, something was with me and all around me; something new, yet something wonderfully comfortable was being shown to me. I was on a journey, with a new appreciation of being guided toward *something*.

> Needless to say, once the process starts, you begin to see the interconnectedness of everything and the succinctness of the points along the path.

Awakening

I could get into great detail, as it excites me to remember and revisit my process, but suffice it to say that I was aware that I was being guided on a specific path, and that my journey was being orchestrated by something beyond my conscious self. Now that I was aware, all I had to do was be willing, open and accepting, to listen, to hear, and most importantly, be willing to follow.

Everyone has that inner voice, although some like to put it off as imagination, wishful thinking, or fate rather than have the courage to run with the delight of it all. I chose to run with delight, to respond to the little nudges here and there, and discover where they took me.

The Nudge

Where would I be if I hadn't followed the *inner nudge* that took me from the boredom of a conference, and into the vendor/booth section in the Spring of 2000, where I spoke with some folks (I don't even remember what we were talking about) who said, "You need to go talk to the guy at the booth at the end of the next aisle." Well, *that guy* was with The University of Texas, Medical Branch, School of Nursing. He was promoting their doctoral program focused on healing, and I knew immediately why I had entered the exhibitor area that day. I had been considering off-shore medical schools, or perhaps, medical law, but the "aha" just wasn't there. Now, I realized that the change I was looking for was to pursue a PhD–not just any PhD, but one from this particular university. For, as I was to find out, mentors (who would later become friends and colleagues) were already in place to provide the safe nurturing environment necessary for my fledgling awareness to grow, develop, and most of all, thrive.

Now, mind you, this is from a nurse who always created jobs outside the box, never working within the parameters of traditional Nursing services because of the restrictions and constraints I always found within that setting. So, to think I would get a *PhD in Nursing* was kind of amusing. I loved my work as a nurse practitioner, and had previously been unable to see how another degree in Nursing would serve me.

But the difference this time was that I listened to my inner self, understanding that it was for a greater purpose–a grander plan that I did not yet understand, but just knew.

Looking Ahead

So, once again–off I went–that is after exploring other doctoral programs closer to home at the behest of my spouse who thought surely something closer would suffice. I did my due diligence with husband in tow. When I exited the Nursing facility in Galveston, he took one look at my beaming face and said, "This is the place, huh?" Interestingly, he had been out looking for places for me to stay during my travels to school; seems he had some inner knowing of his own that I would be making that journey.

At this point, I had an awareness of something, of being guided in a specific way; I had tapped into my inner-knowing without yet understanding what was taking place. Thankfully, though, I proceeded with gusto—the understanding would follow.

Understanding

To really see and feel the warmth of illumination, we must rid ourselves of a lot of baggage that gets in the way. This is because baggage just keeps us from moving along the path, holds us back from being propelled on our journey, and camouflages wonderful and exciting places along the way. The lesson is to disclose our baggage–recognize it, acknowledge it, and get beyond it. Along with many others, that was one of my most important lessons the first semester of my doctoral program.

Integration

One of the exercises in my doctoral program was to describe, in detail, three or four most pertinent stories from our nursing practice. Well, of course, I found this frustrating and irritating, because I thought I had hundreds of experiences from, at that point, my twenty-five year career, but nothing that rose to the criteria of *pertinent*. But after much angst and wrestling with this assignment, *those experiences* finally began to distill, and when they did, I was thrilled–actually in awe–and quite incredulous that maybe, just maybe, I was making another very important discovery for the nurse within.

> "*...I have no stories...*" and so begins the journey of healing, growth toward knowing....

To help the reader understand, I offer my stories. I have italicized those parts of the story that are drawn from my deeper memory.

Case 1

I was a fairly young nurse working in the intensive care unit one evening, caring for a seventeen year-old boy. He had been in the unit a few days and was in a coma, on the ventilator, as a result of a failed suicide attempt. I don't believe that he had left a note, but was found with the rifle in such a position that there could be no other explanation.

Earlier in the day during this particular shift, it had been determined that he was brain dead with no chance of survival. I was told that the mother would be coming to say good-bye, and that we would turn off the life-support that evening. I had never been in this type of situation before and I remember feeling a strange sense of apprehension about the coming event.

Oddly enough, I don't really remember a great deal of detail although the impact of the situation has always stayed with me...

...he was lying quietly in the first bed to the left of the nurse's station, his face swollen and somewhat eccymotic from the effect of the wound. It had entered under the chin and exited out the back of the head, so it wasn't readily visible. He was still and quiet–only the rhythmic sound of machines and beeps from various monitoring devices were heard amid the constant chaos of the ICU. People's lives were moving around him while his lay silently dependent on technology. There was a picture of him above the bed...dressed up, smiling, young...not recognizable here, now, on the ventilator with no response. I couldn't imagine what must have driven him to this fate, and I felt profoundly sorry for the family. Perhaps they had an idea, but what if they didn't? The shock, confusion and grief must have been overwhelming. My time with him was short and I did not get the opportunity to interact with family–only him, and he was already essentially gone.

The mother arrived, and oddly enough, I don't remember saying much to her—although I suppose I must have. The emotion was thick, and I didn't know what to do, but just "be." When she was ready, the machines were turned off, and I stood with her, quietly, my hand touching her back, as we waited and watched until his heart stopped and all essence of her son was gone.

I can't imagine the grief; the sadness was heavy...

I know that from that point I must have pulled all the lines and removed the endotrachial tube, preparing his body for the morgue, but I have no memory of those activities.

Case 2

There had been a rash of seriously ill children in the ICU. We were all quite distressed. It was always draining to be in such a highly charged and intense environment; having innocent children as the victims made it worse. Strained by the emotional toll of so many hopeless cases so close together, we talked about it amongst ourselves, trying to give each other emotional support. At that point we had suicide, child abuse and incurable illness to deal with.

On this particular evening, I was caring for a two-year-old boy who was now terminally ill following encephalitis. He was on the ventilator, no response, brain dead. His family had made the heart-wrenching decision to turn off the life support, but had also decided to have his organs donated. The retrieval was to happen on my shift, and I was asked to accompany him to the operating room…

...he was so tiny and still amid the white sheets–a sterile environment that should have been strewn with toys, dirty fingerprints and treasures that only little boys can find from the out of doors. Dwarfed by the machines that kept him alive, he lay quietly with plump little fingers limp on my own. There was no response as I softly stroked the little hand—torn by the thought that he would not live to experience life, but trying to think of the lives he would be able to save. Soft blond hair curled around his face, long lashes brushed against his ruddy little cheeks–he looked like a sleeping cherub. It was so unfair. He was only slightly older than my own daughter, and I was so thankful and grateful that this wasn't her.

I don't recall ever seeing the parents although I may have, but I couldn't begin to feel their loss–I only know how profound the emotion was for me as I recall the moments, wheeling him in his bed along with the various life-supporting machines, taking him to the waiting room in the operating-suite where his little life would inextricably end. I remember feeling somewhat like I was betraying him although I told myself this wasn't the case. Intellectually, I knew that his short little life was at an end, but I was responsible for caring for him this particular night, and I did not relish the responsibility of taking him to his ultimate and final death.

The hall seemed long; the room was cold and sterile–an air of tenseness was palpable. Everyone was preparing; a recipient was waiting; he was dying. His small body was placed on the table and prepped for the procedure. When all was in readiness, the surgeon's knife poised and ready, the ventilator was turned off. We all waited and watched as the heartbeat finally slowed, time of death was called out, and the incision was made...the heart had not yet completely stopped...

What stayed with me beyond the intense emotion of the experience was the fact that he was not completely legally dead. I knew that the heartbeat was supposed to completely stop, but it didn't. Even though the few seconds between what was supposed to happen and what did happen were really inconsequential in the scheme of things, the preciousness of "life" was not completely respected, and that bothered me.

I remember saying something quietly to someone later, but those details elude me. What sticks with me is the profound emotion of the ending of his life.

Case 3

This story occurred while I was a Nursing student in OB/GYN. I was working in Labor and Delivery and, as usual, it was busy. We had an impending delivery and I was to be assisting with a physician I liked and respected…

...I was the usual nervous, but excited, student. My tray was in readiness at the proper position to the patient's left side above the left stirrup. The patient was ready and the doctor in position. I had worked with him successfully before, so I was calm, but energized for the impending birth.

He looked at me and said, "Do you want to do this delivery?" I laughed nervously thinking he was joking (I think I even said something like, "Oh, yeah, right!"), but he said, "I'm serious, come down here and do this."

I looked around the room at the other nurses for some help because, after all, I was only a student, and I didn't know if I was allowed to do what he was asking. All I recall is some shrugging of shoulders in response. It was a weekend, so the instructor was not around.

The next thing I knew, the physician pulled the tray down, asked me to change positions, and firmly placed me in position to deliver the baby. He was calm and encouraging telling me exactly what to do. I remember the excitement of the moment as well as a healthy fear of the "What ifs..?" I remember feeling the physician's presence over my right shoulder as he guided me step by step in the delivery. I did everything–including the episiotomy.

It was absolutely amazing! I remember not being able to find the words to express how I felt when that new little life burst upon the scene, drawing her first breath and crying lustily. I was so incredibly excited that I could hardly wait for the shift to end, so I could share the excitement and joy of the experience.

I was ecstatic and filled with such wonder and awe and giddy excitement that I felt like I was floating.

Case 4

I was working as a nurse practitioner at a long-term care facility and admitted a 62 year-old man with terminal cancer. He had had colon cancer many years ago and had just been diagnosed with multiple areas of metastases. The one of most concern to him was the one to the brain. This had left him with a seizure disorder which was disconcerting as he was aware of them, and they were painful.

When we met, I introduced myself, explained my role and told him that I would be participating in his care. He asked if I knew about his case—that he was here to die. I told him that I had had the opportunity to review his medical record, so I was aware of his medical condition. More importantly, I told him, I was interested in how he felt about it, how he was doing, how he was coping.

He was very calm and engaging and spoke without hesitation or discomfort. He didn't seem surprised that I asked such a question, and responded readily. He said that he had had a good and full life and that he was prepared for the end. He expressed his desire to keep his mental capacities and to not have pain. He was aware that these two issues were in his future, knew they would have to be addressed, and expressed his desire that they be minimalized as much as possible.

He told me about parts of his life–how he was a marathon runner, loved the outdoors, and rode motorcycles. Interestingly, he did not tell me about his work–only those things that were meaningful, those things that he enjoyed. He expressed concern regarding his family and what they were going through, but overall, he was so calm and accepting that I was intrigued.

I stopped in to see him often, even if only for a quick hello to see how he was doing. He always looked at me directly and calmly, and it was as if there was always an inner connection that superseded our vocal conversations.

Something passed between us that was understood, but went unsaid.

As time passed, he experienced pain and the seizures increased. We talked about it and discussed the type of medications available, their strength, and the potential side effects that might interfere with his ability to think clearly. I always let him know that I was mindful of his wishes and would do my best to honor and respect them. With information that I provided, he would choose what he thought was the appropriate medicine for his pain at that time. His pain increased, but as it accelerated, thankfully, the end came. He was coherent and alert until the event that abruptly led to his death.

His spirit left on a weekend. I was told he was peaceful–just as he had wished.

As I sat back and read the words that had flown off my fingertips and felt the emotionality and depth of these experiences, it was as if blinders simply fell off. I found myself looking at my passion–working with patients making the most significant life transitions of all. I had stories that heralded both birth and death, significant experiences that started as a fledgling nurse, occurred just prior to the "story" exercise, and have continued to this day.

> Was it really *soul transition* work in whatever capacity it chose to exhibit? *What a warm sense of excitement!*

Acceptance

A calm, secure purpose-of-being settled in when I realized that there was so much more to life than that which I had known or understood thus far. Things that were within, that were happening every day, went unrecognized, leaving the personal rewards withering in the depths of a nurse's soul, lost to the fullness of the cause that had once driven it into this profession. This new understanding brought with it validation of my existence, my worth as a healing practitioner, and the role I was here to fulfill.

Now there was much more fulfillment in life experiences, completeness to encounters, and depth of satisfaction—overlooked for far too long. That which was elusive had become real, tangible, and rewarding. A sense of renewed appreciation for nursing brought with it a fresh perspective for practice and a deeper strength of passion toward the care of others.

Soul Work

It was at about this time that I experienced the most amazing awakening of all–one that I can only describe as a true message of enlightenment–one that left me with a simple clarity that I was working on something much greater than a PhD. I was doing exactly what I was called to do. I was in exactly the right place, and was in perfect harmony moving in synchronicity with the Universe. When this sort of moment happens it is exhilarating, dumbfounding, exciting and incredulous–and I found myself in true awe of being called into service fully, wholly, Soul-ly.

There was absolutely no doubt, no question and no trepidation–the transformation into full understanding of inner knowing was not only immediate, but especially amazing, mostly because it did not bring with it an understanding of the how or why—so the lesson became acceptance of what "is" with an excited energy focused on "what" it will be. What a change from how I usually attended to something–my usual approach would be to have to know how, when, where, and with whom. Here, I had none of that–it did not even occur to me to question the process. This was a time when I had no preconceptions, but was just open for what was to come because I just knew it would. I really didn't spend any time trying to figure it out, but just went along my path of work and school with a deep sense of knowing with a little spice of excitement tossed in, wondering what was opening before me.

Clarity

One of the most exciting revelations was that of nature's clarity. I remember driving along the highway and all of a sudden realizing that I could actually see the leaves on the trees and hear the birds rather than let the countryside go by in a blur. It was as if mother earth in all her glory were chiming in to show her support of my newly-awakened self. I found myself exclaiming with glee and talking to beautiful nature that was proudly showing up for my new-found attentiveness. Beautiful wild flowers along the road were heralded for the depth of their hues, the variety of their species, and the tenacity of their adherence to the sometimes precarious roadsides. I was able to experience feeling connected and seeing the world in a whole new light–through a new lens.

Another major insight into the opening of a higher level of consciousness and knowledge of the inner-connectedness occurred the day of 9/11. What a devastating event–one that I felt on the soul level, as I had a clear sense of 880 souls being released and soaring home. That's the only way I know to explain it–I just felt the change at a very deep level–I don't know why I felt that specific number–I just did, and I just knew…and as it so happened, I was driving to Galveston that day–and as I was, I had the profound sense of the changes occurring at the soul level and the adjustments that even nature and the earth were experiencing to begin the alteration to such a catastrophic loss–for after all, we are One, so we were all experiencing this profound loss.

Connectedness

Interestingly enough, during this time frame, we had sold our home in Austin and moved to Houston where my husband had been working for the last year—and what a year that was. We had our home in Austin, his corporate apartment in Houston, and my student condo in Galveston! We would often talk on our cell phones as we were making our commutes until we saw each other on the highway. Then we would wave and blow kisses as we passed each other, feeling connected in even that small way. We often laughed about the situation, but both of us felt like we were where we were supposed to be.

The Catalyst. Soon thereafter, we experienced two devastating financial catastrophes. Not unlike many others at that time, we experienced financial loss and my husband's job was absorbed with an international purchase of the company he had headed.

These unexpected events certainly presented me with an opportunity to run amuck or chase down another avenue, looking to replace what was lost. But that did not even enter the picture as an option. While it certainly presented its share of challenges, we viewed it as a *catalyst* that would move both of us together along the path. In fact, this point could have been devastating to our home and relationship, but instead I found it to be a time of bonding and strengthening–one where we pulled together in support of one another.

Communion. By that time, I was having pretty regular conversations communing with God, nature, angels, and my higher self as I made my way back and forth to Galveston, and it was a time of solidifying the nature of this type of communication–how it could happen with simple thought and openness to the reality of the Divine. Hearing, listening to, and honoring your inner voice, knowing that you are connected to the Universe waylays impatience and fills you with joyful anticipation of what is to come–and as Deepak Chopra says—be invested in the process, not the outcome.

The Vision

In actuality, what occurred in the midst of what seemed to be chaos and disarray was an opening of the vision and a peek into what lay ahead–what I was to do. *It came with clarity in a dream, and while I had no idea how, I simply knew that I would build a healing sanctuary, and that it would be for individuals seeking personal and/or interpersonal healing working through life transitions.* I almost immediately sketched out the property layout and marveled that I was called upon for such a task.

Synchronicity. My husband's field is marketing and advertising. He had always been either the owner of his business or the top executive. He felt that it was unlikely that he would have ever willfully exited the corporate world without the big nudge of international acquisition. While certainly taking some adjustment, it gave him the opportunity to return to more grass roots marketing that we thought would better prepare him to partner with me as the vision unfolded.

I found the time at UTMB working on my doctorate to be one of incredible personal and professional growth. Incredulously, I felt nurtured, supported, encouraged, and cared for–so very different from my early experiences as a nurse that had left me empty and unfulfilled nearly driving me from the profession. It was really one of the most exciting and fulfilling times of my life, and as this growth occurred, so did the vision–and as the vision unfolded, it was so deliciously right. The clarity was without comparison and I found that I had acquired a deep sense of calm and knowingness about the fact that "it" would come to pass.

Close on the heels of that revelation came the understanding that I was to include, somehow, a peaceful living environment for our elders, one that did not function under the traditional medical model, but one that supported the mind, body, and spirit as both families and individuals prepared for the final life transition; one that openly honored the spiritual nature of this event.

I had experienced the importance of this in practice when my elderly patients who were nearing death would whisper to me about their deceased loved ones who had arrived to help them get ready. Somehow they knew that I would understand and not think them delusional or psychotic. I was so blessed that our spirits recognized within one another acceptance of this process—a process that exhibits such a thin veil between our worlds. I just wished that I could physically see what my patients were seeing and experience this beautiful event as they did. They did not look upon it with fear and trepidation, but with longing, and a little bit of excitement; they were completely comfortable and grounded in the reality of what they were experiencing.

What a joy–if only we could more proactively assist in this transition as it is supposed to occur–allow and support the spirit to soar and fly free on its journey, rather than burden it by holding the body down with the process of medical knowhow–just because it is available doesn't mean it is justified. That's another story, but hence my desire to create a beautiful setting to support this transition that is as pivotal as birth–the circle of life.

Spiritual Growth

Along with the unfolding vision came opportunities for learning–opportunities to stretch my capacity of spiritual growth, to investigate and experience learning on a higher plain–one that embodied a deeper sense of clarity and understanding. It seems like it was a test to my commitment, because it came at a time when we experienced financial loss, and at a time when I would once have said, "We really can't afford to do that." But times had changed for me and they were no longer bound by previous constraints.

So with my husband's blessing, I set out on an adventure to study *Angel Therapy* with Doreen Virtue, an experience that expanded my awareness of all things spiritual, and cleansed my soul in preparation for the journey laid out before me. Beautiful moments of deep peace and understanding were coupled with the unfolding of new ways of knowing that finally resonated to the depth of my soul and affirmed my soul's work with life transitions.

Letting Go

As my journey progressed, I came to understand that *letting go* and *forgiveness* were paramount to *opening of self*, and necessary for soul work. I didn't have to drive the ship any longer–for who was I kidding–I hadn't been driving all along! I had been floating along buffeted hither and yon by life's whims and experiences while learning lessons along the way and making progress on my life journey.

Illumination

It seemed like once the illumination occurred, I was being thrown at warp speed along the trail—there was so much to learn and so much to know that while I continued to add arrows to my quiver of knowledge, it seemed like I could only skim the surface when what I wanted to do was hunker down and sink my teeth deeper into a fuller sense of understanding of each lesson that came my way.

However, it came to me that these lessons were being presented for recognition and understanding, not necessarily for mastery. I discovered that those with a broader scope and deeper level of understanding merged into my path to offer reference and strength of foundation to this process. I began seeing how when the time was right, messengers would be sent to offer encouragement or share like dreams and journeys that would keep me invigorated and energized.

TRUSTING THE VISION

So, more on the story…I finished my doctoral work and soon after we moved back to Austin. Bear in mind, that at this point I held the vision, but still had no earthly idea how or when it would take place–I just knew it would. I went about my life, taking care of the elderly as a nurse practitioner and teaching at the university, all the while wondering how this was going to come about. It was 2004, and while I did not have a glimmer of how it would materialize–I just had a deep confidence that it would–and around the holidays that year I just knew that something pivotal would happen in 2005 to begin bringing the vision to fruition.

Of course, I'm thinking…I must be going to meet someone, a benefactor or someone with a like vision with income to sustain such a project…or perhaps I would win the lottery (but that didn't seem the way). Anyway, here's what happened.

The Dream

I had a dream that tapped into my inner knowing, and I understood. I woke up on that Friday morning in August 2005 with a clear sense that I needed to open a healing center as the first step–an integrative practice that would care for patients from the mind, body, spirit perspective, and one that would nurture and provide a place for healing. I went downstairs and told that to my husband—that I needed to open a healing center, and from it everything else would flow.

Intention

Looking back, it seems like I might have thought "Wow! That's too daunting of a task." But, you know, that never entered my mind! It was simply a given–I had been told and I instantly set off to do it!

I knew what it needed to look like, so we set out that morning exploring neighborhoods for appropriate space. We settled on the second place that we seriously considered and worked through the contract, signed the lease and began the building process. I was having a marvelous time manifesting the dream and creating the center. I envisioned it to be warm, inviting, nurturing, beautiful, peaceful, and healing. And that is exactly what transpired. The intention was held without waver during the months of building, and I lived the "Secret" before I knew it had a name and a process!

Watching the ebb and flow of the process was exhilarating and exciting! To feel so connected with Spirit and so engaged with the process of my life plan was phenomenal. So, 14 months after I had dreamed of building a healing center, and 8 months after signing the contract and starting the office construction, we were ready to open!

Before any client or patient came through the door, we had an intimate, beautiful blessing ceremony with just the practitioners and a Spiritual leader in attendance. Each space and each participant were anchored and blessed while the entire space was cleansed with the intention set to deliver healing care for the highest good of each person who entered our space. At the same time, I had requested simultaneous prayer go up from family and friends who participated in this blessing with us. Prayers were anchoring us from Florida, California, Oklahoma, and northern Texas. It was a very moving time, and I was overflowing with gratitude and filled with wonder that I had been given this task—it was just me, after all–and a multitude of angels, both on earth and in heaven.

The Challenge

Staying the Course

Now, the doors were open. What came next was the challenge of maneuvering a spiritual practice in the physical world. Now the bills had to be paid, and the practice had to be managed! I soon found that the business of running a practice was just that–a business–and really not what I signed up for! However, it had to be done, and I was the only one to do it. There is a lesson in there somewhere; I just know it!

As this was a new venture, I continued to work and care for patients in Skilled Nursing Units, Assisted Living, and Long-Term Care. While I was very thankful for income from my outside jobs, I was left with little time to work on the growth of the healing center. Sometimes, I wondered if lack of faith that the healing center would grow rapidly enough for financial concerns kept me tied to the other jobs, but there was no choice at that time. I have since come to realize that time has allowed me to continue to learn and further educate myself to care for patients in the new setting in the new way that was needed; and to know myself more fully.

Self-Knowing. I had a strict upbringing in a home heavily influenced by religion and control based on guilt and punishment. The ensuing philosophy was the epitome of a modernistic paradigm. There really was only one way, and it was the right way. I grew, but I did not flourish.

I floundered while trying to live my life from this perspective, and thus, I became adept at ignoring philosophy even while secretly struggling with my soul. What I actually struggled with was the whole concept of religion and its influence, without realizing that there was an overall philosophy to be understood. I didn't have to worry about paradigm because I could not articulate what one was!

I am touching on personal issues because I do not feel that I am what I am or can know what I am or know what I know without acknowledging the most human of all components—my Self.

Philosophical disarray creates chaos. Nowhere was this more evident than in my life. I thought I knew that what I had been taught in my upbringing was right. At least I had been told that it was the only way, and that if anyone tried to teach another religion or philosophy, it was wrong. Don't be fooled they would say–it's just the devil in sheep's clothing leading you astray!

It was difficult to keep that influence at bay while trying to be open to new ideas and philosophies. I am, however, comfortable with my self and the direction I am heading. I can now own the feelings of ambiguity with a sense of knowledge from personal history. What I now know is that my historical philosophy may be right for those who taught me, but it is not right for me.

Of course, I am not dismissing all aspects of my upbringing, but am now aware that I don't have to buy the whole bushel of apples to get one good one. I can pick and choose, and keep or discard information as I answer the most intriguing of all questions, "What is right for me?" From what perspective do I live my life, and what philosophical paradigm resonates with me? What is useful to my life and to my practice?

It was a confusing struggle for some time as I tried to get some sense of my self, and this impacted all aspects of my life. I struggled with the question, "What do I really know?" because what I know and what I am supposed to know are two different things. Coming to this realization was a deep relief and a sense of release to explore new options.

Self-Integrity. After my healing center had been open a couple of months, I realized that I had a little nagging–dare I say–doubt? No, there was never any doubt, but I did acknowledge what is really best described as a *strange little fear* deep in my gut about just what I was trying to do–about being successful, and at some level I wondered if I was dragging my feet and not going for the gusto because I was afraid of being a success?

Now, how weird does that sound after all I've already said? Well, its honesty and I have found that above all else we must walk our journey with integrity and perform our healing work for the highest good of others, not for what we think is important, but for what their spirit needs and has presented itself to claim. So, above all else we *must* be honest with ourselves! After all, what type of preparation did I have to run a business? What type of training did I have to undertake such a task?

Folks who had felt called to do similar type of work would ask me at times how I knew what to do, had I taken some course or followed some business plan—and indeed these same questions would be thrown at me at a later time when issues of business management caused some greater challenges for me on a personal level.

My answer is, "Nothing formal, only life lessons and the faith to follow that inner voice—my higher self at the deepest level of inner knowing—knowing at my core—that this was my passion, my journey, my destiny to fulfill on this earthly plane."

Self-direction. I talked to myself and tried to keep upbeat and focused with the intention set for growth and healing success for the practice. Let me tell you, this can be an issue when constantly confronted by financial constraints, but I was so confident that what I was doing had been asked of me, and what was given to me was really from God, that I held my head high, looked ahead with calm confidence and worked harder to support the vision.

Self-reflection. As I continued on the path of personal growth, I found myself taking a deep look inside to understand where any misplaced fear about the success of the practice was coming from. Incidentally, this was at a time when I had signed up to take a class with Sonia Choquette on being a sixth sensory practitioner–understanding and following your voice at a higher level and being able to understand and connect beyond our five usual senses.

Just like the Doreen Virtue class, I almost didn't go because of financial constraints, but felt compelled, and once again followed that feeling and went. And oh my! What an experience—one of the best of my life–and one where I was able to understand where that little seed of fear came from–and once I understood, that let me know how to begin working with it and putting it aside with the confidence that I was indeed on the right track.

I also experienced more blessings of understanding how my spiritual guides were assisting and supporting this process. It was like fine-tuning at a higher level of consciousness. It was a time to be with like spirits, to celebrate self and our life journeys, to see the interconnectedness of the universe and to be thankful for my place in it all.

The Dark Times

I needed those joyous times of kindred fellowship to lift my spirits and fill my emotional tank because the "work"–while exhilarating when able to look forward and up, could also be quite depleting at times. Periods of carrying the burdens alone made me bend over, barely able to just look at one step at a time–seeing no further than each step ahead. But if that's what it took, that's what I did. I refused to be beaten–not because I was stubborn, but because I could not fail my life-plan–that which was given as my duty to fulfill. Now that I knew, there was no option or choice of quitting. Knowing that we are spiritual beings here in this space and at this time for a purpose did not allow for any other overall response. I now know when I'm aligned with God and Spirit and when I'm not—that feeling of being slightly askew without really knowing how or why, helps me attend to the path.

In retrospect, I must acknowledge periods of frustration, and sometimes overwhelming pressure, as I tried to juggle all I was doing while holding everything up and in its proper place. It would feel very heavy at times, trudging along, often feeling quite alone on a path that was (at that moment) feeling narrow and hazardous. During those times, my pace may have been slowed, but my spirit remained determined.

The Need for Others

What is found on this journey is a gathering of like-spirits moving along with synchronicity that completes the picture, filling up those missing bits of knowledge in a loving, willing way. These beautiful like-minded journey-partners extend helping hands and lift us, at times, over rough spots, merge together to carry us through dark times, and whose own strengths and beliefs sustain us.

The Reward

Sharing the daunting darker places of the journey is part of the honesty in sharing the story. Nothing is without work or without struggle, for it is in those times that we find our strength, learn the depth of our fortitude, and find the ability to shine even brighter as we forge through the fire. We come around the bend not broken of spirit, but with a lighter, more sure-footed step, a thicker skin perhaps, but with a deeper glow of contentment as we draw closer to fulfillment.

I have been provided a map and have been given sustenance for my journey. The path has been illuminated by knowledge and the enlightenment for change has created a stored energy source for the future. There is now a proportional escalating response in relation to knowledge and growth. As I learn, I grow. As I grow, my ability to illuminate others develops. I have likened this to the example of a simple flashlight. They come in various sizes with varying degrees of illumination depending on the bulb and the strength of the light source.

I started as the tiniest of lights with the smallest of batteries and have grown a few sizes to a brighter bulb with an intermediate light source. I have grown as a result of input from multiple knowledge sources that have illuminated my path enabling me to grow stronger and more self-sufficient. I still do not have adequate light source to independently see all that lies ahead, or to be able to share the journey in its entirety with others. However, I can now see my path more fully and there is sufficient light to be able to share the path with others.

> The enlightenment had occurred. The wonder and fascination of the journey continued.

We cannot "make" this happen, we cannot manipulate a true vision into fruition, but we *can* know that we are spiritual beings in human bodies moving together with open hearts in loving gratitude of understanding. We are One; we are built the same, but our journeys are unique. Claim those differences. If it seems difficult, push through and emerge with a radiant understanding and deeper sense of knowing that will enlighten your path and forge the journey ahead.

I do know that I have opened my *self* to the clear and beautiful energy of the Heavens available to each of us and have made discoveries that I had not even the slightest inkling about a few short years ago. I celebrate the glorious moments, acknowledge the ones that make me stronger, and honor the wisdom of the Universe that is available for the asking.

I have learned that none of this is about me. It is about being an open and willing vessel available for use by the master potter–that molding is pivotal for strength and clarity; both are paramount for holding the vision and staying the course.

AN ANALYSIS

Once I understood that I was truly being guided on a journey, I could see that it was not a meandering trail, but rather an ever-upward spiraling path, filled with both beauty and challenging obstacles along the way–all to be considered lessons provided to hone our skills, lessen our burdens, and heighten our commitment.

Now, I must say that temptation presented itself–little side roads that one could run down or veer off on…and while I'm not saying there wasn't some sightseeing along the way, or an eagerness to jump to the end and see what's around the corner, I found that in doing so, the journey was only waylaid, the lessons weren't fully learned and the foundation would weaken.

What is it that keeps us steadfastly on the path focused toward the unfolding of our life work? I must say it is the strength of vision and commitment to fulfill it, once known. For I have held the vision with calm assuredness and have had the strength to forge ahead even when times were tough. If we actually listen to our inner voice and respond, the path illuminates–and it's much easier to maneuver in the light!

Reflecting

Where do I begin? Twenty-four years is a long time to be in a profession without having the realization of the impact that was being made, both personally and professionally, or having the Ways-of-Knowing to fully understand and explore the process. Carper's identification of the four patterns of knowing helped to shed light on this.[1]

Having been developed in 1975, this frame of reference for Nursing practice was not taught in the mid-1970s when I was in Nursing school, although the first pattern, *empirics*, was the acceptable way of knowing at that time. Carper posits that empirics, defined as the science of Nursing, is knowledge that is systematically organized into theories and laws. Empirical knowledge explains, describes, and predicts phenomena in Nursing. Nursing was presented more from this frame of reference as well as from the task point of view. Measurable and observable data are considered empirical in nature.

The *aesthetic* way-of-knowing is described as the art of Nursing and includes the concept of empathy, explaining the capacity for participating in someone else's feelings. The art of Nursing is in the moment. It is how we are and how we know what we know. It is expressive rather than descriptive or formal. The *ethical* pattern is the moral component. Herein arise dilemmas with ambiguity and uncertainty. These are matters of obligation, and this is where Nursing focuses on what ought to be done.

---

[1] While discussed more fully in Chapter 2, I offer it here as the context for my thoughts.

Finally, the *personal* way-of-knowing is heralded by far to be the most difficult one to master while being the most essential in understanding the meaning of health as it pertains to the individual and to their well-being. It is through personal knowing that we gain insights into how our philosophy impacts our ability to care for others and to adequately facilitate a healing environment, from their perspective (Nicoll, 1997).

> Through uncovering my personal knowledge, I came to know what I really know and was propelled along the path toward discovering the *how of knowing*.

Personal Knowing

Being unaware of the essence from the lived experiences of my earlier days is only acceptable now because they have been awakened as wonderful memories that can be drawn upon for reflection, growth, and learning. It is profound to think that they were buried so deeply that *realization of their presence*—let alone their meaning—was absent. We must make every effort to see that this does not continue to happen to our future nurses. They must know their heritage and have the opportunity to embrace it to the fullest extent.

Dearth, stagnation and staleness of *being* were replaced by a fresh sense of wonder regarding daily practice, a stirring of excitement for future discoveries and a renewed sense of *well-being* regarding the profession of Nursing. I have gleaned the rarest of pearls from this experience. I have been given back the *why* of becoming a nurse, and not a day or encounter goes by without a thought about *what is really going on here* as I connect in the experience and engage with the patient accordingly. The path was illuminated; detail intricately displayed; the intrigue of discovery was beckoning.

> To understand that there is meaning to practice and significant implications for future practice is marvelously invigorating.

Certainly, the perspective from which I was functioning was haphazard at best. If it was from any particular paradigm, it was borrowed or pressed upon me from elsewhere. I had not made a conscious decision or discovery of my own regarding the perspective that was right for me. It was something that I kept in the back of my mind while struggling silently along the way with ambiguity, and without a knowledge base from which to begin to facilitate a change. I came to understand that the philosophy from which I lived was a hodgepodge of rules and regulations, learned family dynamics and religious influence that had previously sculpted my life.

I was never comfortable in those shoes, but had never been given permission to get new ones. There was only one style available that was right and correct, and it was the only one to be worn, regardless of fit. If they caused pain, then pain was a necessary evil, caused most assuredly, by the one wearing the shoe – not the shoe itself!

As Kuhn (1996) says, it is time to discard and move on when the current paradigm no longer works or is unable to answer your questions. He explains that when multiple questions or anomalies occur which impact the paradigm, it causes unrest and subsequent revolution resulting in the destruction of the old paradigm and the emergence of the new one. I think this is quite apropos to what was at work in my life, and although I did not adhere to the rigidity of Kuhn's thinking, the principle is similar.

Certainly, multiple issues were present that questioned the historical paradigm and called for change. A new paradigm was rising through the rubble and there was certainly no looking back as it emerged, especially since there was no ownership with the old one. There was, however, ownership with the change.

I look back because it is the knowledge of our personal history that translates into the basis of who we are. It may be that the knowledge begets change, which is relevant to this case. I am who I am by virtue of what I have been, what I have been through and how that has affected me in my lifetime. I look back, so that I can learn from my mistakes and from my experiences whether positive or negative.

I reflect upon the wealth of memories that have accumulated, so I can grow from the knowledge that exudes from them. I look back and savor the time spent with patients, savor my role as the nurse who had the ability to truly impact their healing journey, and be content in the place in which I find myself.

Holistic Knowing

Nursing has been a part of me, as well as been infused through me. Caring, nurturing, helping, giving, loving, and creating healing environments is something I see myself doing in all aspects of life. It is like a dimension of my self that is more than that defined by a profession.

It is my sense of well-being that springs from helping others. I believe that these attributes and concepts cannot be isolated to only one component of life if the goal and desire is to assist others on their healing journey. I do not think it is possible to encapsulate this to only one life compartment.

The Impeders

I have spent a lot of time in the Nursing profession, trying to change and trying to be anything but what I was, simply because I had had such negative experiences within the profession by those who served as models. Those who should have been positive mentors most certainly were not. In my previous experience, there was no room for autonomy, thinking outside the box, or developing new roles that were on the edge for nursing practice, but still well within the scope of Nursing.

There was a negative sense of competitiveness and a striking component of rigidity that I did not wish to associate with. I was drawn away from the profession and found myself on the cusp between medicine and Nursing, functioning in an advanced practice role. I was comfortable functioning in the medical model, as this was the model I was initially trained under although it did not meet my needs from the nursing perspective that I had grown to appreciate for myself. Having not been able to find a level of comfort and satisfaction within my own profession, I actively sought, at several junctures, to go to medical school. I had been readily accepted by physicians, and finally thought that entering that paradigm would be the best option.

The Facilitators

Finding the program at UTMB with its central construct of healing was the overall enlightenment toward the illumination of my soul and resurgence of a love and connection for the profession I originally began. With the program philosophy geared toward a process of mutuality and the belief that all of us have unique and varied talents that are valued equally, I began to feel that I had finally come home. I had found my niche among those of like mind and spirit.

An Emerging Practice Model. Earlier I spoke about my stories–about the stories I didn't think I had, but stories that once uncovered will inform the rest of my life experience. Learning about my personal practice and what was important to me through my stories was a remarkable experience. Every nurse should have the opportunity to participate in this enlightening experience, for not only did it open a world of soul discovery, it informed the creation of a model that delineates my personal healing practice and depicts what I believe is happening and is pivotal in the nurse-patient relationship.

Being introduced to the Modeling and Role Modeling (MRM) Nursing theory was like coming home in a way. You might have already gleaned from all that I have said…I was not a proponent of Nursing theory–except for what I "endured" while in school. Previously, I thought, what does that have to do with practice? When will I ever utilize that information? Well, here I stood with all of my discoveries and enlightened world-view and I finally got it. It is the pattern of personal knowing that became obvious through my syntheses of cases that enabled me to develop the Stabilization Model for Transcendent Healing (SMTH).

Linked to the grand theory of Modeling and Role-Modeling, my synthesized practice model operates from the following assumptions and propositions shown in Tables 15.1 and 15.2, respectively. Related concepts are described below.

Table 15.1 Philosophical beliefs: The Stabilization Model for Transcendent Healing.

Life is an ongoing process. A state of health is desired. When illness occurs, there is no longer a state of health. Without a state of health, a need exists. Nursing is a nurturing profession that strives to help those in need. Nurses help when illness occurs.

Table 15.2 Propositions: The Stabilization Model for Transcendent Healing.

Life is a journey that is transcendent in nature. The journey consists of constantly active interactions. Human beings have a life force that is interactively connected. Connection occurs knowingly or not with subsequent cause and effect–often of unknown magnitude. Health is desired and is a state of dynamic equilibrium. Illness results in disrupted equilibrium. Nursing interactively facilitates and mobilizes stabilization of the environment, so that healing can occur. Healing transcends illness to allow a return to equilibrium.

Connection occurs when the nurse recognizes disrupted equilibrium within a client and begins to view the disruption from within their framework and perspective.

Engagement occurs as the nurse begins to acquire an understanding of the client's world by developing a mirror image of the situation from their perspective. The nurse engages the client in the process as information is gathered (intuitive or concrete) and synthesized while being mindful to evaluate the situation from the theoretical perspective.

Stabilization is the process by which the nurse plans and implements interventions to create a healing environment unique to the client. It is an interactive process between the client and the nurse, whose recommendations are developed with respect to the theoretical base for the practice of nursing.

Transition is the state in which the client successfully fulfills the mutual plan developed in concert with the nurse, and equilibrium occurs.

Transcendence continues as the client separates from the stabilizing environment to proceed along the life journey having transcended the disruption.

Linkages to MRM
The linkages to the MRM grand theory are described as follows:

Modeling is exhibited during the phases of *Connection* and *Engagement.* The *act* of modeling begins as the nurse makes the connection with the client and views the perceived need from within their framework. The *art* of modeling occurs as the nurse engages the client and develops an understanding of the client's world by developing a mirror image of the situation from their perspective. The *science* of modeling occurs during the engagement process as information is gathered (intuitive or concrete) and analyzed, while the nurse evaluates the situation from the theoretical perspective.

Role-Modeling occurs during the *Stabilization* phase. During this process, the *art* and *science* of role-modeling are developed as the nurse creates a healing environment unique to the client while planning interventions with respect to the theoretical base for the practice of nursing. This allows for the return of equilibrium (Erickson, 1990).

Looking forward

Revisiting my practice model has been an enlightening experience. The SMTH is the perfect model for my healing practice and needs to be brought to the fore in this process. I plan to further the development of this model and bring it to mainstream Nursing as I proceed on this journey. It has potential for Nursing education, research and practice. If we can find a way to impact our profession at the entry level with development of the personal way-of-knowing, then I believe that Nursing can and will be impacted in a very powerful way. People are hungry for connection and interaction and I believe those of us in the healing profession are there for much the same reason.

I have learned so much, and yet, there is so much to learn. I have been awakened to my vision, am on a path of enlightenment, and have experienced subsequent change along the way. The old paradigm is gone and in its place is the growth of a new one. There is a lifetime of work to do, of learning, of knowing, of being, of sharing. Isn't it convenient that that is exactly what I have before me–a lifetime?

SUMMARY

Writing my story has brought forth nostalgia, laughter, and at times, tears. It has also re-invigorated and re-energized my desire to create and maintain true healing environments for those I encounter on this life journey. Focused on honoring the Spirit in each of us, I welcome the friends and guides who join me along the way as I continue to press toward full implementation of the vision given to me to fulfill.

It is interesting that as I move through this process it becomes ever clearer that I am simply the willing conduit for this work. Life is about movement, growth, expansion of heart, transcendence of spirit, and attending to tasks pertaining to our unique journeys. Learn from the past, engage in the present and seek out opportunity for the future. “What ifs” don’t exist, so spend time fully present in the moment, open to the wisdom and flow from the Universe. And embrace the Journey……Namaste.

EPILOGUE

Helen L. Erickson

THE PURPOSE

This book was designed to advance discussions among nurse educators and nurse leaders regarding three key questions:

> *How do we advance the discipline of Nursing so that we close the gap between knowledge and practice?*
>
> *How can we prepare novices of our profession so that they are not only competent, ethical practitioners, but also assertive, altruistic members of the profession, able to utilize Nursing's knowledge base?*
>
> *What can we do, as educators, to facilitate nurses to become integrated holistic professionals?*

Each section was intended to focus on one of these questions; each also built on the other, to some extent. Interestingly, as usual, this work has taken on a life of its own. This is because the contributing authors rose to the occasion, and went beyond my expectations. While I had laid out the questions I hoped to address, some responded with work that *just needed to be printed.* As a result, the work presented herein has exceeded my expectations.

I know that each author struggled at times, aiming to write something profound, only to discover that it is difficult to write what we know to be true in our hearts, but sometimes don't have words to express. Each wished to write words of wisdom, only to learn that wisdom is not just cognitive knowledge, but also *knowing* drawn from within, and for some, from a higher source. Perhaps this is what Christopher Johns calls *What I know to be true, but not for certain.* In any case, each author aimed to offer you something of worth, something that will help you go beyond their words to a new level of *knowing*.

I launched this book with a discussion of systems and system characteristics, indicating that we view Nursing as a system, interacting with others, and all existing within the context of a larger system or suprasystem. I had hoped that you would be able to carry those thoughts with you as you read the following chapters. Perhaps, the most important concepts discussed were those that described the characteristics of systems. Specifically, the concepts of *power bases, driving, and restraining forces* are significant considerations for anyone wishing to use what is written in this text and become more proactive in Nursing. As I said in that first chapter, Nursing is a "sleeping bear." I stated in the second chapter that *our philosophy is the driving force behind our actions* and either stated or implied that our philosophy determines how we exert power, how decisions are made, strategies designed, and people selected as colleagues. I would be thrilled if this book nudges just one more nurse to rise from hibernation and speak out for a more compassionate model of healthcare.

Throughout the book, we've reminded the reader that students or novice nurses are *human beings, with feelings and needs.* They are vulnerable because they usually lack power in the system, yet they encounter challenging, and sometimes traumatic experiences in the normal course of practice. Unfortunately, the current norm is to ignore or discount these experiences, leaving the nurses to deal with them by themselves. A related issue, discussed throughout, is the role of the educator in creating strong, competent professional nurses.

Faculty and other nurse leaders don't always stop to think about their students or colleagues as *active learners*, but instead, they are often perceived as *passive recipients* of their teaching. Stressed by the responsibility to *teach Nursing,* nurse educators often focus on what students *must learn* or *haven't learned*, rather than how they can facilitate them *to learn and think.*

Sometimes when this happens, faculty interacts with students in ways that have the potential to be hurtful. As a result, rather than facilitating them to learn, become more skilled and informed, *and* find meaning in their experiences, some faculty's attitudes and behaviors have the effect of impeding growth. Usually, these educators are not mean or bad people, they have simply lost sight of the bigger perspective. They fail to remember that students are humans, trying to do their life-work, and that educators are responsible for facilitating them on their journey.

Since these events often happen during the usual course of the *teaching-learning* experiences, some novices conclude that this is normal, that they need to be able to detach from their clients, ignore the humanity of those in their care, be tough and *do their job.* Others decide that they are incompetent or not worthy. We concluded with one nurse's life-journey, impacted negatively by individuals and systems, but able to find her way when facilitated by faculty and peers; an experience that usually occurs when the *teacher* views his or her role as a *mentor*. How wonderful it would be if all nurse leaders and educators would view themselves as mentors, ready to guide the young, novice nurse (including formal students) or mentee, into a more humane, compassionate healthcare environment.

We hope that you, the reader, will take our work for what it is meant to be—*a source of knowledge, a stimulant for knowing, and a catalyst for self-discovery.* If you are able to read our work, nod your head at least one time, perhaps, smile knowing that you already knew what is being stressed, and know in your heart that you have learned something more—or if you wish to share any part of this work with one other person—then we will know that we have accomplished our goal.

Thank you for your interest in our work. We welcome feedback and dialogue, knowing that there is much to learn when we are open to discovery.

Best always,

Helen L. Erickson,
Editor

BIBLIOGRAPHY

INTRODUCTION

Cruess, S. R., Johnston, S., & Cruess, R. L. (2004). Professionalism: A working definition for medical educators. *Teaching and Learning in Medicine, 16* (1), 74-76.

Cruess, S. R., Cruess, R. L., & Steinert, Y. (2008). *Teaching Medical Professionalism.* Cambridge, UK: Cambridge University Press.

Sullivan, W. M., & Shulman, L. S. (2004). *Work and Integrity: The crisis and promise of professionalism in America.* New York: Jossey-Bass.

Iwasiw, C., Goldenberg, D., & Andrusyszyn, M. A. (2009). *Curriculum Development in Nursing Education.* Sudbury, MA: Jones and Bartlett Publishers.

Locsin, R. C., & Purnell, M. J. (Eds.). (2009). *A contemporary nursing process: The (un)bearable weight of knowing in nursing.* New York: Springer Publishing.

CHAPTER 1

American Holistic Nurses Association. (2007). *Holistic nursing: Scope and standards of practice.* American Holistic Nurses Association: Silver Springs, MD.

American Nurses Association. (1980). *Nursing: A social policy statement.* Washington, DC: American Nurses Association.

Auger, J. (1976). *Behavioral Systems in Nursing*. Inglewood Cliffs, NJ: Prentice.

Duncan W. J. (1978). *Essentials of Management* (2nd ed.). New York: Dryden.

Erickson, H. (1985, March/April). New challenges for nurses. *DCCN,* 99-100.

Erickson, H., Tomlin, E., & Swain, M. A. (1983/2009). *Modeling and role-modeling: A theory and paradigm for nursing.* Englewood Cliffs, NJ: Prentice-Hall. Second-ninth printing, 1988-2009; Cedar Park, TX. EST Co.

Hall, A. D, & Fagen, R. E. (1968). Definition of a system. In W. Buckley (Ed.), *Modern Systems Research for the Behavioral Scientist.* Chicago: Aldine Publishing Co.

Ludwig von Bertalanffy, K. (1968). *General System theory: Foundations, Development, Applications*. New York: George Braziller.

Maslow, A. H. (1968). *Toward a Psychology of Being* (2nd ed.). New York, NY: Van Nostrand.

Nightingale, F. (1873). A subnote of interrogation. *Fraser's Magazine*, 567-577.

Santayana, G. (1905-6). Reason in Commonsense. In G. Seldes (Ed.), *The Great Thoughts* (p. 367). New York: Ballantine Books.

World Health Organization. (1947). *Chronicle of the World Health Organization* (Vol. 1). New York: United Nations.

Young, P. L., & Olsen, L. (2009). *The healthcare imperative: Lowering costs and improving outcomes. Workshop summary* (p. 4.). Washington, DC: The National Academies Press.

CHAPTER 2

Abdellah, F. G. (1957). Methods of identifying covert aspect of nursing problems. *Nursing research, 6*(4), 118-124.

American Holistic Nurses Association. (2007). *Holistic nursing: Scope and standards of practice.* American Holistic Nurses Association: Silver Springs, MD.

American Nurses Association. (1980/2003). *A Social policy statement* (Rev. ed.). Washington, DC: American Nurses Association.

American Nurses Association. (2008). *Guide to the Code of Ethics for nurses.* Washington, DC: American Nurses Association.

Cody, W. (1995). About all those paradigms: Many in the universe, two in nursing. *Nursing Science Quarterly, 8*(4), 144-147.

Dickoff, J., James, P., & Wiedenback, E. (1968). Theory in a practice discipline. Part 1: Practice-oriented theory. *Nursing Research, 17*(5), 415-435.

Erickson, H. (1985). *Synthesizing clinical experiences: A step in theory development.* Ann Arbor, MI: Biomedical Communications, The University of Michigan.

Erickson, H., Tomlin, E., & Swain, M. A. (1983/2009). *Modeling and role-modeling: A theory and paradigm for nursing.* Englewood Cliffs, NJ: Prentice-Hall. Second-ninth printing, 1988-2009; Cedar Park, TX: EST Co.

Fawcett, J. (1992, February). Conceptual models and nursing practice: The reciprocal relationship. *Journal of Advanced Nursing, 17*(2), 224-228.

Fawcett, J. (1984/1995). *Analysis and evaluation of conceptual models of nursing* (3rd ed.). Philadelphia: F. A. Davis.

Fry, V. S. (1953). The creative approach to nursing. *American Journal of Nursing, 53,* 301-302.

Gebbie, K., Rosenstock, L., & Hernandez, L. (Eds.). (2003). *Who will keep the public health?* Washington, DC: The National Academies Press.

Henderson, V. (1960). *Basic principles of nursing care.* Washington, DC: American Nurses Association.

Huch, M. H. (1995). Nursing and the next millennium. *Nursing Science Quarterly,* 8(1), 38-44.

Institute of Medicine. (2001). Crossing the quality chasm: A new health system for the 21st century. Committee on Quality of Health Care in America. Washington, DC: The National Academies Press.

Institute of Medicine. (2003). Health professions education: A bridge to quality. Washington, DC: The National Academies Press.

Leeman, J., Jackson, B., & Sandelowski, M. (2006). An evaluation of how well research reports facilitate the use of findings in practice. *Journal of Nursing Scholarship.* Sigma Theta Tau, International, 38(2), 171-177.

Leininger, M. M. (1978). *Transcultural nursing: Concepts, theories, and practices.* New York: Wiley.

McCain, F. R. (1965). Nursing by assessment—not intuition. *American Journal of Nursing, 65*(4):82-83.

McCaughan, D., Thompson, C., Cullum, N., Sheldon, T., & Thompson, D. (2002). Acute care nurses' perceptions of barriers to using research information in clinical decision-making. *Journal of Advanced Nursing, 39*(1), 46-60.

McCleary, L., & Brown, T. (2003). Barriers to pediatric nurses research utilization. *Journal of Advanced Nursing, 42*(4), 364-372.

McKenna, H. P. (1997). *Nursing Models and Theories* (pp. 144-146). London: Routledge.

McKibbon, K. A. (1998). Evidence-based practice. *Bulletin of the Medical Library Association, 86*(3), 396-401.

Orlando, I. J. (1961). *The dynamic nurse-patient relationship: Function, process, and principles.* New York: G. P. Putnam's Sons.

Nightingale, F. (1915). *Florence Nightingale to her nurses.* London: McMillian and Company.

Parse, R. R. (1987). *Nursing science: Major paradigms, theories, and critiques* (pp. 208-210). Philadelphia: W. B. Saunders.

Ryan, P., & Lauver, D. (2002). The efficacy of tailored interventions. *Journal of Nursing Scholarship, 34*(4), 331-337.

Rogers, M. E. (1983). *An Introduction to the Theoretical Basis of Nursing.* Philadelphia: F. A. Davis.

Schim, S. M., Benkert, R., Bell, S. E., Walker, D. S., & Danford, C. A. (2007). Social justice: Added metaparadigm concept for urban health nursing. *Public Health Nursing, 24*(1), 73-80.

Sidani, S., Doran, D. M., & Mitchell, P. H. (2004). A theory-driven approach to evaluating quality of nursing care. *Journal of Nursing Scholarship, 36*(1), 60-65.

Silva, M. C. (1999). The state of nursing science: Reconceptualizing for the 21st century. *Nursing Science Quarterly, 22*(3), 43-50.

Smith, J. A. (1981). The idea of health: A philosophical inquiry. *Advances in Nursing Science, 3*(3), 43-50.

Watson, J. (1979). *Nursing: The philosophy and science of caring.* Boston: Little Brown.

Yura, H., & Torres, G. (1975). Today's conceptual frameworks within baccalaureate nursing programs. In *Faculty-curriculum development Part III: Conceptual framework—Its meaning and function* (pp. 17-25). New York: National League for Nursing.

CHAPTER 3

American Nurses Association. (2003). *A social policy statement.* Washington, DC: American Nurses Association.

Benoliel, J. Q. (1987). Response to "Toward holistic inquiry in nursing: A proposal for synthesis of patterns and methods." *Scholarly Inquiry for Nursing Practice: An International Journal.* 1(2), 147-152.

Boykin, A. (2009). Foreword. In R. Locsin, & M. Purnell (Eds.), *A Contemporary nursing process: The (un)bearable weight of knowing in nursing* (pp. xvi-xvii). New York, NY: Springer Publishing.

Calabria, M. D., & McCrae, J. A. (Eds.). (1994). *Suggestions for thought by Florence Nightingale: Selections and commentaries.* Philadelphia, PA: University of Pennsylvania Press.

Carper, B. A. (1978). Fundamental patterns of knowing in nursing. *Advances in Nursing Science, 1*(1), 13-23.

Cowling, W. R. (2007). A unitary participatory vision of nursing knowledge. *Advances in Nursing Science. 30*(1), 61-70.

Cowling, W. R., & Repede, E. (2008). Consciousness and knowing: The pattern of the whole. In R. C. Locsin, and M. J. Purnell (Eds.), *A Contemporary Nursing Process: The (Un)Bearable Weight of Knowing in Nursing* (pp.73-98). New York, NY: Springer Publishing.

Erickson, H. L. (2006a). Connecting. In H. L. Erickson (Ed.), *Modeling and role-modeling: A view from the client's world.* (pp. 300-323). Cedar Park, TX: Unicorns Unlimited.

Erickson, H. L. (2006b). Searching for Life Purpose: Discovering Meaning. In H. L. Erickson (Ed.), *Modeling and role-modeling: A view from the client's world* (pp. 5-32). Cedar Park, TX: Unicorns Unlimited.

Erickson, H. L., & Erickson, M. (1995). The Metaparadigm and Ways-of-Knowing. Unpublished manuscript.

Erickson, H., Tomlin, E., & Swain, M. A. (1983/2009). *Modeling and role-modeling: A theory and paradigm for nursing*. Englewood Cliffs, NJ: Prentice-Hall. Second-ninth printing, 1988-2009. Cedar Park, TX: EST Company.

Hamric, A., & Hanson, C. (2003). Educating advanced practice nurses for practice reality. *Journal of Professional Nursing, 19*(5), 262-68.

Henderson, V. (1961). *Dynamic nurse-patient relationships.* New York, NY: G.P. Putnam's Sons.

Johns, C. (1995). Framing learning through reflection within Carper's fundamental ways of knowing. *Journal of Advanced Nursing*, 22; 226-34.

Johns, C. (2004). *Becoming a reflective practitioner* (2nd ed.). Oxford: Cambridge.

Johns, C. (2005/2007). Expanding the gates of Perception. In C. Johns and D. Freshwater (Eds.), *Transforming nursing through reflective practice* (2nd ed.). Oxford: Blackwell Publishing.

Leebov, W. (2008). *Wendy Leebov's essentials for great patient experiences: No nonsense solutions with gratifying results.* Chicago, IL: Health Forum, Inc.

Munhall, P. L. (1993). Unknowing: Toward another pattern of knowing. *Nursing Outlook, 41,* 125-128.

Munhall, P. L. (2009). Unknowing: Towards the understanding of multiple realities and manifold perceptions. In R. C. Locsin, and M. J. Purnell (Eds.), *A Contemporary nursing process: The (Un)Bearable weight of knowing in nursing* (pp.153-173). New York, NY: Springer Publishing.

Nightingale, F. (1859/2003). *Notes on Nursing*. New York, NY: Barns & Noble Books.

Phenix, P. H. (1964). *Realms of meaning: A philosophy of the curriculum for general education.* New York: McGraw Hill.

Purnell, M. (2009). Pheonix Arising: Synoptic Knowing for a Synoptic Practice of Nursing. In R. C. Locsin, and M. J. Purnell (Eds.), *A Contemporary nursing process: The (Un)bearable weight of knowing in nursing* (pp.3-16). New York, NY: Springer Publishing.

Rogers, M. E. (1970). Introduction to the theoretical basis of nursing. *Nursing Research, 19*(6), p. 541.

Silva, M. C., Sorrell, J. M., & Sorrell, C. D. (1995). From Carper's patterns of knowing to ways of being: An ontological philosophical shift in nursing. *Advances in Nursing Science,* 18 (1), 1-13.

Schön, D. A. (1983). *The reflective practitioner: How professionals think in action.* New York, NY: Basic Books.

Smith, J. (1981). The idea of health: A philosophical inquiry. *Advances in Nursing Science, 3*(3), 43-50.

Watson, J. (1979). *Nursing: The philosophy and science of caring.* Boston: Little Brown

White, J. (1995). Patterns of knowing: Review, critique, and update. *Advances in Nursing Science, 17*(4), 73-86.

CHAPTER 4

American Holistic Nurses Association. (2007). *Holistic nursing: Scope and standards of practice.* Silver springs, MD. American Nurses Association.

American Nurses Association. (2001). *Code of Ethics for nursing with interpretive statements.* Washington, DC. American Nurses Association.

American Nurses Association. (2004). *Nursing: Scope and standards of practice.* Washington, DC. American Nurses Association.

Anderson, L.W., & Kratwohl, D. R. (Eds.). (2001). *Taxonomy for Learning, Teaching, and Assessing: A revision of Bloom's Taxonomy of educational objectives.* New York, NY: Longman.

Bloom, B. S. (Ed.). (1956). *Taxonomy of educational objectives, the classification of educational goals—Handbook 1: Cognitive Domain.* New York, NY: McKay.

Brekke, M., & Schultz, E. (2006). Energy theories: Modeling and Role-modeling. In H. L. Erickson (Ed.), *Modeling and role-modeling: A view from the client's world* (pp. 33-66). Cedar Park, TX: Unicorns Unlimited.

Carper, B. A. (1978). Fundamental Patterns of knowing in nursing. *Advances in nursing science, 1* (1), 13-23.

Chinn, P. L., & Kramer, M. K. (1995). *Theory and Nursing* (4th ed.). Saint Louis, MO: Mosby.

Chinn, P. L., & Kramer, M. K. (2004). *Integrated knowledge development in nursing.* Saint Louis, MO: Mosby.

Clements, P. T., & Averill, J. B. (2006). Finding patterns of knowing in the work of Florence Nightingale. *Nursing Outlook, 54* (5), 268-274.

Erickson, H. L. (2006a). Searching for life purpose: Discovering meaning. In H. L. Erickson (Ed.), *Modeling and role-modeling: A view from the client's world* (pp. 5-32). Cedar Park, TX: Unicorns Unlimited.

Erickson, H. L. (2006b). Connecting. In H. L. Erickson (Ed.), *Modeling and role-modeling: A view from the client's world* (pp. 300-323). Cedar Park, TX: Unicorns Unlimited.

Erickson, H. L. (2006c). The healing process. In H. L. Erickson (Ed.), *Modeling and role-modeling: A view from the client's world* (pp. 411-444). Cedar Park, TX: Unicorns Unlimited.

Erickson, M., Erickson, H. L., & Jensen, B. (2006) Affiliated Individuation and self-actualization: need satisfaction as prerequisite. In H. L. Erickson (Ed.), *Modeling and role-modeling: A view from the client's world* (pp. 182-207). Cedar Park, TX: Unicorns Unlimited.

Erickson, H., Tomlin, E., & Swain, M. A. (1983/2009). *Modeling and role-modeling: A theory and paradigm for nursing.* Englewood Cliffs, NJ: Prentice-Hall. Second-ninth printing, 1988-2009; Cedar Park, TX: EST Co.

Glaser, B. G., & Strauss, A. L. (1967). *The Discovery of Grounded Theory: Strategies for Qualitative Research.* Chicago, IL: Aldine Publishing Co.

Heath, H. (1998). Reflection and patterns of knowing in nursing. *Journal of Advanced Nursing, 27* (5), 1054-1059.

Hertz, J., & Baas, L. (2006). Self-care: Knowledge, resources, and actions. In H. L. Erickson (Ed.), *Modeling and role-modeling: A view from the client's world* (pp. 97-120). Cedar Park, TX: Unicorns Unlimited.

Johns, C. (1995). Framing learning through reflection within Carper's fundamental Ways-of-Knowing. *Journal of Advanced Nursing, 22*, 226-34.

Johns, C. (2002). *Guided reflection: Advancing practice.* Oxford, UK. Wiley-Blackwell.

Johns, C. (2004a). *Becoming a reflective practitioner* (2nd ed.). Oxford: Cambridge.

Johns, C., (2004b). Becoming a transformational leader through reflective practice. *Reflections on Nursing Scholarship,* 30 (2), 24-26.

Johns, C., (2005/2007). Expanding the gates of perception. In C. Johns and D. Freshwater (Eds.), *Transforming nursing through reflective practice* (2nd ed.). Oxford: Blackwell Publishing.

Kinney, C. (2006). Heart-to-heart nurse-client relationships. In H. L. Erickson (Ed.), *Modeling and role-modeling: A view from the client's world* (pp. 277-299). Cedar Park, TX: Unicorns Unlimited.

Kratwohl, D. R., Bloom, B. S., & Masia, B. B. (1964/1973). *Taxonomy of educational objectives, classification of educational goals-Handbook II: Affective domain.* New York, NY: McKay.

McCain, F. R. (1965). Nursing by assessment, not intuition. *American Journal of Nursing,* 65 (4), 82-83.

McCaffrey, M. (2009). Clinical knowing in advanced practice nursing. In R. C. Locsin, and M. J. Purnell (Eds.), *A Contemporary nursing process: The (Un)Bearable weight of knowing in nursing* (pp.329-356). New York, NY: Springer Publishing.

Munhall, P. (1993). Nursing research: a qualitative perspective, (4th ed.). Sudbury, MA: Jones and Bartlett Publishers.

Nightingale, F. (1915). *Florence Nightingale to her nurses*. London: MacMillian and Co.

Polanyi, M. (1962). *Personal knowledge: Towards a post-critical philosophy.* Chicago, IL: The University of Chicago Press.

Schaefer, J. (Ed.). (2006). *The poetry of nursing: poems and commentaries of leading nurse poets.* Kent, OH: Kent State University press.

Schön, D. A. (1983). *The reflective practitioner: How professionals think in action.* New York, NY: Basic books.

Schön, D. A. (1987). Educating the reflective practitioner. Address to the 1987 meeting of the American Educational Research Association.

Silva, M. C., Sorrell, J. M., & Sorrell, C.D. (1995). From Carper's patterns of knowing to ways of being: an ontological, philosophical shift in nursing. *Advances in nursing science,* 18 (1), 1-13.

Smith, M. (2009). Holistic knowing. In R. C. Locsin, and M. J. Purnell (Eds.), *A Contemporary nursing process: The (un)bearable weight of knowing in nursing* (pp.133-152). New York: Springer Publishing.

Watson, J. (1979). *Nursing: The philosophy and science of caring.* Boston, MA: Little Brown.

Watzlawick, P. (1967). *Pragmatics of human communication: A study of interactional patterns, pathologies, and paradoxes.* New York, NY: W. W. Norton.

White, J. (1995). Patterns of knowing: review, critique, and update. *Advances in nursing science, 17*(4), 73-86.

CHAPTER 5

American Nurses Association. (2001). *Code of Ethics for nursing with interpretive statements.* Washington, DC. American Nurses Association.

American Nurses Association. (2004). *Nursing: Scope and standards of practice.* Washington, DC. American Nurses Association.

Bloom, B. S. (Ed.). (1956). *Taxonomy of educational objectives, the classification of educational goals—Handbook 1: Cognitive Domain.* New York: McKay.

Bruner, J. S. (1965). The growth of the mind. *American Psychologist, 20,* 1007-1017.

Bruner, J. (1966). *Toward a theory of instruction.* Cambridge, MA: Harvard University Press.

Bruner, J. (1967). Education as a social construction. In W. Huckins & H. Bernard (Eds.). *Readings in Educational Psychology.* New York: Wirkl Publishing.

Bruner, J. (1986). Actual minds, possible worlds. Cambridge, MA. Harvard University Press.

Bruner, J. (1996). *The culture of education.* Cambridge, MA. Harvard University Press.

Erickson, H., Tomlin, E., & Swain, M. A. (1983/2009). *Modeling and role-modeling: A theory and paradigm for nursing.* Englewood Cliffs, NJ: Prentice-Hall. Second-ninth printing, 1988-2009; Cedar Park, TX: EST Co.

Nightingale, F. (1915). *Florence Nightingale to her nurses.* London: McMillian and Company.

Piaget, J. (1967/1971). *Biology and knowledge.* Chicago: University of Chicago Press.

Rogers C. (1961). *On Becoming a Person.* New York: Norton.

Selye, H. (1976). *The stress of life* (Rev. ed.). New York: McGraw-Hill Book Company.

Wood, D., Bruner, J., & Ross, G. (1976). The role of tutoring in problem solving. *Journal of child psychology and psychiatry,* 17, 89-100.

CHAPTER 6

Bruner, J. S. (1965/1971). *Some elements of discovery. The relevance of education* (pp. 68-81). Oxford, UK: W. W. Norton.

Erickson, H. L. (Ed.). (2006a). *Modeling and role-modeling: A view from the client's world.* Cedar Park, TX: Unicorns Unlimited.

Erickson, H. L. (2006b). Connecting. In H. L. Erickson (Ed.), *Modeling and role-modeling: A view from the client's world* (pp. 300-323). Cedar Park, TX: Unicorns Unlimited.

Erickson, H. L. (2006c). Search for life purpose: Discovering meaning. In H. L. Erickson (Ed.), *Modeling and role-modeling: A view from the client's world* (pp. 5-32). Cedar Park, TX: Unicorns Unlimited.

Erickson, H.L. (2006d). Nurturing growth. In H. L. Erickson (Ed.), *Modeling and role-modeling: A view from the client's world* (pp. 324-345). Cedar Park, TX: Unicorns Unlimited.

Erickson, H. L. (2006e). Facilitating development. In H. L. Erickson (Ed.), *Modeling and role-modeling: A view from the client's world* (pp. 346-391). Cedar Park, TX: Unicorns Unlimited.

Erickson, M., Erickson, H., & Jensen, B. (2006). Affiliated-individuation and self-actualization: Need satisfaction as prerequisite. In H. L. Erickson (Ed.), *Modeling and role-modeling: A view from the client's world* (pp. 182-207). Cedar Park, TX: Unicorns Unlimited.

Johns, C. (2004). *Becoming a reflective practitioner: A reflective and holistic approach to clinical nursing, practice development, and clinical supervision* (2nd ed.). Oxford, UK: Blackwell Publishing.

Johns, C. (2010). *Guided reflection: Advancing practice.* Oxford, UK: Blackwell Publishing.

Nightingale, F. (1915). *Florence Nightingale to her nurses.* London: McMillian and Company.

Watzlawick, P. (1967). *Pragmatics of human communication: A study of interactional patterns, pathologies, and paradoxes.* New York, NY: W. W. Norton.

Wood, D., Bruner, J., & Ross, G. (1976). The role of tutoring in problem solving. *Journal of Child Psychology and Psychiatry*, 17, 89-100.

CHAPTER 7

Aristotle. Metaphysics, Book II, Chapter 1, 993b, lines 20, 22. In Seldes, G. (Ed.), *The Great Thoughts* (p.18). New York, NY: Ballantine Books.

Benson, D. (2006). Adaptation: Coping with stress. In H. L. Erickson (Ed.), *Modeling and Role-Modeling: A view from the client's world* (pp. 240-276). Cedar Park, TX: Unicorns Unlimited.

Brekke, M. & Schultz, E. (2006). Energy theories: Modeling and role-modeling. In H. L. Erickson (Ed.), *Modeling and Role-Modeling: A view from the client's world* (pp.33-66). Cedar Park, TX: Unicorns Unlimited.

Chinn, P. L., & Kramer, M. K. (2004). *Theory and nursing* (4th ed.). St. Louis, MO: Mosby.

Engel, G. L. (1968). A life setting conducive to illness. *Annals of Internal Medicine*, 69, 293-300.

Erickson, H. (1976). Identification of states of coping utilizing physiological and psychological data. Masters thesis, 1976:16. Ann Arbor, MI: The University of Michigan Ann Arbor.

Erickson, H. (1984). Self-care knowledge: Relations among the concepts support, hope, control, satisfaction with daily life, and physical health status. *Dissertation Abstracts International.* 1984: 46, 06B: 136, University Microfilms No. 84-12 18.

Erickson, H. (1988). Modeling and role modeling: Ericksonian approaches with physiological problems. In J. Zeig, & S. Langton (Eds.), *Ericksonian pychotherapy: The state of the art* (pp.477-490). New York, NY: Brunner/Mazel.

Erickson, H. (1990a). Theory-based practice. In H. L. Erickson, & C. Kinney (Eds.), *Modeling and role-Modeling: Theory, practice and research* Vol. 1(1), 1-27. Society for Advancement of Modeling and Role-Modeling.

Erickson, H. (1990b). Self-care knowledge: A exploratory study. In H. L. Erickson, & C. Kinney. (Eds.), *Modeling and Role-Modeling: Theory, practice and research* Vol. 1(1), 178-202. Society for Advancement of Modeling and Role-Modeling.

Erickson, H. (1990c). Modeling and role-modeling with psychophysiological problems. In J. K. Zeig & S. Gilligan (Eds.), *Brief Therapy: Myths, methods, and metaphors* (pp. 473-491). New York: Brunner/Mazel.

Erickson, H. (2002). Facilitating generativity and ego integrity: Applying Ericksonian methods to the aging population. In B. B. Geary & J. K. Zeig (Eds.), *The Handbook of Ericksonian Psychotherapy.* Phoenix, AZ: Zeig Tucker Publications.

Erickson, H. L. (Ed.). (2006a). *Modeling and role-modeling: A view from the client's world.* Cedar Park, TX: Unicorns Unlimited.

Erickson, H. (2006b). Facilitating developmental processes. In H. L. Erickson (Ed.), *Modeling and role-modeling: A view from the client's world* (pp. 208-237). Cedar Park, TX: Unicorns Unlimited.

Erickson, H. (2006c). Connecting. In H. L. Erickson (Ed.), *Modeling and role-modeling: A view from the client's world* (pp. 300-323). Cedar Park, TX: Unicorns Unlimited.

Erickson, H. (2006d). Searching for life purpose: Discovering meaning. In H. L. Erickson (Ed.), *Modeling and role-modeling: A view from the client's world* (pp. 5-32). Cedar Park, TX: Unicorns Unlimited.

Erickson, H. (2006e). The healing process. In H. L. Erickson (Ed.), *Modeling and role-modeling: A view from the client's world* (pp. 411-443). Cedar Park, TX: Unicorns Unlimited.

Erickson, H. (2006f). Nurturing growth. In H. L. Erickson (Ed.), *Modeling and role-modeling: A view from the client's world* (pp. 324-345). Cedar Park, TX: Unicorns Unlimited.

Erickson, M. (2006a). Attachment, loss and reattachment. In H. L. Erickson (Ed.), *Modeling and role-modeling: A view from the client's world* (pp. 208-237). Cedar Park, TX: Unicorns Unlimited.

Erickson, M. (2006b). Developmental processes. In H. L. Erickson (Ed.), *Modeling and role-modeling: A view from the client's world* (pp. 121-181). Cedar Park, TX: Unicorns Unlimited.

Erickson, H. & Swain, M. A. (1990). Mobilizing self-care resources: A nursing intervention for hypertension. *Issues in Mental Health Nursing,* Vol. 11 (3), 217-236.

Erickson, M., Erickson, H., & Jensen, B. (2006). Affiliated-individuation and self-actualization: Need satisfaction as prerequisite. In H. L. Erickson (Ed.), *Modeling and role-modeling: A view from the client's world* (pp. 182-207). Cedar Park, TX: Unicorns Unlimited.

Erickson, H., Tomlin, E., & Swain, M. A. (1983/2009). *Modeling and role-modeling: A theory and paradigm for nursing.* Englewood Cliffs, NJ: Prentice-Hall. Second-ninth printing, 1988-2009; Cedar Park, TX: EST Co.

Erikson, E. (1963). *Childhood and society.* New York: W. W. Norton.

Finch, D. (1987). Testing a theoretically based nursing assessment. Unpublished Masters thesis. Ann Arbor, The University of Michigan.

Frisch, N., and Frisch, L. (2006). *Psychiatric mental health nursing.* New York, NY: Delmar Publishers.

Halldorsdottir, S. (1991). Five basic modes of being with another. In D. A. Gaut, & M. M. Leininger (Eds.), *Caring: The compassionate healer* (pp. 37-49). New York, NY: National League for Nursing.

Kinney, C. (2006). Heart-to-heart nurse-client relationships. In H. L. Erickson (Ed.), *Modeling and role-Modeling: A view from the client's world* (pp. 277-299). Cedar Park, TX: Unicorns Unlimited.

Kinney, C. & Erickson, H. (1990). Modeling the client's world: A way to holistic care. *Issues in Mental Health Nursing, 11* (2), 93-108.

Rogers, S. (1996). Facilitative affiliation: nurse-client interactions that enhance healing. *Issues in mental health nursing, 17,* 171-184.

Rogers, S. (2002). Nurse-patient interactions: What do patients have to say? Unpublished dissertation, The University of Texas at Austin.

Scheela, R. (1992). The remodeling process: A grounded theory study of adult male incest offenders' perceptions of the treatment process. *Journal of Offender Rehabilitation, 18,* 1-2.

Selye, H. (1976). *The stress of life* (Rev. ed.). New York, NY: McGraw Hill.

Walker, M., & Erickson, H., L. (2006). Mind-body-spirit relations. In H. L. Erickson (Ed.), *Modeling and role-Modeling: A view from the client's world* (pp. 67-94). Cedar Park, TX: Unicorns Unlimited.

Chapter 8

Bruner, J. S. (1966). *Toward a theory of instruction.* Cambridge, MA: Harvard University Press.

Bruner, J. S. (1967). *On knowing: Essays for the left ha*nd. Cambridge, MA: Harvard University Press.

Bruner, J. S. (1983). *In search of mind.* New York, NY: Harper & Row.

Bruner, J. S. (1984). *In search of mind: Essays in autobiography* (Alfred P. Sloan Foundation Series). New York: HarperCollins.

Bruner, J. S. (1996). *The Culture of Education.* Harvard University Press. Cambridge, MA. Retrieved October 4, 2009 from website: http://www.des.emory.edu/mfp/brunerculture.html

Carper, B. (1978). Fundamental patterns of knowing in nursing. *Advances in Nursing Science*, *1*, 1: 13-23.

Maslow, A. H. (1968). *Toward a psychology of being.* New York: Van Nostrand Reinhold.

Schön, D. A. (1983/1991). *The reflective practitioner: How professionals think in action.* New York: Basic Books, Inc.

CHAPTER 9

American Nurses Association. (2003). *A social policy statement.* Washington, DC: American Nurses Association.

Bruner, J. S. (1965/1971). *Some elements of discovery: The relevance of education* (pp. 68-81). Oxford, UK: W. W. Norton.

Erickson, H. (1982). Helping students synthesize clinical experiences: A step in theory development. (Audiobook on tape: Lectures, speeches). Nursing Resources National Conference and Exhibition, Spring: San Francisco.

Erickson, H. L. (1985). Synthesizing clinical experiences: a step in theory development. The University of Michigan Medical Center: Ann Arbor, MI. Biomedical communications, The University of Michigan Medical Center.

Johns, C. (1995). Framing learning through reflection within Carper's fundamental ways of knowing. *Journal of Advanced Nursing, 22*, 226-34.

Johns, C. (2010). *Guided reflection: Advancing practice* (2nd ed.). Oxford, UK: Wiley-Blackwell. (in press).

Johns, C. (2004). *Becoming a reflective practitioner* (2nd ed.). Oxford, UK: Cambridge.

Johns C (2009). *Becoming a reflective practitioner* (3rd ed.). Oxford, UK: Wiley-Blackwell.

Lee, E.A.D. (2006). Finding your model of caring practice. *Journal of Christian Nursing, 23* (3), 14-19.

Nightingale, F. (1915). *Florence Nightingale to her nurses.* London: McMillian and Company.

Schön, D. A. (1983/1991). *The reflective practitioner: How professionals think in action.* Aldershot, England: Ashgate.

Schön, D. A. (1987). *Educating the reflective practitioner: Towards a new design for teaching and learning in the professions.* San Francisco, CA: Jossey-Bass.

Schön, D. A. (1991). The *reflective turn: case studies in and on educational practice.* New York, NY: Teachers press, Columbia University.

Thorne, S., Kirkham, S. R., & MacDonald-Emes, J. (1997). Interpretive description: A noncategorial qualitative alternative for developing nursing knowledge. *Research in Nursing & Health*, 20, 169-177.

Chapter 10

Bond, L. A. (1996). Norm- and criterion-referenced testing. *Practical Assessment, Research & Evaluation,* 5(2). Retrieved January 21. 2009 from http://PAREonline.net/getvn.sap?v=5&n=2.

Boston, C. (2002). The concept of formative assessment. *Practical Assessment, Research, & Evaluation,* (9). Retrieved January 21, 2009, from http://PAREonline.net/getvn.asp?v=8&n=9.

Bourke, M. P. & Ihrke, B. A. (2009). The evaluation process. In D. M. Billings & J. A. Halstead (Eds.), *Teaching in nursing* (3rd ed.). St. Louis: Saunders Elsevier.

Erickson, H. (2006). Nurturing growth. In H. L. Erickson (Ed.), *Modeling and role-modeling: A view from the client's world* (pp. 324-345). Cedar Park, TX: Unicorns Unlimited.

Erickson, H., Tomlin, E., & Swain, M. A. (1983/2009). *Modeling and role-modeling: A theory and paradigm for nursing.* Englewood Cliffs, NJ: Prentice-Hall. Second-ninth printing, 1988-2009; Cedar Park, TX: EST Co.

Ertmer, P. A. & Newby, T. J. (1996). The expert learner: Strategic, self-regulated, and reflective. *Instructional Science*, 24, 1-24.

Goldenberg, D., & Dietrich, P. (2002). A humanistic-educative approach to evaluation in nursing education. *Nurse Education Today*, *22*, 301-310.

Greenleaf, R. K. (2002). Essentials of servant leadership. In L. C. Spears & M. Lawrence (Eds.), *Focus on leadership: Servant leadership for the 21st century.* New York: John Wiley & Sons, Inc.

Hayes, J. M. (2007). Evaluation of programmatic learning outcomes. In M. J. Bradshaw & A. J. Lowenstein (Eds.), *Innovative teaching strategies in nursing and related health professions* (4th ed.). Boston: Jones and Bartlett Publishers.

Hertz, J., & Baas, L. (2006). Self-care: Knowledge, resources, and actions. In H. Erickson (Ed.), *Modeling and role-modeling: A view from the client's world* (pp.97-120). Cedar Park, TX: Unicorns Unlimited.

Kirkpatrick, J. M., & DeWitt, D. A. (2009). Strategies for assessing/evaluating learning outcomes. In D. M. Billings & J. A. Halstead (Eds.), *Teaching in nursing: A guide for faculty* (3rd ed.). St. Louis: Saunders Elsevier.

MacNeil, M. S. (2007). Concept mapping as a means of course evaluation. *Journal of Nursing Education, 46* (5), 232-234.

McDonald, M. E. (2007). *The nurse educator's guide to assessing learning outcomes* (2nd ed.). Boston: Jones and Bartlett Publishers.

Mertler, C. (2001). Designing scoring rubrics for your classroom. *Practical Assessment, Research & Evaluation,* 7 (25). Retrieved January 21, 2009, from http://PAREonline.net/getvn.asp?v=7&n=25.

Mezirow, J. (2000). Learning to think like an adult. In J. Mezirow and Associates (Eds.), *Learning as transformation.* San Francisco: Jossey-Bass.

Moskal, B. M. (2003). Recommendations for developing classroom performance assessments and scoring rubrics. *Practical Assessment, Research, & Evaluation,* 8(14), Retrieved January 21, 2009, from http://PARE online.net/getvn.asp?=8&n=14.

National League for Nursing (2004). *Excellence initiatives.* Retrieved July 20, 2009, from http://www.nln.org/excelence/hallmarks_indicators.htm.

Nielsen, A., Stragnell, S., & Jester, P. (2007). Guide for reflection using the clinical judgment model. *Journal of Nursing Education, 46*(11), 513-516.

Nightingale, F. (1915). *Florence Nightingale to her nurses.* London: McMillian and Company.

Nitko, A. J. (2007). Educational tests and measurement: An introduction (2nd ed). New York, NY: Hartcourt, Brace, and Jovanovich.

Novak, J. D., & Canas, A. J. (2008). The theory underlying concept maps and how to construct and use them. PublishersTechnical Report IHMC CmapTools. Retrieved July 26, 2009, from http://cmap.ihmc.us/Publications/ReserachPapers/TheoryUnderlyingConceptMapsHQ.pdf

O'Connor, A. B. (2006). *Clinical instruction and evaluation: A teaching resource.* Boston: Jones & Bartlett.

Robinson, F. P. (2009). Servant teaching: The power and promise for nursing education. *International Journal of Nursing Education Scholarship, 6*(1) 1-15.

Schultz, E. D. (1998). Academic advising from a nursing theory perspective. *Nurse Educator, 23*(2), 22-25.

Van Merrienboer, J., & Paas, F. (2003). Powerful learning and the many faces of instructional design: Toward a framework for the design of powerful learning environments. In E. De Corte, L. Vershcaffell, N. Entwistle & J. Van Merrienboer (Eds.), *Powerful learning environments: Unraveling basic components and dimensions.* Oxford, UK: Elsevier.

White, C. P. (2004). Student portfolios: An alternative way of encouraging and evaluating student learning. In M. Achacoso & M. Svinicki (Eds.), *Alternative Strategies for Evaluating Student Learning: New Directions for Teaching and Learning.* San Francisco: Jossey-Bass.

Worral, P. S. (2003). Evaluation in healthcare education. In S. B. Bastable (Ed.), *Nurse as educator* (2nd ed.). Sudbury, MA: Jones and Bartlett Publishers.

CHAPTER 11

American Nurses Association. (2001). *Code of ethics for nursing with interpretive statements.* Washington, DC: American Nurses Association.

Andrews, M. M., & Boyle, J. S. (2008). *Transcultural concepts in nursing care* (5th ed.). Philadelphia: Wolters Kluwer Health/Lippincott Williams & Wilkins.

Berggren, V., Bergstrom, S., & Edberg, A. K. (2006). Being different and vulnerable: Experiences of immigrant African women who have been circumcised and sought maternity care in Sweden. *Journal of Transcultural Nursing, 17*(1), 50-57.

Brekke, M. & Schultz, E. (2006). Energy Theories: Modeling and role-modeling. In H. L. Erickson (Ed.), *Modeling and Role-Modeling: A view from the client's world* (pp.33-66). Cedar Park, Texas: Unicorns Unlimited.

Brennan, J. (1999). Reconciling immigrant values. In V. D. Ferguson (Ed.), *Case studies in cultural diversity: A workbook* (pp. 179-184). Boston: Jones and Bartlett.

Capers, C. F. (1992). Teaching cultural content: A nursing education imperative. *Holistic Nursing Practice*, 6(3), 19-28.

Erickson, H. C. (1990). Self-care knowledge: An exploratory study. In H. Erickson & E. Kinney (Eds.), *Modeling and Role-Modeling: Theory, research and practice.* monograph, 1 (1), (pp. 178–202). Austin, TX: The Society for Advancement of Modeling and Role-Modeling.

Erickson, H. L. (2006a). Connecting. In H. L. Erickson (Ed.), *Modeling and role-modeling: A view from the client's world* (pp. 300-323). Cedar Park, TX: Unicorns Unlimited.

Erickson, H. L. (Ed.) (2006b). *Modeling and Role-Modeling: A view from the client's world.* Cedar Park, Texas: Unicorns Unlimited.

Erickson, H., Tomlin, E., & Swain, M. A. (1983/2009). *Modeling and role-modeling: A theory and paradigm for nursing.* Englewood Cliffs, NJ: Prentice-Hall. Second-ninth printing, 1988-2009; Cedar Park, TX: EST Co.

Frisch, N. C., & Frisch, L. E. (1998). *Psychiatric mental health nursing: Understanding the client as well as the condition.* Albany: Delmar.

Heath, H. (1998). Reflection and patterns of knowing in nursing. *Journal of Advanced Nursing, 27* (5), 1054-1059.

Health and Human Services Office of Minority Health. (2000). *National Standards for Culturally Linguistically Appropriate Services (CLAS)*. Federal Register 65(247), 80865-80879. Department of Health and Human Services, U.S. Public Health Service. Washington, D.C. Retrieved February 7, 2009, from www.diversityrx.org;www.hablamosjuntos.org, and www.hhs.state.ne.us/minorityhealth/docs/CLASBrochure.pdf. (Unavailable from commonly cited www.omhrc.gov websites.)

Hertz, J. E. (1996). Conceptualization of perceived enactment of autonomy in the elderly. *Issues in Mental Health Nursing, 17* (3), 261-273.

Hertz, J. E., & Baas, L. (2006). Self-Care: Knowledge, resources, and actions. In H. L. Erickson (Ed.), *Modeling and Role-Modeling: A view from the client's world* (pp. 97 – 120). Cedar Park, TX: Unicorns Unlimited.

Hwang, H., Lin, H., Tung, Y., & Wu, H. (2006). Correlates of perceived autonomy among elders in a senior citizen home: A cross-sectional survey. *International Journal of Nursing Studies*, *43*(4), 429-437. Retrieved March 30, 2009, from CINAHL database.

Jackson, L. E. (1993). Understanding, eliciting, and negotiating clients' multicultural beliefs. *Nurse Practitioner 18* (4), 30-43.

Leininger, M. (1991). The theory of culture care diversity and universality...sunrise model. *Culture care diversity and universality: A theory of nursing* (pp. 5-68). New York: National League for Nursing.

Leininger, M. (1996). Culture care theory, research, and practice. *Nursing Science Quarterly*, *9*(2), 71-78.

Leininger, M. (2007). Theoretical questions and concerns: Response from the theory of culture care diversity and universality perspective. *Nursing Science Quarterly*, *20*(1), 9-13.

Luckmann, J. (1999). *Transcultural communication in nursing*. Albany: Sage.

Matsui, M., & Capezuti, E. (2008). Perceived autonomy and self-care resources among senior center users. *Geriatric Nursing*, *29*(2), 141-147. Retrieved March 30, 2009, from CINAHL database.

Munhall, P. L. (1993). 'Unknowing': Toward another pattern of knowing in nursing. *Nursing Outlook, 41*, 125-128.

Nailon, R. E. (2006). Nurses' concerns and practices with using interpreters in the care of Latino patients in the emergency department. *Journal of Transcultural Nursing, 17*(2), 119-128.

Nance, T. A. (1995). Intercultural communication: Finding common ground. *JOGNN, 24*, 249-255.

National Council on Interpreting in Health Care. (2005). *National Standards of Practice for Interpreters in Health Care*. Retrieved February 7, 2009, from www.ncihc.org.

National Institute of Health. (2010). *Re-engineering the clinical research enterprise: Translational research.* Retrieved February 24, 2010 from http://nihroadmap.nih.gov/clinicalresarch/overview-translational.asp.

Outlaw, F. (1994). A reformulation of the meaning of culture and ethnicity for nurses delivering care. *Medsurg Nursing, 3*(2), 109-111.

Purnell, L. (2005). The Purnell model for cultural competence. *Journal of Multicultural Nursing & Health, 11*(2), 7-15.

Rogers, M. (1970/1981). *An introduction to the theoretical basis of nursing.* Philadelphia: F.A. Davis.

White, J. (1995). Patterns of knowing: Review, critique, and update. *Advances in Nursing Science, 17(4),* 73-86.

CHAPTER 12

American Association of Colleges of Nursing (AACN) (1996). *The Essentials of Master's Education for Advanced Practice Nursing* (1996). Washington, DC: AACN Publishing.

American Nurses Association (1995). *Scope and standards of advanced practice registered nursing,* Washington, DC: ANA Publishing.

Carper, B. (1978). Fundamental patterns of knowing in nursing. *ANS Advanced Nursing Science*, I, 13-23.

Codman, E. (1916). *A study in hospital efficiency.* Boston, MA: Privately printed.

DiCenso, A., Guyatt, G., & Cliska, D. (2005). *Evidence-based nursing : A guide to clinical practice.* St. Louis: Elsevier.

Dossey, B. (2000). *Florence Nightingale: mystic, visionary, healer.* Springhouse, PA: Springhouse Press.

Donabedian, A. (1966). Evaluating the quality of medical care. *Milbank Memorial Fund Quarterly*, *44* (3 July Supplement), 166-206.

Fawcett, J., & Garity, J. (2009). *Evaluating research for evidence-based nursing practice.* Philadelphia: FA Davis.

Guyatt, G., Cairns, J., Churchill, D., et al. [Evidence-Based Medicine Working Group] (1992). Evidence-based medicine. A new approach to teaching the practice of medicine. *JAMA,* 268, 2420-2425.

Guyatt, G. H., & Rennie, D. (1993). Users' guides to the medical literature. *JAMA*, 270, 2096-2097.

Guyatt, G. H., & Rennie, D. (2002). *Users' Guides to the Medical Literature: A Manual of Evidence-Based Clinical Practice*. New York: McGraw Hill.

Hertz, J. E., Rossetti, J., Koren, M. E., & Robertson, J. F. (2005). Management of relocation in cognitively intact older adults. Iowa City, IA: The University of Iowa Gerontological Nursing Interventions Research Center, Research Translation and Dissemination Core. Retrieved January 29, 2010 from http://www.guideline.gov/summary/summary.aspx?ss=15&doc_id=8110&nbr=4517.

Horsley, J. A., Crane, J., Crabtree, M. K., & Wood, D. J. (1983). *Using research to improve nursing practice: A guide, CURN project.* New York: Grune & Stratton.

JCAH. (2009). Joint Commission on Hospital Accreditation Organization History. Retrieved January 29, 2010 from http://www.jointcommission.org/AboutUs/joint_commission_history.htm.

JCAHO. (2010). Joint Commission on Hospital Accreditation Organization History. Retrieved, January 14, 2010 from http://www.jointcommission.org/AboutUs/joint_commission_history.htm.

National Association of Clinical Nurse Specialists. (1998). *Statement on Clinical Nurse Specialist Practice and Education* (1998). National Association of Clinical Nurse Sepecialists.

NIH Partners in Research Program: Pathways for Translational Research. Retrieved February, 24, 2010 from http://www.ninr.nih.gov/ResearchAndFunding/DEA/OEP/FundingOpportunities/Challenge_Grants.htm.

Pivens, M. L. S. (2005). Detection of depression in the cognitively intact older adult. Iowa City (IA): University of Iowa Gerontological Nursing Interventions Research Center, Research Dissemination Core. Retrieved February, 24, 2010, from http://www.guideline.gov/summary

Smith, L. (2010). Models for evidence-based practice in holistic nursing. Unpublished manuscript.

Westfall, J. M., Mold, J., & Fagnan, L. (2007). Practice based research–"Blue Highways" on the NIH roadmap. *JAMA, 297,* 403-406.

Chapter 13

American Nurses Association. (2004). *Code of Ethics for nursing with interpretive statements.* Washington, DC. American Nurses Association.

Aycock, N., & Boyle, D. (2009). Interventions to manage compassion fatigue in oncology nursing. *Clinical Journal of Oncology Nursing, 13*(2), 183-191.

Baird, K., & Kracen, A. C. (2006). Vicarious traumatization and secondary traumatic stress: A research synthesis. *Counseling Psychology Quarterly, 19*(2), 181-188.

Bush, N. (2009). Compassion fatigue: Are you at risk? *Oncology Nursing Forum, 36*(1), 24-28.

Bruner, J. S. (1965/1997). *Some elements of discovery in the relevance of education* (pp. 68-81). Oxford, UK: W.W. Norton

Brekke, M. & Schultz, E. (2006). Energy Theories: Modeling and role-modeling. In H. L. Erickson (Ed.), *Modeling and Role-Modeling: A view from the client's world* (pp.33-66). Cedar Park, Texas: Unicorns Unlimited.

Ceslowitz, S. B. (1989). Burnout and coping strategies among hospital staff nurses. *Journal of Advanced Nursing, 14,* 553-557.

Clayton, D., Erickson, H., & Rogers, S. (2006).Finding meaning in our life journey. In H. L. Erickson (Ed.), *Modeling and Role-Modeling: A view from the client's world* (pp. 391-410). Cedar Park, Texas: Unicorns Unlimited.

Corley, M. C. (2002). Nursing moral distress: A proposed theory and research agenda. *Nursing Ethics, 9,* 636-650.

Cronin-Stubbis, D., & Rooks, C. A. (1985). The stress, social support, and burnout of critical care nurses: The result of research. *Heart & Lung, 14*, 31-39.

Devilly, G., Wright, R., & Varker, T. (2009). Vicarious trauma, secondary traumatic stress or simply burnout? Effect of trauma therapy on mental health professionals. *Australian & New Zealand Journal of Psychiatry, 43*, 373-385.

Dominguez-Gomez, E. & Rutledge, D. N. (2009). Prevalence of secondary traumatic stress among emergency nurses. *Journal of Emergency Nursing, 35*(3), 199-204.

Duquette, A., Kerouac, S., Sandhu, B., & Beaudet, L. (1994). Factors related to nursing burnout: A review of empirical knowledge. *Issues in Mental Health Nursing, 15*, 337-358.

Erickson, H. L. (2006a). Searching for Life purpose: Discovering meaning. In H. L. Erickson (Ed.), *Modeling and role-modeling: A view from the client's world* (pp. 5-32). Cedar Park, TX: Unicorns Unlimited.

Erickson H. L. (2006b). Connecting. In H. L. Erickson (Ed.), *Modeling and role-modeling: A view from the client's world* (pp. 300-323). Cedar Park, TX: Unicorns Unlimited.

Erickson, H., Tomlin, E., & Swain, M. A. (1983/2009). *Modeling and role-modeling: A theory and paradigm for nursing.* Englewood Cliffs, NJ: Prentice-Hall. Second-ninth printing, 1988-2009; Cedar Park, TX: EST Co.

Figley, C. (1995). *Compassion fatigue: Coping with secondary traumatic stress disorder in those who treated the traumatized.* New York: Brunner-Routledge.

Frank, A. W. (1995). *The wounded storyteller.* Chicago: The University of Chicago Press.

Gunther, M., & Thomas, S. (2006). Nurses' narratives of unforgettable patient care events. *Journal of Nursing Scholarship, 38*, 370-376.

Haeckel, E., H. (1899). The riddle of the Universe. In G. Seldes (Ed.), *The Great Thoughts* (p. 170). New York: Ballantine Books.

Halbenleben, J. R. B., Wakefield, B. J., Wakefield D. S., & Cooper, L. B. (2008). Nurse burnout and patient safety outcomes: Nurse safety perception versus reporting behavior. *Western Journal of Nursing Research, 30,* 560–577.

Harris, P. L. (1984). Burnout in nursing administration. *Nursing Administration Quarterly, 8*, 61-70.

Hertz, J., & Baas, L. (2006). Self-care: Knowledge, resources, and actions. In H. L. Erickson (Ed.), *Modeling and Role-modeling: A view from the client's world* (pp. 97-120). Cedar Park, TX: Unicorns Unlimited.

Jameton, A. (1984). *Nursing practice: The ethical issues.* Englewood Cliffs, NJ: Prentice Hall.

Jenkins, R., & Elliott, P. (2004). Stressors, burnout and social support: Nurses in acute mental health settings. *Journal of Advanced Nursing, 48*, 622-631.

Joinson, C. (1992). Coping with compassion fatigue. *Nursing, 22*(4), 116, 118-120.

Laposa, J. M., & Alden, L. E. (2003). Post traumatic stress disorder in the emergency room: Exploration of a cognitive model. *Behaviour Research and Therapy, 41*, 49-65.

Maslach, C., & Schaufeli, W. (1993). *Historical and conceptual development of burnout. Professional burnout: Recent developments in theory and research* (pp. 1-16). Philadelphia: Taylor & Francis.

McCann, L. & Pearlman, L. A. (1990). Vicarious traumatization: A framework for understanding the psychological effects of working with victims. *Journal of Traumatic Stress, 3*(1), 131-149.

McElroy, A. M. (1982). Burnout: A review of the literature with application to cancer nursing. *Cancer Nursing, 5*(3), 211-217.

Meadors, P., & Lamson, A. (2008). Compassion fatigue and secondary traumatization: Provider self-care on intensive care units for children. *Journal of Pediatric Health Care, 22*(1), 24-34.

Mulder, J. (2000). Transforming experiences of wisdom: Healing amidst suffering. *Journal of Palliative Care, 16*(2), 47-54.

Sandelowski, M. (1991). Telling stories: Narrative approaches in qualitative research. *Research in Nursing and Health, 16,* 213-218.

Walker, M., & Erickson, H. (2006). Mind-body-spirit relations. In H. L. Erickson (Ed.), *Modeling and Role-modeling: A view from the client's world* (pp. 67-94). Cedar Park, TX: Unicorns Unlimited.

CHAPTER 14

Boyd, E. and Fales, A. (1983). Reflective learning: key to learning from experience. *Journal of Humanistic Psychology, 23*(2), 99-117.

Carper, B. (1978). Fundamental patterns of knowing in nursing. *Advances in Nursing Science*, *1*(1), 13-23.

Hepworth, B. (2010). Retrieved Jan 12, 2010, from http://www. brainyquote.com/quotes/authors/B/Barbara_Hepworth.html

Hansen, F. J. (2008). Phronesis and eros–the existential dimension of phronesis and clinical supervision of nurses. In C. Delmar, & C. Johns (Eds.), *The Good, the Wise, and the right clinical nursing practice.* Oxford, UK: Blackwell publishing.

Jarrett, L. & Johns, C. (2007). Constructing the reflective narrative. In C. Johns, and D., Freshwater (Eds.), *Transforming nursing through reflective practice.* (2nd ed., pp. 162-179). Oxford, UK: Blackwell publishing.

Johns, C. (1995). Framing learning through reflection within Carper's fundamental ways of knowing. *Journal of Advanced Nursing*, *22*, 226-234.

Johns, C. (2002). *Guided reflection: Advancing practice.* Oxford, UK: Wiley-Blackwell.

Johns, C. (2004). *Becoming a reflective practitioner* (2nd ed.). Oxford, UK: Cambridge.

Johns, C. (2006). *Engaging reflection in practice: A narrative approach.* Oxford, UK: Blackwell publishing.

Johns, C. (2009a). Journeying with Alice: Some things I know but not for certain. *Complementary Therapies in Clinical Practice*, *15*(3), 133-135.

Johns, C. (2009b). *Becoming a reflective practitioner* (3rd ed.). Oxford, UK: Wiley-Blackwell.

Johns, C. (2010). *Guided reflection: Advancing practice* (2nd ed.). Oxford, UK: Wiley-Blackwell. (in press).

Johns, C., & Freshwater, D. (Eds.). (2007). *Transforming nursing through reflective practice* (2nd ed.). Oxford, UK: Blackwell publishing.

Jones, R., & Jones, G. (1996). *Earth Dance Drum*. Salt Lake City, UT: Commune-a-Key.

Margolis, H. (1993). *Paradigm and barriers: How habits of mind govern scientific beliefs*. Chicago: University of Chicago Press.

Rael, J. (1993). *Being and vibration.* Council, OK: Oak books.

Sangharakshita, U. (1998). *Know your mind.* Birmingham: Windhorse.

Schön, D. A. (1983/1991). *The reflective practitioner: How professionals think in action.* Aldershot, UK: Ashgate.

Wheatley, M. J. (1999). *Leadership and the New Science: Discovering Order in a Chaotic World*. San Francisco: Berrett-Koehler.

Chapter 15

Cameron, J. (2002). *The Artist's Way: A Spiritual Path to Higher Creativity.* New York: Penguin Putnam Books.

Erickson, H. (1990). Theory-based practice. In H. Erickson & C. Kinney (Eds.), *Modeling and Role-modeling: Theory, Practice, and Research, 1*(1) 1-27. Austin, TX: Society for Advancement of Modeling and Role-modeling.

Erickson, H., Tomlin, E., & Swain, M. A. (1983/2009). *Modeling and role-modeling: A theory and paradigm for nursing.* Englewood Cliffs, NJ: Prentice-Hall. Second-ninth printing, 1988-2009; Cedar Park, TX: EST Co.

Kuhn, T. S. (1996). *The Structure of Scientific Revolutions* (3rd ed.). Chicago: The University of Chicago Press.

Nicoll, L. H. (Ed.). (1997). *Perspectives on Nursing Theory* (3rd ed.). Philadelphia: Lippincott.

APPENDIX A

NEW CHALLENGES FOR NURSES

Helen Erickson
Unpublished manuscript, 1985

THE PROBLEM

Nurses are confronted with new challenges every day. Generally, these are due to an individual patient's unique problems. Recently, however, many have found themselves torn by demands secondary to the implementation of the prospective payment system while simultaneously challenged by colleagues to practice more efficiently. Hospital administrators, eager to maintain system solvency, have focused on nursing as major expenditures within the system. Nurses have been told that they will have to practice more efficiently and more effectively. Since nursing care provided in critical care units is more expensive than care provided in general care units, critical care nurses have been identified as those who can make the greatest impact if they become more efficient and effective.

Several possibilities have been proposed. In general, there are two major themes among these: either nurses are asked to alter the client-nurse ratio or they are asked to decrease hospital length of stay. While these two measures seem to have potential for effecting immediate savings, it is important to consider the potential long-term cost-benefit as well. Each is explored below.

Altered client-nurse ratios

Since it is generally assumed that a 6:1 patient/nurse ratio is less expensive than a 5:1 or 3:1 ratio, at first view it would appear that this change would decrease the cost of nursing care in intensive care units. It is possible, however, that increasing the number of patients that a nurse is responsible for would ultimately increase the average length of hospital stay, thus increasing cost of hospital stay.

Obviously, an increased client-nurse ratio would mean that nurses would have less time to spend with each client. When nurses are unable to spend time necessary to prevent complications or identify early signs of impending complications, the predicted result is *an increase in complications.* The number of complications is directly related to length of hospital stay. This situation is compounded by the fact that the increase in length of stay may be due to an extended stay in the critical care unit. That is, complications might not only increase hospital stay, but require a transfer to an intensive care. If this should happen, the total cost of care would be markedly increased, not decreased.

Another factor to consider when determining whether or not to alter the client-nurse ratio is the potential for increasing staff frustration, fatigue, and burnout, thus increasing staff sick-time and turnover. Presumably, if nurses are expected to assume responsibility for more patients than time permits, their stress level increases and job satisfaction decreases. Unrelenting stress results in an increase in frustration, fatigue, illness and ultimately, burnout; factors all related to staff turnover. As staff turnover increases, cost related to orientation of new staff increases. Thus, while altering client-nurse ratios for care has the potential for decreasing the cost of health care, simultaneously, there are factors to consider that might ultimately increase health care cost.

Decreased Length of ICU Stay

The second commonly proposed measure for saving money is to move patients through intensive care units more quickly than current practice. However, this approach also has disadvantages. Consider, as an example, the potential for discharging patients from the intensive care unit in two days, rather than the current three days. Patients who previously had the advantages of intensive care nursing for three days, would now be dependent on the unit nurses for their care on the third post-operative day. Unless these individuals achieve a state of health in two days that equals the health status currently achieved in three days, they could be at high risk. That is, unless staffing is increased on the general care units, sicker patients could be sent to units with insufficient staffing to accommodate their needs. Nurses would not be able to give them the individualized care necessary to prevent complications and/or identify phenomena that indicate early stages of complications. Thus, the same difficulties exist with this approach: the potential for an increase in client complications, sick-time and turnover, as well as potential for a decrease in staff job satisfaction.

Theory-based nursing

At first appearance, it might seem that there are no ready solutions; nurses will just have to practice more efficiently or more effectively. I propose, however, that nurses do have options, and can make a major change that would be cost effective and would decrease staff turnover. Simply stated, nurses who practice from a theory consistent with their own philosophy will be more efficient. I propose that nurses who practice purposefully and systematically within the context of a holistic, health-oriented nursing theory base, could result in shorter hospital visits and decrease the number of readmissions—the two major reasons for the escalation of health care costs.

However, initially, practice from a holistic, health-oriented theory base is difficult. It requires that nurses learn the theory and practice continuously within its parameters. Before nurses can do this, they must consider their philosophy of nursing and conceptualize their beliefs about mankind, (1) and then determine whether the theory they aim to use is consistent with their own philosophy and belief system.

Finally, they must seek the support necessary (within the system) for implementing the theory base since implementation always effects changes within the system. These changes include philosophical issues as well as practice issues. Each is very important, each is related to the other; neither can be successfully implemented without the other.

PHILOSOPHICAL ISSUES

Most critical care settings have been established to provide specialized care for particular medical problems. There are coronary care units, respiratory intensive care units, and so forth. As a result, many nurses have become specialists in health problems that relate to medical problems. Nurses in coronary care units have become very proficient in reading monitors, interpreting blood chemistries, assessing the cardiovascular system and recognizing early signs of cardiac failure. Nurses in other intensive care settings have developed expertise related to the particular medical problem associated with the setting. Although many of these nurses have also developed practice models for individualizing nursing care, since intensive care nursing is traditionally determined by the medical problem, holistic, personalized nursing care is discounted. Nursing care is often aimed at meeting the biophysical needs of the clients with minimal consideration of the mind-body relationships. Care is focused on the current state of the biophysical subsystem without much consideration for stressors that preceded the current health problem or the effect that the current health status might have on the psyche, and thus, ultimately on the individual's ability to recover. Many professionals state that the physiological needs of these patients are so great that they must be attended to in order to save the individual's life, and that meeting these needs is the role of the intensive care unit nurse. They also state that these demands require so much nursing time that there is no time left for meeting other needs. This perspective has merit, but needs to be reconsidered given current challenges and recent findings.

Evidence of mind-body relationships

Several have provided evidence that psychosocial needs are related to the biophysical status. Thiel and colleagues (2) studied fifty subjects with myocardial infarcts and a control group of fifty healthy subjects and found that those with myocardial infarcts reported higher anxiety and depression scores than healthy people; many reported that they experienced these feelings before they had the myocardial infarct. Friedman and colleagues (3) studied a population of healthy people and found that those who reported feeling blue, were experiencing low energy and having sleep difficulty were high risk for heart attacks. Thomas and Greenstreet (4) studied a group of medical students and also found that those who were tired when they woke up were at a high risk for heart attacks. Others have found that there's a relationship between depression and sudden death (5), increased life events, and sudden death (6), high depression scores before cardiac surgery and postoperative death (7), depression before surgery and increased rates of mortality (8), and high psychosocial stress post-hospitalization for myocardial rehospitalization (9). An interesting aspect of this latter study was that rehospitalization could not be predicted by biophysical symptoms at the time of discharge. Instead, rehospitalization was predicted by *psychosocial symptoms at the time of discharge.*

Others have also provided evidence that a mind-body relationship exists. LeShan (l0) described relationships between perceived loss of dependency relationships and the onset of cancer. Parkes (11) found that those widowed had a much higher incidence of illness the first year after their losses than a comparable population of people who had not experienced the loss of a spouse. Sime (12) found that those who experienced high levels of preoperative fear needed more analgesics and had longer recovery rates than those with low preoperative fear. Kinsman and Dahlem (13) studied a group of people with asthma and found that those who demonstrated panic and fear symptomotology had longer hospitalization and were discharged home with more medications.

Several found relationships between psychosocial stress and specific biophysical responses. Among these are stress related to cardiac arrythmias (14), increased cholesterol levels (15, 16), blood clotting time (l7), uric acid levels (18), decreased immune response (19) and hypertension (20). Stress, discussed by many authors, has often been related to feelings of loss of control. Stotland and Blumenthal (21) described anxiety as an intermediate between feelings of loss of control and increased autonomic responses. Engel (22) described a Giving-up: Given-up Complex that resulted in vasovagal syncope or vasodepressor response, leading to ventricular fibrillation. Erickson (23) tested a model relating perceived support with perceived control, satisfaction-with-daily-life and physical health status, and found that feelings of satisfaction-with-daily-life predicted for the number of health problems experienced by subjects. The concept satisfaction-with-daily-life in this last study was similar to Engel's Giving-up: Given-up Complex (24). As dissatisfaction with life develops, the phenomena described by Engel in the Giving-up: Given-up Complex emerged. According to Erickson, satisfaction-with-daily-life decreases accordingly.

To summarize, the state of mind seems to be related to one's risk for onset of physical illness and, once ill, seems to be a factor in terms of one's ability to recover from illness. Psychosocial stressors can cause biophysical responses and can impede one’s ability to mobilize the coping resources needed to contend with biophysical stress states. The potential impact of a psychosocial stressor is dependent on the individual's perception of that stressor and therefore, the individual's perceptions will influence his health status. Thus, health is a dynamic, ongoing process that precedes the point of hospitalization and continues after discharge. Disease, on the other hand can be conceptualized as a state that can be singled out in time and addressed without consideration for past or future life events. Since nursing is "the diagnosis and treatment of human responses to actual or potential health problems" (25) not the diagnosis and treatment of the problem or disease itself, there are several issues that relate to the practice of nursing.

PRACTICE ISSUES

If psychosocial distress is related to illness onset, then it is important for nurses to consider the stressors that cause psychosocial distress as they plan care for the acutely ill person. Otherwise, nurses plan interventions that address the stress state (the outcome of the stressors) rather than the source of stress (the stressors), thus leaving the stressors to cause further stress and jeopardize the individual's potential for recovery (26).

Consideration of these relationships may be key when contemplating a different approach to providing nursing care in critical care settings. Schmidt and Wooldridige (27) studied the effect of working with a group of twenty-five preoperative subjects to discuss fears and concerns. This group of surgical patients slept better, had less anxiety the morning of surgery, recalled more detail but fewer fearful or unpleasant experiences during the day of surgery, had less postoperative urinary retention, required less anesthesia, less pain medication, resumed oral intake faster and was discharged home sooner than a matched control group. Mumford, Schlesinger, and Glass (28) analyzed thirty-four controlled studies to determine the effect of psychological intervention on recovery from surgery and heart attacks. They reported that in the thirteen studies that used hospital days post-surgery or post-heart attack as outcome indicators, hospitalization was reduced an average of two days below the control group's average of 9.92 days. While most interventions in these studies were not planned to meet specific needs of particular patients, interventions were planned to meet psychosocial needs in general.

These authors concluded that in the studies where interventions were designed to the coping style of the individual, the effects of psychosocial interventions were further enhanced (29-33). If nurses take these findings seriously, they might decide that the most efficient way to purposefully design interventions that match an individual's coping style would be to systematically practice from a holistic theory base that incorporates the clients' perceptions as primary data. One theory base that includes mind-body relations and focuses on stressors as perceived by the client is Modeling and Role-Modeling (34).

Modeling and Role-Modeling

The theory and paradigm for nursing, Modeling and Role-Modeling, was derived from integrating many years of clinical practice and research; clinical practice which ranged from pediatric to adult care, acute care settings to private practice. Basic to Modeling and Role-Modeling is the belief that each human has a unique model of his or her world and that the nurse must operate within this model. In order to plan interventions consistent with the client's view, the nurse must first develop a model of her client's world, and then analyze that model within the context of the theory base of Modeling and Role-Modeling. "The act of modeling is the process the nurse uses as she develops an image and understanding of the client's world—an image and understanding developed within the client's framework and from the client's perspective. Modeling contains the art and science of nursing. The art of modeling is the development of a mirror image of the situation from the client's perspective. It requires communication skills basic to nursing. These skills will help the nurse put one foot into a world foreign to herself. The science of modeling is the scientific aggregation and analysis of the data collected about the client's model.

Role-modeling cannot occur until the nurse has modeled her client's world and has aggregated and analyzed the constructs of that world. Role-modeling is the facilitation of the individual in attaining, maintaining, or promoting health through purposeful interventions. These interventions are planned based on the data analyses. Role-modeling is also both an art and a science. The art of Role-modeling occurs when the nurse plans and implements interventions that are unique for her client. The science of role-modeling occurs as the nurse plans interventions with respect to her theoretical base for the practice of nursing (35).

The practice of modeling and role-modeling requires an understanding of the theory bases of the model and acceptance of some of the underlying premises. While some nurses seeking alternative approaches to critical care nursing may choose to develop an understanding of the theoretical aspects of this model, others may choose to practice from a conceptual (rather than theoretical) framework. In either case, if critical care nurses are to seriously address mind-body relationships, there are a few issues that merit consideration. These factors distinguish nursing from other professions. They can be listed as: holism versus wholism, nursing process as an interpersonal relationship versus nursing process as a problem-solving format, caring versus curing, client versus patient, nurturing versus controlling, and facilitating versus regulating.

Holism implies that the whole is greater than the sum of the parts. "Human beings are holistic beings who have multiple interacting subsystems. Permeating all subsystems are the inherent bases. These include genetic makeup and spiritual drive. Body, mind, emotion, and spirit are a total unit and they act together. They affect and control one another interactively. The interaction of the multiple subsystems and the inherent bases creates holism." (36) Wholism is different in that it is a state in which the whole is equal to the sum of the parts. "Wholism suggests that man is an aggregate of the biophysical, psychological, social, and cognitive subsystems with inherent bases throughout; it does not imply dynamic relationship among these subsystems" (37).

The nursing process can be thought of as a problem-solving process similar to the process used by all professionals to assess, diagnose, and resolve client problems or it can be thought of as an "ongoing, interactive exchange of information, feelings, and behavior between the nurse and the client, wherein the nurse's goal is to nurture and support the client's self-care" (38). It is the latter definition of the nursing process that is important for nurses to consider as they try to plan interventions that are holistic in nature.

When nurses refocus nursing from a problem-solving approach to an interpersonal approach that is systematic and purposeful, they simultaneously refocus from curing to caring. When nurses are concerned with curing, they focus on the disease or illness problem, and the related organ and/ or system. Nursing care is planned to address related problems. On the other hand, nursing that is concerned with the interpersonal problem, and the human responses to actual or potential problems will take into account the medical problem, but will primarily focus on the client's responses to the problems. Thus, demonstrating a focus on caring rather than curing. Such an approach has another implication: these nurses consider their recipients of care as active members of the health care team. They approach their consumers as clients rather than as patients. A client is one "who is considered to be a legitimate member of the decision-making team, who always has some control over the planned regimen, and who is incorporated in his or her own care as much as possible." A patient is one "who is given aid, instruction and treatment with the expectation that such services are appropriate and that the recipient will accept them and comply with the plans" (39).

As nurses work with clients, aiming for holistic health, they nurture the individual in mobilizing and using resources need to cope with the stressors related to their health problem. This approach is different from controlling the administration of the resources needed. When the nurse nurtures the individual, she must consider the client's needs, from the client's perception. These perceptions are considered the client's self-care knowledge (40). On the other hand, when she controls administration of resources, it is not necessary to know or understand the recipient's perspective; it is merely necessary to understand the medical and nursing care plans. Often, it is difficult for health care consumers to mobilize their own self-care resources needed for self-care actions (41). Nurses assist them in this process as they facilitate them to identify, mobilize, and develop their own strengths and assets. When nurses regulate their individual's resources, they are not concerned with self-care resources, self-care knowledge, or self-care actions. Their concern is with the resources identified by health care providers as necessary to contend with the illness or disease problem.

Conclusions

Nurses will be challenged to become increasingly efficient, to practice quickly and wisely. One way to master this challenge is to practice more purposefully by using a holistic nursing theory base that promotes client well-being. When care is focused on nurturing and facilitating clients, so that they can mobilize the resources needed to cope, they will get well faster and stay well longer. Nurses who work toward this end will not only be more efficient in their work setting, they will also find that their ability to cope with work-related stressors will increase. As their coping ability increases, they will also experience an increased sense of satisfaction with the practice of professional nursing (43).

REFERENCES

1. Erickson, H., Tomlin, E., & Swain, M. A. (1983). *Modeling and Role-Modeling: A Theory and Paradigm for Nursing*. Englewood Cliffs, N.J: Prentice-Hall, pp.9-24.

2. Thiel, H., Parker, D., & Bruce, T. (1973). Stress factors and the risk of myocardial infarction. *Journal of Psychosomatic Research.1*, 7: 43-57.

3. Friedman, G., Uty, H., Klatsky, A., & Siegelaub, M. (1974). A psychological questionnaire predictive of myocardial infarction. *Psychosomatic Medicine.* 36:327-343.

4. Thomas, C., & Greenstreet, R. (1973) Psychobiological characteristics in youth as predictors of five disease states: suicide, mental illness, hypertension, coronary heart disease, and tumor. *Johns Hopkins Medical Journal.* 132:16-43

5. Greene, W., Goldstein, S., &. Moss, A. (1972). Psychological aspects of sudden death. *Archives of Internal Medicine,* 129:725-731.

6. Rahe, H., & Lind, E. (1971). Psychosocial factors and sudden cardiac death: a pilot study. *Journal of Psychosomatic Research.* 15:19-24.

7. Zheutlin, S., & Goldstein, S. (1977). The prediction of psychosocial adjustment subsequent to cardiac insult. *Journal of Clinical Psychology*. 33:706-710.

8. Kimball, C. (1977). Psychological responses to the experience of open heart surgery. In: Moos, R. (Ed) *Coping With Physical Illness*. New York: Plenum, pp.113-133.

9. Prince, R., & Miranda, S. L. (1977). Monitoring life stress to prevent recurrence of coronary heart disease episodes. *Canadian Psychiatric Association Journal*. 22, 6:161-168

10. LeShan, L. (1959). Psychological states as factors in the development of malignant disease: A critical review. *Journal of National Cancer Institute*. 22: 1-18.

11. Parkes, C. (1972). *Bereavement: Studies of Grief in Adult Life*. New York: International University Press.

12. Sime, A. (1976). Relationship of pre-operative fear, type of coping, and information received about surgery to recovery from surgery. *Journal of Personal Social Psychology*. 34:716-724.

13. Dahlem, N., Kinsman, R., & Horton, D. (1979). Requests for as needed medications by asthmatic patients: Relationships to prescribed oral corticosteroid regimens and length of hospitalization. *Journal of Allergy Clinical Immunology*. 63:23-27.

14. Lown, B., and Verrier, R. (1976). Neural activity and ventricular fibrilation. *New England Journal of Medicine*. 294:1165-1170.

15. Gore, S. (1973). The influence of social support and related variables in ameliorating the consequences of job loss. Doctoral dissertation, University of Pennsylvania.

16. Rosenman, R., & Friedman, M. (1974). Neurogenic factors in pathogenesis of coronary heart disease. Medical Clinics of North America. 58:269-179.

17. Theorell, T., Lind, E., Froberg, J., Karlsson, C., Levi, L. (1974). A longitudinal study of 21 subjects with coronary heart disease: Life changes, catecholamine excretion reactions. *Psychosomatic Medicine*.

18. Kasl, S., Cobb, S., & Brooks, G. (1968). Changes in uric acid and related biochemical cholesterol in men undergoing job loss. *Journal of American Medical Association*. 206:1500-1507. 34:505-516.

19. Bartrop, R., Lazarus, L., Luckhurst, E., Kiloh, L., & Penny, R. (1977). Depressed lymphocyte function after bereavement. *The Lancet*. 1:834-836.

20. Friedman, M., Rosenman, R., and Carroll, V. (1958). Changes in serum cholesterol and blood clotting time in men subjected to cyclic variation of occupational stress. *Circulation*. 17:852

21. Stotland, E., & Blumenthal, A. (1964). The reduction of anxiety as a result of the expectation of making a choice. *Canadian Review of Psychology*. 18(2):139-145.

22. Engel, G. (1978). Psychological stress, vasodepressor (vasovagal) syncope, and sudden death. *Annals of Internal Medicine*. 89:403-412.

23. Erickson, H. (1984). Self Care Knowledge: Relations among the concepts hope, support, control and satisfaction with daily life. Unpublished dissertation, Ann Arbor, Michigan: University of Michigan.

24. Engel, G. (1968). A life setting conducive to illness: The giving-up given-up complex. *Annals of Internal Medicine.* 69:293-299.

25. American Nurses' Association: Social Policy Statement. (1980)American Nurses' Association. Kansas City, MO. pp. 9-10.

26. Erickson, H., & Swain, M. A. (1982). A model for assessing potential adaptation to stress. *Research in Nursing and Health.* 5:93-101.

27. Schmidt, E., & Wooldridge, P. (1973). Psychological preparation of surgical patients. *Nursing Research.* 22:108-L16.

28. Mumford, F., Schlesinger, H., and Glass, G. (1982). The effects of psychological intervention on recovery from surgery and heart attacks: an analysis of the literature. *American Journal of Public Health,* 1972:141-151.

29. Sime, A. (1976). Relationship of pre-operative fear, type of coping, and information received about surgery to recovery from surgery. *Journal of Personality in Social Psychology.* 34:716-724.

30. Feltotr, G., Huss, K., Payne, E., et al., (1976). Preoperative nursing intervention with the patient for surgery: outcomes of three alternative approaches. *International Journal of Nursing Studies.* 13:83-96

31. Lindeman, C., Van Aernam, B. (1971). Nursing intervention with the presurgical patient; the effects of structured and unstructured preoperative teaching. *Nursing Research.* 20:319-322.

32. Delong, R. (1971). Individual differences in patterns of anxiety arousal, stress-relevant information and recovery from surgery. Dissertation. Los Angeles: University of California, I970. Dissertation Abstracts. I97l; 32: 5548.

33. Levitan, S., Kornfeld, D. (1981). Clinical and cost benefits of liaison psychiatry. *American Journal of Psychiatry.* 138: 790-793.

34. Erickson, H., Tomlin, E., and Swain, M. A. (1983). *Modeling and Role-Modeling: A Theory and Paradigm for Nursing.* Englewoods Cliff, NJ: Prentice-Hall.

35. pp. 94-96

36-37. p. 45-47

38. p.103

39. p. 254

40-41. p. 48

42. World Health Organization. (1947). Constitution of the World Health Organization. The Chronicle. 29-43.

43. Claus, K., & Baily, J. (1980). *Living with stress and promoting well-being.* St. Louis: The C.V. Mosby Company.

APPENDIX B

Helen L. Erickson

PROSPECTIVE PAYMENTS, THE NURSING PROFESSION, AND NURSING EDUCATION: 1985

ABSTRACT

As the healthcare system evolves, threats of solvency emerge. In response, many talk about necessary changes in Nursing. Nurses seem to respond to the inevitability of cost containment as either a threat or a challenge. The first group is more reactive to change, the second is proactive. The purpose of this article is to discuss some issues related to these two world views. Special considerations are given to the differences between these views as they relate to the educational process and nursing in the healthcare system. Three major issues will be addressed. They include: l) issues discussed in respect to planning curricula for the future, 2) impact on relationships between schools and service agencies, and 3) evaluation considerations. The intent of this paper is to help nurses understand differing views, so we can learn to accept diversity, a prerequisite to building cohesion in the profession.

REACTIVE VERSUS PROACTIVE PERSPECTIVES

A major topic for discussion among nurses today is the potential relationships among the Prospective Payment System, professional nursing, and nursing education. I've have noted that nurses tend to take one of two positions. Some seem to perceive the Prospective Payment System (PPS) as a threat, while others perceive it as a challenge. The first group tends to respond reactively, the second proactively.

These responses are mixed among educators, administrators, staff, and community nurses; no group seems to respond more one way than the other. There are however, distinct differences in their views. Those who respond reactively focus on the agency. They are concerned with the impact of the Diagnostic Related Grouping (DRG) model on the system, and seem to have an underlying concern that their agency will not be able to handle the financial-burden that is inevitable. They tend to talk about the PPS as though the DRG model is the most important aspect of the plan. They identify the profit-making programs in the agencies, want to market those programs and diminish, if not delete, the programs that lose money. They address ways that nurses can help the agencies save money, argue that nurses will have to be more alert to medical charting, and note when complications are diagnosed, to be certain that these are recorded for the purpose of the DRGs. They also state that nurses will have to increase their service-orientation. For example, they argue that nurses will have to assume responsibility for more patients and move patients through intensive care units faster.

The proactive nurses recognize some of the same issues, but simultaneously perceive these changes as a potential for future change. They identify ways that nurses and Nursing can change in order to facilitate clients to get well faster and to stay healthy longer. They talk about relationships among the DRG model, the patterning of observations, and the essence of caring. They believe that nursing care must be more theory-based and more person-centered. They argue that the only way to effect the changes mandated is to change the focus of nursing care from a disease-orientation to a health focus.

They also believe that nurses need to assume proactive leadership in the healthcare team. They argue that we must help people get better in a shorter period of time, rather than merely moving people through the intensive care unit faster. Otherwise, we will merely be "dumping" sicker people onto units unprepared to provide care. The ripple out affect would be an increase in complications, and an increase in hospital stay. As discussions have evolved, controversy about appropriate curricula for the future has grown.

CURRICULAR ISSUES

When discussing curricula, there are three ways to consider the differences between those who respond reactively and those who respond proactively. The first is to consider the concerns that provide a base for the curricula, the second is to consider the focus of the curricula, and the third is the specific content that would be incorporated in the curricula depending on the view.

Base of Knowledge

Nurses who are reactive (see Table 1) tend to be agency-oriented, and are concerned that we should incorporate content into the curricula that will help students understand the impact of the DRGs on the system. They are concerned that we teach students how to help agencies stay in business by saving money for the agency. Thus, they argue that the students should be taught how to be good managers, and how to practice low-cost care. Since most agencies are disease-oriented, low-cost care is closely linked to disease-oriented care by these nurses.

On the contrary, proactive educators are concerned that we prepare students to be health-care oriented, to understand the role of the nurse in society, to be a leader and provider of holistic care for individuals, families, and groups. They believe that holistic, person-centered, health-oriented care must be provided for all people, in primary, secondary, and tertiary care systems. They want to teach students how to take leadership roles *throughout society*, not just in the healthcare system agencies. Table 1. outlines key differences between the two orientations of nursing education.

Table 1. Differing curricular issues based on orientation

REACTIVE VIEWS	PROACTIVE VIEWS
1. Maintain agency solvency.	1. Provide holistic health care.
2. Help agencies stay in business by teaching nurses how to provide low cost care.	2. Help nurses develop professionally, become generalist-prepared to practice in varied settings.
3. Teach students to be good managers and practice efficiently.	3. Teach students to be leaders who also manage efficiently.
4. Practice cost-effective, disease-oriented care.	4. Practice holistic, person-centered, health-directed care.
5. Be technically-competent professionals.	5. Be systematic and purposeful in professional practice.

Goal of Education

As nurses develop strategies to contend with changes in healthcare (secondary to the changes in financing), their orientation affects their plans (Table 2). Reactive nurses tend to give priority to agencies that will be impacted first by the changes in financing. They focus on the impact of the PPS on the system with an emphasis on the DRGs. From their view, this perspective is both appropriate and necessary, *since the concern is maintaining* agency solvency. They believe that major efforts must be taken to maintain the system so that people can be nursed properly and so that nurses will have jobs. They emphasize the students' clinical experiences and argue that students need more in-hospital clinical practice. Their goal is to prepare the technically-proficient student.

On the other hand, proactive educators are more concerned with *the role of the nurse in health care delivery* than they are with the delivery system. They try to find ways to teach students *to learn and to be able to think* about what has been learned (1). These faculty want students to be able to differentiate their professional activities from those of other professions, including medicine, social work, nutrition, and so forth. They believe that nurses must be able to clearly articulate *what they do that is unique to health care delivery*, before they will be able to contribute as leaders in the healthcare delivery system. They are concerned that students learn how to negotiate collaborative roles and positions, so they have the potential to affect change. They argue that nurses will only be able to help systems if they are able to provide such leadership. While, they also recognize the need to assist systems in the adjustment to change, their strategies are very different from those described above.

These proactive nurses focus on increasing the students' communication expertise. They believe that students need to learn how to communicate with colleagues verbally and in writing, how to document care professionally and from a holistic nursing perspective, how to communicate with clientele therapeutically, and how to use computers to facilitate communication.

These nurses also focus on teaching students how to analyze systems so that they can understand the multiple factors that impact health care in general and nursing practice in particular. They perceive that the system, as a whole, is greater than the sum of the parts of the system. Stated in another way, they want to teach students to understand the gestalt of the system.

Table 2. Educational goals based on differing world views.

REACTIVE VIEWS	PROACTIVE VIEWS
1. Teach students what to do as efficiently as possible.	1. Teach students how to learn and how to think about what has been learned.
2. Teach content of PPS; focus on DRGs.	2. Teach students how to differentiate nursing from medicine.
3. Increase hospital clinical experiences.	3. Prepare students with knowledge needed to negotiate collaborative roles and positions.
4. Prepare technically-proficient students.	4. Help students develop expertise in: •communication •system theory •system utilization & analysis •nursing concepts and theories •clinical judgment, critical thinking.

They argue that students must be taught how to analyze the system so that they can effect changes in the system. They perceive that these skills are necessary if nurses are to assume leadership roles. Underlying these aims is the prerequisite aim of teaching students how to practice from a base of Nursing knowledge. Some believe that this base of knowledge should be a conceptual framework; others say it should be a theory base, and still others argue for a combination of the two. In any case, all seem to argue that learning should be focused on the goals of Nursing as opposed to the goals of medicine (2, 3, 4).

Curricular Content

The content that faculty want to teach also differs depending on their views. While all faculty members want to prepare students well, the amount of time and emphasis placed on various courses is related to the faculty's perception of the future of the profession and the future role of the professional (see Table 3).

Reactive nurses tend to want to teach specific content. They argue that students should learn basic facts, develop specific skills, and be able to apply content in specific situations. As stated above, these individuals want to increase the amount of time students spend in clinical practice. They argue that this is necessary in order to prepare the clinically-competent nurse. They stress that they should teach students how to identify and differentiate abnormalities and problems, focusing primarily on the pathology of the individual. The language they use when discussing "nursing problems" is similar to the language used when discussing medical problems.

These nurses often want to teach Nursing using the systems of the body as a framework. The basic sciences are emphasized as a theory base for understanding functional relations within the biophysical subsystem. Outcome goals are usually defined within the context of arresting, controlling or curing a medical problem as opposed to promoting holistic health. When discussing curricular content that will prepare the nurse as a member of the system, these individuals emphasize content that will prepare the nurse as a cost-effective manager. They support inclusion of specific content such as the cost of supplies, unnecessary treatments, and inefficient staffing. Their aim is to teach students how to be an advocate for the system. On the other hand, those primarily concerned with preparing the undergraduate nurse for a generalist position will take an alternative approach to education. They argue that we must prepare students by facilitating their learning of concepts rather than focusing on teaching specific content. They also argue that Nursing concepts and theories for professional practice must be emphasized.

Table 3. Curricular content supported by differing orientations.

REACTIVE VIEWS	PROACTIVE VIEWS
1. Content teaching.	1. Concept teaching.
2. Basic sciences with emphasis on pathophysiology.	2.Nursing theory with scientific bases including: •inductive and reductive research skills. •system analyses (power bases, communication lines, budget issues, organizational lines). •PPS (DRG, quality assurance, patterning). •values and philosophy clarification.
3. Money saving issues; for e.g., cost of supplies, BSN as manager of other nursing staff.	3. Cost-effective budget issues (primary nursing, budget resources).
4. Nursing problems articulated within context of medical model.	4. Nursing problems articulated within context of nursing theory.
5. System advocate.	5. Client advocate.

They include the basic sciences in the required program, but emphasize the need to integrate this knowledge with knowledge acquired from the behavioral sciences. They argue that integrated knowledge provides a holistic framework for understanding the normal, healthy client. These nurses believe that students should be prepared to apply Nursing theory in clinical settings, both in agencies and in the community. While they support the need for students to learn pathology related to the basic and behavioral sciences, their emphasis is placed on using this knowledge to help clients regain health, prevent illness, and promote holistic well-being.

These nurses argue that we should teach students both deductive and inductive research skills. These skills enable the student to aggregate clinical experiences, integrate it with past learning and synthesize their knowledge into a new whole for professional practice (5, 6). They also want to teach students how to analyze systems with specialconsideration of the relationship between the system's philosophy, mission and goals and the nurses own philosophy and mission in life. Their perspective of the content to be emphasized as the students analyze systems includes the power bases within the system, formal and informal organizational structures of the systems, communication lines among system members, and budget issues including source of budget, budget control, budget planning and related implications of these issues. These faculty members believe that it is necessary to inform students of the Prospective Payment pl an. However, they believe that content should include all the issues related to the PPS including the concepts of patterning, quality assurance, and the DRG model. Finally, these faculty members argue that the nurse should be a client advocate, concerned with providing holistic, person-centered nursing.

SCHOOL-AGENCY RELATIONSHIPS

Relationships among the nurse educators and nurse administrations in clinical agencies are impacted by the approach taken while adapting to these changes in society. Those who respond reactively tend to have one set of concerns while those who respond proactively tend to have another. As stated earlier, there are reactive and proactive educators, administrators, and clinicians. No one group responds entirely one way or another. Table 4. outlines these differences. Those who are concerned about the impact on the system tend to take a stance that the students in the clinical areas take time from the nurses in those areas. This view is followed by a perspective that time costs the system money. These perceptions are often supported by statements that agencies have been generous in the past, but given the future financial constraints, agency staff may not be able to afford such generosity. Thus, nursing staff may not be able to accommodate students in the same manner as previously. There are discussions regarding necessary future negotiations with the schools in order to "recoup" the costs of nursing education.

This argument is supported by the fact that although medical education is considered as a pass-through expense in the PPS, nursing education is not. Therefore, the systems will have to find alternative ways to accommodate this expense. These individuals often argue that faculty will have to become more clinical-competent in order to decrease the amount of agency staff time spent working with students. They perceive faculty practice as a means for ensuring that faculty will be technically-competent.

These attitudes differ from those who are concerned with the long-range impact of current changes in society and the healthcare delivery systems. These individuals perceive that students are nursing resources needed to assure solvency in the agencies in the future. They talk about cost-effectiveness. While they recognize the cost of providing learning opportunities for nursing students, they perceive the cost of student education as a necessary investment in the future, rather than merely a cost for today. They perceive the need to negotiate and provide environments conducive to mentoring these future nurses.

They also believe that the mentoring of these nurses is their professional responsibility. While these individuals recognize the need to combine practice, education, and research, their view of faculty practice is different from that above. They believe that faculty practice is necessary to develop, implement, and test nursing theory. The focus of conversation among these nurses differs depending on the view taken. Those who are agency-oriented discuss cost-benefit contracts. They are concerned with the benefit for the agency as it relates to the cost incurred when students are placed in the agency. They discuss issues that focus on service that the agencies get from students, want students to be technically-proficient, urge faculty to increase the technical learning experiences, and the time spent practicing functional nursing in the clinical arena.

Table 4. Faculty-agency relations based on differing orientations.

REACTIVE VIEWS	PROACTIVE VIEWS
1. Students take time; time costs money.	1. Students are tomorrow's resources; a critical investment in the future.
2. Limited acceptance of baccalaureate nursing students.	2. Increased interest in baccalaureate nurses.
3. Negotiations to "recoup agency costs."	3. Negotiations to provide an environment conducive to mentoring future nurses.
4. Cost-benefit contracts.	4. Cost-effective contracts.
5. Service for agencies.	5. Collaborative relationships between service and academia.
6. Teach technical care.	6. Teach how to learn and how to use knowledge; prepare competent, professional students.
7. Management as major focus.	7. Leadership with management skills as major focus.
8. Faculty practice means technically-competent faculty.	8. Faculty practice-development, implementation, and testing of nursing theory.

They also want students to be taught how to be good system managers. They argue that the agency can no longer afford expensive orientation and phase-in programs for the graduates—that students will have to be prepared to assume charge of numbers of clients upon completion of their program.

These attitudes differ from those who approach our future from a proactive perspective. These nurses argue that we need to develop cost-effective contracts, but that the aim of the effectiveness is in respect to the long-range cost as opposed to short-range expenses. They argue that the major issue is for schools and agencies to learn how to negotiate collaborative relationships, build cohesion among the nursing community, and provide environments to prepare competent, professional students. Their focus is on teaching the student how to learn and how to use knowledge, with an expectation that this type of learning will be most cost-effective in the long run.

While these nurses argue that nurses need to learn management skills, this knowledge is developed within the context of learning how to be a leader; the major concern is learning leadership skills with management skills embedded within them.

Evaluation

Reactive agency nurses tend to want different evaluation processes from those who respond proactively. These differences (Table 5) relate to the evaluation of the student as well as evaluations in the agency.

Those who approach these changes reactively tend to argue that students should be evaluated based on their ability to recognize and recall content. They are interested in competency-based nursing. Quality of care is determined based on the length of hospital stay as it relates to the DRG. Episodic care is emphasized.

Table 5. Evaluations based on differing orientations

	REACTIVE VIEWS	PROACTIVE VIEWS
STUDENTS	1. Recall and recognition of content.	1. Integration and synthesis of concepts.
	2. Competency -based practice with a focus on technical proficiency.	2. Application of concepts and related skills; focus on clinical judgment.
AGENCY	1. Length of stay.	1. Health status at discharge. (patterning of individual's use of agency)
	2. Episodic care.	2. Distributive care.

These views differ from those who argue that the integrations and synthesis of concepts is more important than the memorization of content. They argue that evaluation should occur in respect to the students' ability to apply nursing concepts and theory bases. Their major concern is the students' ability to exercise professional judgment while applying knowledge aimed at promoting holistic, health-oriented care. They perceive quality of care as being measured by the clients' health status at the time of discharge as opposed to their length of stay. This view requires that nurses have some way of diagnosing health status at the time of admission to the agency. In this light, these diagnoses have to be within the context of a nursing theory or conceptual framework that addresses the holistic person, his needs, concerns, and responses to actual and potential health problems (7). While there are few who are entirely reactive or proactive in their perceptions of these issues, people do seem to hold one set of views more than the other. Given this, there are differing potential outcomes of changes that will occur.

Diversity and Cohesion are Important

Lazarus (8) has stated that we tend to respond to stressors depending on our perceptions of the stressors. Crisis theory states that there are two aspects to a crisis: danger and opportunity (9). Today is certainly a time of change, and thus filled with stressors. Many perceive that it is also a time of crisis. If we were to extrapolate, we could say that how we experience a crisis will determine our primary responses. That is, we will probably respond differently if we experience the situation to be an inherent danger or an opportunity for change. Those who perceive the danger will probably respond primarily reactively while those who perceive the opportunity will respond primarily proactively.

I think that it will be important for all nurses to maintain a view of both the risks and the opportunities in order to plan most appropriately. Clearly changes are underway. The major trends identified by Naisbitt (10) reflect these changes. Naisbitt has predicted an increased interest in humanism. Coupling this with the national trend toward holistic self-care and behavioral health as opposed to behavioral medicine (11), nurses need to also recognize that *changes will occur whether or not nurses choose to be influential in shaping the outcomes.*

Key differences in the two approaches described above include focusing on learning as opposed to teaching, addressing concept-learning as opposed to content-teaching, developing curricula that include all the cognitive domains as defined by Bloom (5) as opposed to focusing on the first three domains and preparing managers rather than leaders who can manage. Those who approach planning for the future reactively perceive a lack of understanding from colleagues who do not support their view and vice-versa. However, because the first group has aligned with the agency more than with the professional, they feel an increasing necessity to align with agency non-nurse administrators. In some cases, these administrators urge that these nurses take on a "service" orientation rather than a "professional" orientation. As a result, there is a limited acceptance of nurses prepared in proactive baccalaureate programs.

Since they perceive that students are a cost to the agency, some talk about the need to charge clinical fees for placement of students in the agency. These nurses often argue that schools must either prepare "technically-proficient" (not merely competent) nurses or the nurses will not be able to find jobs. Those who tend to take the other view argue that the students need to have varied clinical experiences that include both inpatient and outpatient care. They view the current changes as an opportunity to restructure the healthcare delivery system. They are eager to encourage cohesion among nurses and ways to negotiate exchanges in services. They urge that we simultaneously identify our particular strengths and diversities and discourage conformity in the profession.

In either case there are some important considerations for the profession and the professionals. We must work closely together over the next few years in order to increase cohesion among nurses. In this respect, we will benefit from understanding one another, working together in order to reach toward the future with anticipation and expectation for nurses and nursing. We need to continuously work within the context of total health care and with an aim toward holistic health. Without this, we might well become more disseminated rather than more cohesive. It will be important during this time that we are able to address both the risks and the opportunities of the inevitable changes of the 80s, but that we also shape the form of the next century, just around the corner.

REFERENCES

1. Bruner, J. (1966). *Toward a theory of instruction.* Cambridge, MA: Harvard University Press.

2. The American Nurses Association. (1980). *Nursing: A social policy statement.* Kansas, MO: ANA.

3. Dickoff, J., James, P., & Wiedenback, E. (1968). Theory in a practice discipline: Part I. practice-oriented research. *Nursing Research*, 17 (415-435).

4. Diers, D., & Dye, M. (1969). Situation producing theory. *American Nurses' Association: Second Nursing Theory Conference.* pp. 33-44.

5. Bloom, B. (1967). Cognitive Domain. In *Taxonomy of educational objectives: Handbook I.* New York: David McKay Company. pp 204-207.

6. Erickson, H., Pesut, D., & Swain, M. A. (1984). Synthesis of clinical experiences: A step in theory development. Unpublished manuscript.

7. The American Nurses' Association. (1980). *Nursing: A social policy statement.* Kansas, MO: ANA. p. 10.

8. Lazarus, R. (1966). *Psychological stress and the coping process.* New York: McGraw-Hill.

9. Aquillera, D., & Meesick, J. (1982). *Crisis intervention: Theory and methodology.* St Louis: The C.V. Mosby Company.

10. Naisbitt, J. (1982). *Megatrends.* New York: Warner Books.

11. Matarazzo, J. (Feb 4, 1984). *Behavioral sciences in health.* Speech presented at conference sponsored by The University of Michigan. Ann Arbor, Michigan.

Appendix C

Table 3.5 The Expanded MWK Model with Holistic paradigm.

	NURSING	HEALTH
Empirical knowing	Knowledge that describes and explains the nursing process as a problem-solving approach, and the scientific methods used to study holistic concepts relevant to Nursing.	Science and scientific processes which explore factors that affect health outcomes.
Esthetical knowing	Clarification of Nursing's philosophy.	Knowledge acquired, consciously and unconsciously, that facilitates or impedes health and well-being.
Ethical knowing	Nursing's Standards & Scope of practice.	Nursing's responsibility to promote, restore and maintain client's health and well-being.
Personal knowing	Awareness of Self as a member of the nurse-client relationship and the health care team.	Clarification of personal definition of health: clinical, role-performance, adaptation, or eudemonistic (Smith, 1981).
Sociopolitical knowing	Nursing's Scope of Practice within society at large.	Skills and strategies required to serve as advocates for promotion of health care.
Unknowing	Skills, attitudes needed to be open to discoveries, and unexpected learning.	Openness to client's various interpretations/definitions of health and well-being.
Reflective knowing	Skills, strategies needed to discover "truths" about self and Nursing.	Discovering the meaning of health through Reflective practice.

ENVIRONMENT	PERSON	SOCIOPOLITICAL
Science and scientific processes which explore the interface and interactions, the environment and associated systems with client(s) and nurses.	Science and scientific processes which explore the nature of client within the nursing context.	Science that delineates nursing's role in society.
Knowledge acquired about the nature of environment and environmental manipulation.	Skills and techniques learned by experience that promote client comfort (often thought of as Art of Nursing).	Understanding of systems theory as it relates to Nursing in society.
Nursing's responsibility to identify environmental stressors, disstressors, and to use resources to promote health.	Nurses' responsibilities in facilitating caring and healing processes of the person.	Clarification and delineation of Nursing's Unique Role in Society.
Recognition of environmental stressors, distressors, and use of resources needed.	Beliefs about client as wholistic or holistic being.	Recognition of personal attributes needed to be change agent.
Models that describe Nursing as part of the healthcare system	Models that describe client as member of the healthcare system.	Models that describe healthcare system in society.
Recognition that the environment is in dynamic flux, never constant.	Acceptance that we cannot know all there is to know about other humans.	Understanding that Nursing's role in society is changing, evolving.
Discovering the impact of environment on self and others through Reflective practice.	Discovering the essence of human nature through Reflective practice.	Discovering Nursing's contribution to health care through reflective practice.

Table 3.6 An alternative Expanded MWK Matrix Model with holistic paradigm and some MRM concepts incorporated.

WAYS-OF-KNOWING	Nursing	Health
Personal Knowing	Sense of self	Philosophy of health
Ethical Knowing	Focus and goals of nursing (and holistic nursing); nursing and holistic nursing's Code of Ethics.	Decisions and actions aimed at health maintenance, promotion and restoration.
Unknowing	Openness, learning about self, in relations with others.	Recognize growth potential in all human beings.
Reflective Knowing	Self-reflection with expanding consciousness.	Reflection on clients' definition of health and well-being.
Esthetical Knowing	Nursing's aims of practice; art of nursing, respect for own intuition.	Client's sense of well-being is paramount.
Sociopolitical Knowing	Nursing's role in interdisciplinary setting; system issues.	Focus of nursing versus other disciplines.
Empirical Knowing	Evidence-based practice that includes knowledge that tests, expands holistic discipline consistent with Nursing's constructs.	Science that specifies outcomes within context of eudemonistic health.

Environment	Client	Sociopolitical
Self-awareness; stress management; use of self to change environment.	Personal beliefs, including cultural norms.	Influence of system on own well-being; leaders, managers and system that influence one's well-being; system resources for self-growth.
Creation of a health-oriented, growth producing milieu.	Clients' world-view is primary source of information.	Use of self as a positive driving force in system; change agent as appropriate
Recognition of environmental potential as helpful/harmful.	Openness to clients' expanding self-care knowledge, resources, and actions.	Openness to uncovering driving/restraining forces; serving as client advocate.
Reflection on other resources.	Reflection on data collected from three sources of information.	Reflection on the effects of system and client interface.
Creating a comforting/ caring/ healing environment using common strategies (Erickson, 2006, pp.309-317).	Facilitating client's story (Erickson, 2006, pp. 316-318), while modeling client's world; collection of secondary source of information.	Working within system to collect tertiary sources of information and to accomplish aims of interventions.
Open communications with other disciplines; clear articulation of nursing's role.	Client advocate; clear statements relating clients' views and implications.	Negotiation of various healthcare team plans; care coordinator using system resources.
Science that addresses environmental impact on client well-being.	Science that addresses client view of the world and relations among three sources of information.	Science that addresses sociopolitical issues impacting professional nursing.

Table 3.7 MWK Matrix Model consistent with Wholistic Paradigm.

WAYS-OF-KNOWING	Nursing	Health
Empirical Knowing	Science that tests, expands theory; connects theory and interventions, outcome focused and evaluated objectively.	Science that specifies clinical health outcomes, problem solving related to illness, system problems, symptoms, etc. Understanding of the organ systems of patients, expert in pathophysiology, psychological dimensions etc., Focus on efficacy of interventions.
Ethical Knowing	Metaparadigm; Focus and goals of Nursing; Code of Ethics.	Decisions and actions aimed at clinical health restoration, maintenance.
Sociopolitical Knowing	Nursing as an identifiable and separate discipline within the system.	Interdisciplinary approach to wholistic health restoration and maintenance.
Esthetical Knowing	Goals of practice focus on technical competence and expertise.	Expertise in technical skills, technology, pain management, and other disease/illness focused interventions.
Personal Knowing	EBN care based on objective data; focus on nurse as a professional care-provider.	Philosophy of health based on ADL Performance, absence of disease, or process of adapting to stress.
Unknowing	Open to continuous learning about professional role and skills.	World contains unknown variables to be studied, understood, and manipulated.

Environment	Client	Sociopolitical
Science that addresses environment impact on techniques, roles, systems, pt. outcomes, non-contextual.	Science that addresses factors, aspects or characteristics of patient, or composite of bio-psycho-social-spiritual dimensions, non-contextual.	Science that addresses social-political issues impacting professional nursing.
Awareness and appropriate use of systems that supports desired outcomes.	EBN and system protocol drives decisions, patient's view is secondary source of knowledge.	Use of self as a positive driving force within system rules and policies.
Open communication with other disciplines, Nurses' role within context of the system. Usually non-contextual patient care.	Decisions made based on EBN and expertise of other disciplines, patient *preferences* may be considered but perceptions not usually considered.	Negotiation among Health care providers.
Awareness and competence in using systems resources to provide EBN care, use of other disciplines knowledge to provide care.	Patient seen as wholistic with multiple, separate dimensions requiring multiple skills.	Collaborate with other disciplines to make sure patients' needs are met, with emphasis on physical needs.
Separation of self from environment and environmental impact on client.	Based on nurse's philosophy of nursing. Focus on efficacy & meeting clients technical needs, relationship between nurse & pt functionally based.	System decisions driven by research, focus on maintaining & supporting system efficacy and finances, awareness of sociopolitical systems but not of impact on care.
Environment can be controlled so may need to be explored to enhance efficacy of interventions.	Client care determined by evidence-based nursing. Research findings will answer questions related to patient care; data are objective.	Openness to uncover system's strengths and limitations that may affect patient care.

Appendix D

SYNTHESIZING CLINICAL EXPERIENCES: A STEP IN THEORY DEVELOPMENT INSTRUCTOR'S MANUAL

©Helen L. Erickson
October, 1985

The University of Michigan Medical Center, Biomedical Communications

TABLE OF CONTENTS

PREFACE

There is nothing more central to a discipline than its way of thinking. There is nothing more important in teaching than to provide the learner the earliest opportunity to learn that way of thinking—the form of connection, the attitude, hopes, jokes, and frustration that go with it. In a word, the best introduction to a subject is the subject itself. At the very first breath, the young learner should...be given the chance to solve problems, to conjecture, to quarrel as those are done at the heart of the discipline. But you will ask, how can this be arranged? (Bruner, 1965, p. 118)

BACKGROUND

Over the past ten years nurses have talked extensively about the need to develop theory bases for the practice of professional nursing. Many have argued that such knowledge should be derived from an integration of practice and research. Dickoff, James and Wiedenback (1969) went one step further when they stated that theory bases for professional practice should not only integrate practice and research, but should actually be derived from clinical practice. They emphasized that theory should be derived from clinical practice, tested in research, and reapplied to practice. According to these authors, this continuous "reoccupation" of practice and research is necessary to prevent the "draining off of energies" inherent in the development of theory that is unrelated to the practice of the profession.

In 1980, the American Nurses Association published the first Social Policy Statement specific to the practice of professional nursing. The authors of this document stated that Nursing is the diagnosing and treating of human responses to actual or potential health problems, not the problems themselves. They also stated that theory provides a base for systematic application of the nursing process, including the data collection, diagnostic, treatment and evaluation phases of the process.

The University of Michigan School of Nursing faculty, concerned with these directives, discussed the role of the educator in preparing the professional nurse who could use retroductive reasoning to integrate knowledge and practice. It was clear that while students were taught how to use deductive reasoning *to apply* knowledge to practice, they were not taught how to *derive* knowledge from practice. Ironically, the faculty's experience indicated that most nurses develop personal practice models to guide their own practices, but few learned how to label and articulate this intuitive knowledge, even though they usually derived these models by integrating knowledge acquired formally with knowledge acquired through practice with their personal belief systems.

Paradoxically, such models provide a base for practice, but they are practiced erratically, are difficult to teach to others, and nearly impossible to study. Rather than serving as a consistent base for objective practice and research programs, they cause confusion in the profession, often described as a gap between practice and research. Take as an example, Mary Sjogren, considered by her colleagues and clients as an excellent nurse. When asked by colleagues how she manages to handle difficult clients, she might respond that, "He really wasn't so bad" or, "We just seemed to hit it off."

Many would interpret this to mean that Mary was a "born nurse," with an approach inherent to her; one that cannot be learned by others. On the other hand, Mary herself might have a bad day, and as a result, not be as effective as usual. This might happen because she was too busy or too tired to practice as usual. Without a clear understanding of why she made specific decisions and performed specific actions, Mary has the potential for erratic practice.

Today, nurses are challenged to be more efficient, to do more in less time, and to practice scientifically. This suggests that we need to learn how to teach students to think about their practice as described by Dickoff, James and Wiedenback (1969). This means we need teach students to reflect on their practice, label and articulate phenomena within a case, aggregate data and articulate relations across cases, identify similarities among them and explain differences based on these relations. They also need to learn how to integrate knowledge acquired through these processes with knowledge acquired through other ways of knowing in nursing.

COURSE DEVELOPMENT

Course Description

A course description, consistent with the School's philosophy, mission and goals was written. According to Block (1971), who expanded on Bloom's work, implementation of mastery learning has preconditions that include specification of behavioral objectives, content of instruction, and evaluation processes. He argued that it is important to clarify the intent of the course for both student and faculty. Bloom (1980) stated that students need criteria that facilitate their movement toward mastery, and that realistic performance standards coupled with instructional procedures enable the majority to master content.

Since the cognitive activity of synthesis requires constructing new wholes from previously identified parts, it was decided that students would have to be taught how to think retroductively with an emphasis on inductive thinking first. Since the aim is to help them integrate knowledge unique to their profession, they need to use clinical case experiences as a source for knowledge acquisition. Bruner's discovery-learning model (1968) was considered the best framework for facilitating retroductive reasoning.

According to Bruner (1968), active learning helps the student make the transition from learning to thinking. He stated, "It matters not what we have learned, but what we can do with what we have learned" (p. 2). Snelbecker (1974, pp. 425-426) stated that the discovery-learning model has five benefits:

1. An increase in intellectual patency.
2. A shift from extrinsic rewards to intrinsic rewards.
3. Learning the heuristics of work and working.
4. Development of strategies for making future discoveries.
5. Development of aids for retrieval and retention of information.

Course Planning

Since the entire program was built on Bloom's model and this course was designed based on Bruner's educational model, we decided to use formative evaluation methods. This means that we need to break the content into small units, assess learning at each stage, and help students determine their degree of mastery at each stage. This approach helps students to pace their learning and identify learning difficulties. As students learn how to learn, they develop a sense of learning for its intrinsic reward, and competition among students is decreased and cooperation is increased.

While students need consistent feedback to help them determine whether they are learning what is deemed important by the experts (the faculty), faculty need to have some means of providing such feedback. Faculty must identify what must be evaluated, in advance, and be clear with the students on what is expected.

Faculty carefully selected course readings to ensure that students would grasp the content necessary and the processes expected. According to Bruner, students acquire "effective power" when selected readings help them reorganize and recode past learning. The objective for recoding is to have fewer pieces of information to juggle at any given time as one attempts to problem-solve. "Effective power" is a component of Structuring of Knowledge, one of Bruner's four themes necessary for instructional theory: Predisposition to Learning, Structure of Learning, Sequencing of Knowledge, and Nature and Pacing of Reinforcements.

Preparing to Teach

Prior to teaching the first session, the instructor would benefit from learning about the philosophy of Bruner's Discovery-Learning Methods. For example, Bruner has stated:

> *A curriculum should involve the mastery of skills that in turn lead to the mastery of more powerful ones, the establishment of self-reward sequences...The reward of deeper understanding is a more robust lure to effort than we have yet realized...If there is a way of adjusting to change it must include the development of a metalanguage and metaskills for dealing with continuity in change...It has to do with the need for studying the possible rather than the achieved.* (1967, p. 32)

From these quotes, one might conclude that Bruner believed that the instructor must be interested in helping the student develop robust skills that provide a base for future learning and focus on the process of learning, not on the teaching of content. Thus, the instructor needs to have a basic understanding of Bruner's beliefs about the teaching-learning process, the expected outcomes of discovery-learning of new knowledge, and what is involved in teaching by the discovery method.

Next, the instructor must take into consideration the components of Bruner's model and determine ways to operationalize this model in the classroom. While there are innumerable strategies that might be used, the basic principles remain the same.

Listed below are comments regarding strategies and Bruner's Discovery-Learning Model. These are intended to provide guidelines and/or examples for the instructor interested in using Bruner's model. However, I would hasten to point out that each instructor will want to consider his or her own strengths and then develop teaching strategies that are consistent with them. In any case, instructors will want to keep the major components of Bruner's model in mind, and address them in each teaching-learning session. This is always done with consideration of the learners' past learning experiences, their current situation, and the expected goals for the session.

An example of the layout of the sessions used for this particular course is shown below. This is followed by a description of the course, Synthesizing Clinical Experiences.

UNIT/SESSION/ WEEK	PRESENTER	ACTIVITY
Unit I Sessions 1-4	Faculty	•Present didactic information and examples. •Reinforce student creativity. •Instill curiosity.
5	Students	Demonstrate mastery of content.
6	Faculty	•Present examples of phenomena and functional relationships in familiar theory bases. •Demonstrate modeling of functional relationships.
7-8	Students	•Aggregate 3-4 clinical cases.
9-10	Faculty Students	•Provide feedback on papers. •Synthesize aggregated cases (in groups).
11-14	Students Faculty	•Present group synthesis to peers. •Feedback to peers on group presentations. •Feedback to students on total performance. •Summary of concepts identified in aggregation process.

UNIT I
Session I:
Why Nursing Theory

I Learning Activities

A. Purpose: This session is designed to motivate and initiate the act of learning on the part of the student. The session focuses on:

1. Decreasing student anxiety in respect to course objectives.
2. Increasing student interest and curiosity about course process and outcomes.
3. Decreasing competition among students.
4. Linking past learning with current course learning and future practice by condensing and recoding information.

B. Lecture Content

1. Provide an overview of the course including expectations of student performance, planned sequencing, and required readings.
2. Explain the relationship between this course and other required courses in the program.
3. Discuss the need for knowledge as a base for practicing professional nursing.
4. Discuss the need for a scientific method of development of nursing knowledge.
5. Aggregate clinical cases using the inductive process.

II Instructor Preparation

A. Objectives for Instructor. When teaching this session the instructor will:

1. Utilize learning preconditions as described by Bruner.
2. Decrease competition among students.
3. Increase cooperation among students.
4. Stimulate the student's curiosity about content of the course.
5. Stimulate the student's curiosity about process and outcome.
6. Present content in small conceptually-sequenced units.
7. Encourage intuitive conceptual thought.
8. Initiate discussion regarding need for theory development.

B. Instructor's Notes. According to Bruner,[1] there are four major themes in instructional theory: Predisposition Toward Learning, Structure of Knowledge, Sequence of Knowledge, and the Nature of Reinforcements. Each will be discussed below.

Predisposition Toward Learning

Predisposition toward learning has several subcomponents, one of which is the *act of learning*. The act of learning is characterized by three processes: the acquisition of knowledge, the transformation of knowledge, and the evaluation of acquired knowledge. The experiences associated with each of these processes impact the individual's predisposition toward learning.

Motivation is another subcomponent of predisposition toward learning. Motivation for intrinsic problem-solving is interfered with by extrinsic factors. For example, many students spend a great deal of effort trying to figure out what the teacher wants (i.e., extrinsic problem-solving) rather than learning how to think. Paradoxically, the reward for learning is crossing the gap from learning to thinking.[2] In order to cross this gap intuition must be encouraged as a way of arriving at an "educated guess."[3] This helps students to start thinking about what they already know, but perhaps aren't consciously aware of knowing.

To resolve the conflict between intrinsic and extrinsic problem-solving, students must be encouraged, permitted, reinforced and aided in intrinsic problem-solving.[4] Again, encouraging students to arrive at an "educated guess," and then reinforcing their discoveries helps the student build intrinsic reinforcement. Discrimination learning, a subcomponent of transformation of knowledge (a subcomponent of the act of learning), is facilitated by personalization of knowledge. Knowledge can be personalized by presenting the content and concepts in such a way that the student can identify individual meaning for himself or herself. Discrimination learning is also facilitated by helping students learn to analyze and evaluate their intuitive knowledge.

Predisposition toward learning is facilitated by three cognitive processes: *activation, maintenance,* and *direction.* Activation can be achieved by stimulating the student's sense of curiosity and uncertainty. This can be done without overstressing the student. The role of the instructor is to encourage the student to explicitly comprehend the terminal behavior expected and to "activate" the student in exploratory behaviors. One means of activating the students' learning is to describe how theory can be developed using the inductive method. Maintenance is facilitated by affirmation of learning; direction is facilitated by encouraging further exploration.

Structure of Knowledge

Structure of knowledge includes three characteristics: *mode of representation, economy*, and *effective powers*. Mode of representation refers to the conceptual means of presenting the information. Concepts can be presented in three ways:

1. *Enactively* (i.e., concretely): a set of actions that will achieve the result. For example, a documentation and practice of a skill.

2. Iconically (i.e., graphically): use of summary images or graphics that stand for a concept, but do not fully define it. For example, pictures, diagrams, illustrations, and graphs that represent a concept or a topic.

3. Symbolically (i.e., alpha-numerically): a set of symbolic or logical propositions drawn from a symbolic system that is governed by rules or laws for forming and transforming propositions. For example, hypotheses or formulas to represent concepts.

Both auditory and visual images should be enactively and iconically presented in the first lecture. Economy refers to the amount of information one must "juggle" at any given time to learn the concepts. The instructor's responsibility is to help students "chunk" information into concepts, so that less energy will be used in learning new knowledge. The term "effective powers" refers to the condensing and recoding of information in order to make it more efficient and less difficult to consider.

Sequencing of knowledge

Sequencing the knowledge helps the learner to grasp, transform, and transfer what is being learned. This is done by stating and restating the nature of the problem and describing the process that will be used in moving from the problem to the solution. Movement from concrete behaviors and enactive representation is important in this process.

Finally, the information must be organized if the student is expected to use both past learning and newly acquired knowledge. This means that knowledge is no longer only associated with the specific situations in which the original learning occurred, but instead is condensed and/or recoded as it is learned. In respect to structuring knowledge to be taught, the value of the organization of the learning depends on its ability to simplify information, to generate new propositions, and to increase the student's ability to manipulate the body of knowledge. The way that the knowledge is structured must always be related to the status and gifts of the learner. Therefore, structuring of knowledge relates to sequencing of knowledge, since the instructor first assesses the student's understanding of the knowledge to be learned and then structures the learning process accordingly.

Nature of Reinforcements

The type of reinforcements and how they are used should be consistent with the basic premises of Discovery-Learning. They should be offered consistently, with positive overtones, and should provide direction for future learning.

III Application to Course

The purpose of the course should be stated at the first class session. The specific goals for the class are stated at the outset of the session, so that the student will understand the sequence proposed for meeting course objectives. A discussion of the course syllabus helps students to understand the structure of the knowledge to be incorporated. Students should be given an overview and rationale for the course and a rationale for how this knowledge relates to their future practice. This provides students with a framework for sequencing of the course, initiates the act of learning, and directs the learning process. Throughout the course, the instructor will want to help students refocus their learning goals. The goal is to move from learning *how to do* things to learning *how to think about* things. This includes learning how to think about what they are doing. If students can learn to value their own perceptions and to think about what they are doing and observing, they can be taught how to label and articulate these experiences, either consciously or intuitively.

Explicit statements about past learning and examples of how past learning relates to current expectations (both in the classroom and in clinical practice), assist students to chunk information by condensing and recoding this knowledge. Students need to be encouraged to value their intuitive responses and their observations. They need to understand that one outcome of the entire program is that they will have the skills and knowledge necessary to initiate theory development. Sample statements about past learning and current expectations might include:

1. You already know what you need to know to be successful; now you need to learn how to reorganize what you already know.
2. You have a great deal of knowledge that you haven't begun to think about.
3. You'll have fun.
4. You will learn how to label and articulate what you already know.

5. This course will help you learn how to think about what you already know intuitively.
6. This course will help you integrate and synthesize what you have learned in formal and informal learning environments in the past.
7. Learning how to label and articulate what you already know will help you predict and prescribe nursing outcomes. This means that you can learn to be more systematic and purposeful in practicing nursing.
8. Remember, when one is learning to label and articulate knowledge already known, there can be no failures, *only discoveries*.

Initially, the instructor will focus on the predisposition of learning and try to activate the learning process by motivating the student to acquire new knowledge and to learn for the intrinsic reward that comes from learning, from being able to apply what one knows from his or her clinical practice, and from identification with an esteemed profession. An effort should be made to maintain student curiosity and interest in the learning process.

Questions are an integral part of the class session. In order that students receive constant positive reinforcement for seeking new knowledge, they should be told that there are no dumb questions—only basic questions. Students are told that if they are wondering about something, that others in the class may have the same concern. Since the focus of Bruner's Model is on *learning* rather than teaching, their questions are always treated with respect and viewed as important and worthwhile issues to raise. According to Bruner, this approach to student inquiry is necessary to help the student cross the gap from learning to thinking.

The Structure of Knowledge is addressed repeatedly in this first lecture. The discussion of the purpose of the course includes an explanation of how students will move in their thinking from the enactive mode to the iconic mode. Students are told that they will learn to think systematically and to have fun thinking. The learning process is related to the "unfolding of a tree where there are buds, then flowers, then leaves—leaves that grow and change." This metaphor, coupled with discussion about nursing theory's role in professional practice, helps the student personalize knowledge, a prerequisite for internalizing the reward for learning.

In the discussion, there are two major thrusts designed to help the student economize and use effective powers. The first is a discussion regarding the relationship of this course to other courses in the program. Bloom's taxonomy (see Session 1 Supplement below) is used as a frame of reference for explaining the design of the school's curriculum. A description of this taxonomy of the cognitive domains as described by Bloom helps the student analyze, integrate, and consolidate past learning. Consolidation of learning is a major technique in structuring knowledge. It helps the student accommodate new information by "making room" for new "pieces" of information. Understanding how all courses in a program function together to create a gestalt learning experience, helps students apply new meaning to past learning. Students are repeatedly reminded that the purpose of this course is to help them synthesize past and current knowledge, so that they can label, articulate, reconstruct, predict, and prescribe for the practice of nursing—in other words, to prepare them for thinking differently in the future. Visual aids as well as verbal statements should be used in order to assure that maximum effort is made to address the students' primary mode of stimuli intake (i.e. visual or auditory).

The second attempt to help the student economize and use effective powers is the discussion of professional nursing. The evolution of the nurse's relationship to the physician is discussed briefly using the nurse/physician/client model.[5] This provides a base of reference for discussing nursing today, and in the future. This discussion provides a basis for a later discussion of why professional nurses need a theory base. It also helps the student clearly focus on the nature of the practice of nursing as compared to the practice of other disciplines. Issues addressed include the relationship between theory-based practice and professional nursing, professional nursing and the ANA Social Policy Statement, and several philosophical issues related to nursing practice.[6] As the student is able to "juggle" more pieces of information by "chunking" them together in a way that has personal or individual meaning, it becomes easier to acquire new knowledge and to meet course objectives. In this way, past learning is reinforced, recoded, and reframed. The comparison of the nurse "practice model" and a "scientific model" is an example that is used in class.

Students are told that each nurse develops his or her own model for practice. These models are usually developed intuitively. Thus, the factors of the model are not labeled or articulated. As a result, nurses cannot predict or prescribe consistently or accurately. Furthermore, they cannot teach others how to use their models, derive research questions from their model, or apply research findings to their model. In addition, because these models are developed intuitively, the factors are not labeled or articulated and the nurse's personal state at any given time will affect how consistent she is in carrying out her model. When she is fatigued, overstressed, upset, or experiencing other feelings, she may not carry through with the model (see Slide 6). For example, although she may "know at one level" that it is important to softly touch and quietly speak to anxious patients in order to help decrease their anxiety, nurses may not carry through with these interventions because they have never really labeled and articulated the specific factors. Other examples include illustrations drawn from clinical practice and statements about having confidence in oneself, daring to be different, learning to think, be curious, and wonder.

This session might be summarized by restating the purpose and the specific goals of this class. A model showing the course process (see Slide 7) is used to further condense what has been presented during this session. Students are told that they will work through this process within the next few weeks and to do so they must have confidence in themselves and in their ability to know, learn, and achieve.

Footnotes

1-4. Jerome Bruner in *Readings in Educational Psychology*, Bernard and Huchins, (Eds.). New York, Wirkl Publishing, 1967.

5. This model is shown on page 19 in *Modeling and Role-Modeling: A Theory and Paradigm for Nursing.* Erickson, H., Tomlin, E., Swain, M. A. Englewoods Cliff, NJ: Prentice-Hall, 1983.

6. The American Nurses Association Social Policy Statement proves a base of reference for this discussion. Slides used to direct and facilitate the discussion can be found in Session 1 Supplement.

IV Supplement (Slides used to Facilitate Teaching)

Slide 1: Purpose of the Course

1. Help you learn how to think systematically about nursing.
2. Help you learn how to think about the development of nursing theory.
3. Help you learn to enjoy thinking intuitively about what you experience.

Slide 2: Goals for the Session

1. Introduction to the course.
2. Explore what you will learn.
3. Discuss how you will benefit from the course.
4. Discuss how you will complete course objectives.

Slide 3: Bloom's Taxonomy

Knowledge: Defines, describes, identifies, labels, names
Comprehension: Distinguishes, infers, explains
Application: Changes, relates, demonstrates
Analysis: Breaks down, discriminates
Synthesis: Combines, creates, reconstructs
Evaluation: Appraises, critiques, compares

Slide 4: What Will You Learn?

1. to label
2. to articulate
3. to reconstruct
4. to predict
5. to prescribe

Slide 5: Professional Autonomy (Nurse-Doctor-Client Model)*

*Erickson, H., Tomlin, E., & Swain M. A: *Modeling and Role-Modeling: A Theory and Paradigm for Nursing.* Englewoods Cliff, NJ, Prentice-Hall, 1983.

Slide 6: Intuitive vs. Scientific Models*

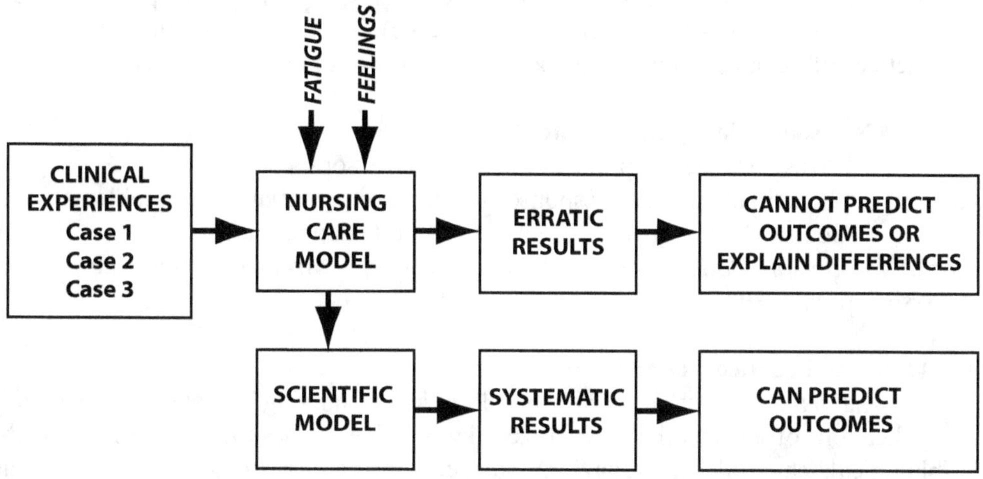

Slide 7: Aggregation-Synthesis Model

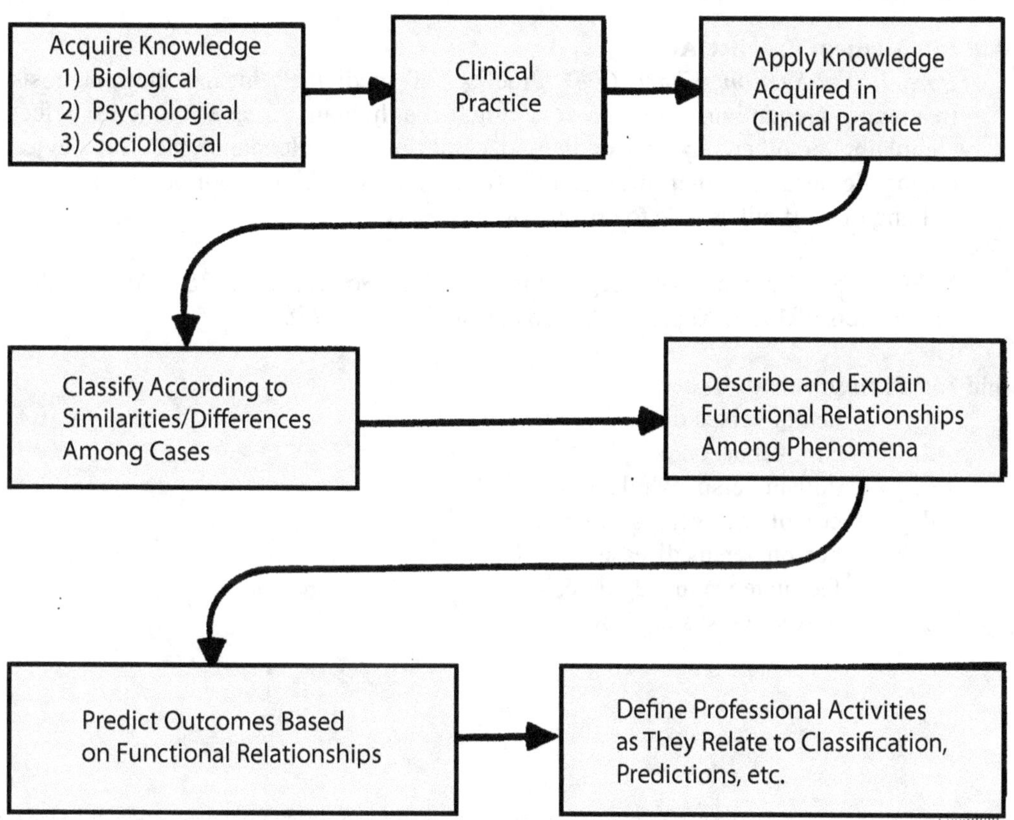

Slides 8 and 9: ANA Social Policy Statement**

Nurses diagnose and treat health-related responses, not the health problem itself. The difference (between nursing and medicine) is where an intermeshing of the practices of nursing and medicine occur. Health is both dynamic and holistic.

Slide 10: ANA Social Policy Statement **

Focus: The health processes of holistic persons.

Phenomena: Human responses to actual or potential health problems.

Goals: Health, growth, development, and adaptation.

***ANA Social Policy Statement.* Kansas City, Missouri, American Nurses Association, 1980.

Slide 11: Nurse Practice Act ***

Part 172. Section 17201 A. "Practice of nursing" means the systematic application of substantial specialized knowledge and skill, derived from the biological, physical, and behavioral sciences, to the care, treatment, counsel, and health teaching of individuals who are experiencing changes in the normal health processes or who require assistance in the maintenance of health and the prevention or management of illness, injury, or disability.

Slide 12: Medical Practice Act***

Part 170. Section 17001 C. "Practice of medicine" means the diagnosis, treatment, prevention, cure, or relieving of a human disease, ailment, defect, complaint, or other physical or mental condition, by attendance, advice, device, diagnostic test, or other means, or offering, undertaking attempting to do, or holding oneself out as able to do, any of these acts.

***State of Michigan, 79th Legislature, Regular Session of 1978. Act Bi, 368, Public Acts of 1987, Approved by Governor, July 25, 1978.

Slide 13: Philosophical Issues

1. health versus disease/sickness.
2. care versus cure.
3. holism versus wholism.
4. compliance versus adherence.
5. person versus disease.
6. facilitate versus regulate.
7. nurture versus control.

Slide 14: Goals of Nursing Related to Nursing Process

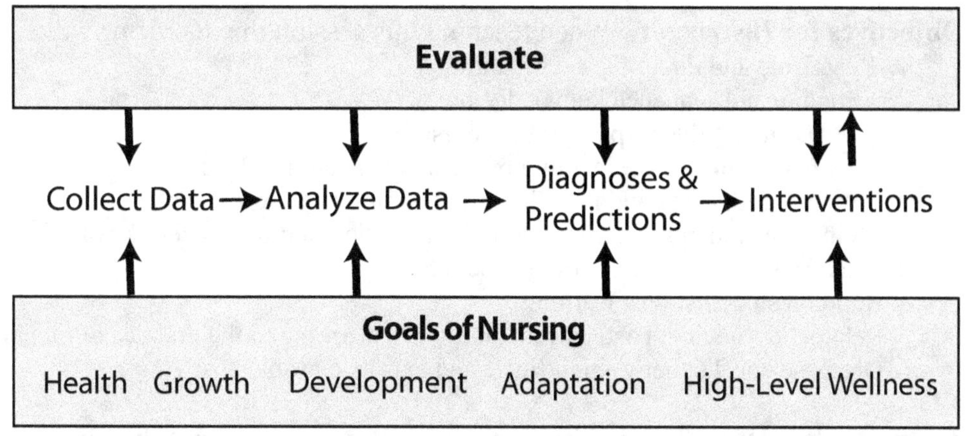

SESSION 2: WAYS-OF-KNOWING AND APPLICATION TO PRACTICE

I Learning Activities

A. Purpose: This session is designed primarily to reactivate and to direct the act of learning.

The act of learning has three subcomponents:

1. acquisition of knowledge,
2. transformation of knowledge, and
3. evaluation of knowledge.

This session focuses on providing structure for knowledge previously learned so that it can be evaluated and transformed. Both enactive and iconic modes are used.

B. Lecture Content

1. Questions regarding course syllabus or course process.
2. Review of last week's presentation.
3. Explanation of why a theory base for professional practice is necessary.
4. How to begin theory development.
5. Overview of the four types of knowledge (i.e. knowledge by tenacity, expert/authority, a priori, and scientific) that are acquired on a regular basis and the advantages and disadvantages of each type.
6. Inductive and deductive reasoning.
7. Relationship between the four types of knowledge and professional nursing practice.

II Instructor Preparation

A. Objectives for Instructor. When teaching this session the instructor will:

1. Reactivate and direct the act of learning.
2. Structure and sequence knowledge by:
   a. Stating the purpose of the course.
   b. Organizing the learning process in a meaningful way.
   c. Condensing and recoding past learning and present discoveries.
3. Reinforce students' learning through discussion and reinforcement of learning derived from formal and informal experiences.
4. Build on students' past learning.
5. Relate the student's past, current, and future learning to the practice of nursing.
6. Decrease conflict between intrinsic and extrinsic problem solving.

B. Instructor's Notes. The session is started with several thoughts in mind:

First, the instructor wants to address the act of learning to assist students to acquire new knowledge that will help them to evaluate and transform previously acquired knowledge. In order to do this the instructor must engage the student's interest in the course and work toward intrinsic rather than extrinsic problem-solving. Consideration is given to allaying anxiety and stimulating curiosity, both prerequisites to facilitating acquisition and transformation of knowledge.

Second, internalizing the learning process is possible only when knowledge has personal meaning. Motivation in this direction can be instilled by encouraging students to be creative, take risks, trust their learning abilities, and to trust that they have already learned considerable knowledge.

Third, activation, maintenance and direction of learning can best be done by simultaneously stimulating the student to think beyond current states of "knowing" while providing a structure for exploration and evaluation of both, knowledge already held and newly-acquired knowledge. As this learning is condensed and recoded, learning is internalized and the student is able to learn how to think about learning. The end result is that the students are able to jump the gap from learning to thinking.

Exploration of alternatives is essential if learning and problem-solving behaviors are to occur. Exploratory behaviors are affected by cultural and motivational factors. The task of teaching is to guide these exploratory behaviors. To get students to explore options, a certain amount of ambiguity is helpful. Too much ambiguity creates anxiety and interferes with learning. To maintain the behaviors, the rewards for exploring have to be greater than the risks of exploring. This can be accomplished by a schedule of intermittent reinforcements for learning. These can take the form of praise for insightful comments or statements that the student is correct or headed in the right direction. Other factors that direct the exploratory behaviors include having a sense of the goal of the task at hand, and having an understanding of the relationship of the alternatives to the achievement of that goal.

III Application To the Course

This course was designed to help students *learn how to think* as opposed to presenting a new set of knowledge (hypothetical versus expository learning). Students are encouraged to be curious and wonder, rather than memorize and recall facts. As students learn how to label and articulate the phenomena identified, they will develop a greater sense of identification with their profession. As the instructor serves as a role model on how clinical cases can be aggregated, students will be able to reorganize their past learning in a way that will facilitate them in the course. Students should be reminded that they already have the observations necessary to succeed in this course. These observations were formed as they practiced nursing over the past three years. Now it is time to label and articulate these observations.

Students are reminded that the only person that can stand in their way is themselves. It is important to stress that there will be no "failures" only "discoveries" during this class. One recommended book (Kohlberg) can be suggested as a resource if and when a student has trouble finding his or her way down the "path of discovery." It is important to stress that you, the instructor, will be available to help them and will direct their path of discovery during this course. Students must therefore be encouraged to be curious, to question, to be aware of being aware, and to allow themselves the pleasure of discovery.

It is important for students to learn to discern between inductive and deductive methods of logic. Deductive methods are used most frequently, resulting in nursing practice being based on theory from other disciplines. In contrast, inductive methods lead to the development of a theory base which arises from the practice of nursing. It should be explained to students that deductively collected data is generally analyzed in terms of a single individual rather than across the population.

As students begin to label and articulate phenomena derived from their observations, they develop a heightened sense of identification with their profession. The goal is learning how to think, not practicing learning by memory and recall. The session can be started by gradually reengaging students in the learning process. It helps to review the syllabus with students. This review provides a restatement of the process that will be used to meet the course objectives. This can be done very quickly, and is most helpful if the student is reassured that each step in the process provides an opportunity for the student to evaluate what has been learned. As the review of the syllabus is done, it is important to make such comments as:

Remember, this is a process course, and in process courses there are no such things as failures-only discoveries. These periodic steps in the course will help you know what you have discovered, and will help you seek the assistance that you need in making future discoveries. As you go through the process of discovery, you will probably learn that there is always something more to discover, to know, to explore. This is what makes learning so much fun! And don't forget, I am here to guide you in your discovery. What you have to do is to give yourself permission to be creative, to learn to be aware, to wonder, and to KNOW that it is okay to have pleasure in learning, knowing, and thinking.

Comments of this nature have additional benefits. They help the student move from extrinsic problem-solving to intrinsic problem-solving. As students learn that they have the capabilities to achieve what is expected, their anxieties decrease. Furthermore, they are motivated to be curious about what they will discover (e.g., what they already know, but aren't aware of knowing).

A brief review of the content of the previous week helps students to remember where they are in the learning process. This activation strategy also provides a frame of reference for maintaining and directing learning and a frame of reference for launching a discussion of why nurses need theory for professional practice. Exploration of the question "Why?" helps stimulate students to identify with the course objectives. This can be done by starting with a discussion of clinical experiences that have left you or your students puzzled, concerned, uneasy, and/or excited. Examples might include: clients that have managed to get well when no one thought that they should or could and clients that seem to give up and die when there is no apparent reason; nurse-nurse communications that seem to be unsatisfactory and/or nurse-physician communications that are unsatisfactory; nurse-other interactions where the nurse in unable to achieve what she is capable of because she does not have the power base, the support, or reinforcement that might be derived from building a common language and knowledge base among nurses. This discussion is designed to help students articulate some of the circumstances they have observed or experienced. It also helps them internalize the need for a common base of knowledge for professional practice.

After several issues that relate to professional practice are identified and articulated, the instructor can discuss how the solution for many of these problems can be found in the development of a theory base for practice. Such comments might include,

Theory is a prerequisite for attaining autonomy as a profession. Theory provides a base for the nursing process. With theory we can be purposeful and systematic in our practice. It directs our data collection, analyses, and evaluation processes, makes possible predictions of outcomes and therefore, specification of nursing interventions. Theory bases also increase communication among nurses. This helps nurses develop a stronger sense of cohesion and build a powerbase needed for proactivity in the health care system. It also improves communication between nurses and clients, and nurses and other professionals.

Statements regarding how theory bases contribute to professional nursing further help students internalize and personalize the need for theory development. The next goal is to help students perceive that they are able to contribute to these processes. This can be achieved by reaffirming that students "know" many things they are not aware of knowing—that they have learned many things using an inductive reasoning process, but that they have not had many opportunities to label and articulate what they already know. A discussion about deductive versus inductive learning helps them grasp the intent. This can be followed by a restatement that students have great knowledge, and that the goal for this class is to identify, label, and articulate all acquired knowledge so that they can use that knowledge to predict and prescribe purposefully and systematically. Since most of the students' formal education is a deductive process, learning inductively needs to be repeatedly reinforced.

Having stated that each student "already has a great deal of knowledge," it is easy to move to a discussion that will help them think about what they know and about what they are learning. This can be done by discussing the four types or categories of knowledge as described by Pierce (1955). The characteristics, advantages, and disadvantages of each type of knowledge can be presented. An example of such knowledge helps students understand (acquire new knowledge) and discriminate among the types. Discrimination is essential if they are to be able to evaluate and transform prior learning. Evaluation and transformation of knowledge are the first steps in moving knowledge acquired by the tenacity method to scientific knowledge.

The relationship between the four types of knowledge and the practice of professional nursing warrants discussion. This helps students further condense all learning to internalize and personalize the need for theory development. It is important to remember to reinforce all past learning and to reiterate that knowledge acquired by the tenacity method provides a base of reference for scientific knowledge. This can be done with statements like:

Remember, there is no good or bad knowledge, only different kinds of knowledge. Each type has its merits, and each can provide a base for building. The real scientist is interested in developing all knowledge to its highest potential. This means that knowledge that you now carry around as intuitive knowledge or expert knowledge can be labeled and articulated in order to move it to a higher level of knowledge. Once it is labeled and articulated, you can study it, refine it, and revise it. Thus, the beauty of the scientific method—it results in self-correction of knowledge.

At this point, positive reinforcement for intuitive knowledge is important. In addition, minimizing negative reinforcements is essential. Any discounting of knowledge moves the student from an intrinsic state to an extrinsic state. The student spends time trying to figure out what the instructor "wants" rather than what she or he is curious about and what can be learned.

The session can be summarized by restating that you would like your students to have an interesting week, have fun, be creative, and find pleasure in thinking and learning.

Session 2 Supplement: (Slides Used to Facilitate Learning)

Slide 15: Four Types of Gaining Knowledge Acquisition

1. Tenacity
2. Expert/Authority
3. A Priori
4. Scientific

Slide 16: Knowledge by Tenacity

Characteristics	Advantages	Disadvantages
1. Based on belief system.	1. Provides structure for quasi-consistency in practice.	1. Biased.
2. Known, because it just is.	2. Promotes cohesion among workers.	2. Value laden.
3. Is not questioned.		3. Not based on data.

Slide 17: Expert/Authority

Characteristics	Advantages	Disadvantages
1. Learned from an expert.	1. Provides team with leadership.	1. Same as tenacity.
2. Often based on knowledge acquired by tenacity.	2. Provides base for decision-making.	2. Data not systematically checked.
3. Can be learned by trial and error.	3. Can be based on data.	3. Erroneous conclusions often result.
		4. Often erroneous generalizations.

Slide 18: A Priori Knowledge

Characteristics	Advantages	Disadvantages
1. Not necessarily based on experience.	1. Based on logic rather than belief system.	1. Biased by experiences and perceptions; world view of nursing.
2. Based on logic or reasoning.	2. Requires that phenomena are identified.	
3. Can be questioned.	3. Encourages identification of functional relations.	

Slide 19: Scientific Knowledge

Characteristics	Advantages	Disadvantages
1. Systematically developed.	1. Supported by data.	1. Time required.
2. Phenomena and relations among them are identified.	2. Self-correcting.	2. Data interpretation and analysis can be biased by world-view.
	3. Comparatively free of bias, values, attitudes.	
	4. More objective than subjective.	

Slide 20: Scientific Process

1. Science: Knowledge gained by systematic study or systematized knowledge in general.
2. System: An assemblage of combination of things or parts forming a complex or unitary whole.
3. Process: Systematic series of actions directed to some end.
4. Scientific Process: A systematic series of actions directed toward acquisition of systematized knowledge.

SESSION 3:
COMMON LANGUAGE IN THEORY DEVELOPMENT

I Learning Activities

A. Purpose: This session is designed to maintain and direct the act of learning and motivate the student to focus on thinking. Emphasis will be placed on the acquisition of a new language, the movement from learning to thinking, and discrimination between learning and thinking.

B. Lecture Content

1. Open session for questions or review as requested by students.
2. Restate the purpose of the course.
3. Reinforce past learning and future potential, encourage curiosity, learning to be aware of being aware.
4. Restate what is needed to move from current knowledge to expected outcomes.
   a. The learning process and what is expected.
   b. That the student already has knowledge that can now be categorized as knowledge by tenacity, expert, a priori, or scientific.
   c. State that the student will be further assisted by learning the language of theory development.
5. Build a language.
   a. Define and discuss conceptual framework and theory base.
   b. Define, discuss, and relate phenomena, concepts, and constructs.
6. Discuss relationship among theory bases, conceptual frameworks, phenomena, concepts, and constructs.
7.

II Instructor Preparation

A. **Objectives for Instructor.** When teaching this session the instructor will:

1. Facilitate cooperation among students.
2. Stimulate student curiosity.

3. Maintain and direct act of learning.
4. Facilitate the acquisition of new knowledge.
5. Facilitate the identification and labeling of intuitive knowledge.
6. Assist the students to sequence new knowledge in respect to previously acquired knowledge.
7. Structure new knowledge to facilitate transformation of previous learning.

B. **Instructor's Notes**. Maintenance and direction are the second and third cognitive processes that facilitate learning. (Activation, the first process, was discussed in Sessions 1 and 2.) Maintenance techniques are those which encourage students to continue exploring alternative solutions for problem solving. Direction techniques are those that help the student gain a sense of the goal of the task as well as the knowledge of the relationship between the information being taught and the goal of the task (Huckabay 1980). Students can be assisted by the instructor who uses maintenance and direction techniques and then reinforces the students at each step of the learning process. Reinforcement was initiated in Session 1 and is continued in each of the following sessions. Explicit reinforcement is emphasized in Session 5.

III Application to Course

To help students structure and sequence learning for this session, goals for the session are stated at the outset of the hour. For example, goals might include:

1. To clarify any issues raised to this point.
2. To discuss the process we will use in this course.
3. To help the students integrate and consolidate their knowledge so that it can be used effectively.
4. To help students develop a new language.
5. To provide examples of theorists who have used an inductive process for theory development.

The session may begin by asking for questions, points of clarification, and concerns. The instructor may wish to make facilitating statements that will give students the security to explore. For example,

I wonder what you have been thinking about, wondering about, or curious about this past week in regard to this class?

Or, if you prefer to ask the question more directly,

Are there any questions about what we have talked about up to this point in time? Remember, there is no such thing as a dumb question, there are only basic questions. Also, if you have a question, you can be assured that one or more of your colleagues has a similar question.

Any questions asked provides you an opportunity to both answer the question directly and to further stimulate the student's curiosity by raising unasked questions relating to either the process or the expected outcomes. This provides an opportunity fro the instructor to restate the purpose of the course and to reinforce students' ability to achieve course objectives. For example (following the answering questions),

And that is why we need a theory base for the practice of professional nursing. That is also why you are working toward the development of nursing theory by aggregating and synthesizing what you already know with what you are learning about your clinical practice. Isn't it exciting to KNOW that you are in the process of becoming scientists? That you are in the process of making discoveries and learning how to think about those discoveries? Remember, if you feel more anxious than excited, it might help you to either refer to Kohlberg or to come and talk with me about what is happening to you and where you are going.

Reiteration of the first few steps in the process will help students break the entire process into small achievable units. This is done by stating something like,

By the end of the term you will have gone through the entire process and will have met each of the course objectives. However, these objectives are like everything else in life- it's nice to know where you are going, but you only have to take one step at a time. Thus, let's focus first on how to achieve the first phase of the course. That can be done by thinking about the issues that we have been discussing in class. These are the issues that are important at this point in time. If you understand what we've been talking about, then you'll be ready to move into the next phase. If, at the same time, you are eager to begin to move into the next phase- the aggregation of you clinical experiences- start to be aware of cases that merely come to your mind because you have been curious about them, wondered about them, or have simply been bugged by them. As you become aware of these cases, make a few notes about what you remember. Why do these cases stand out in your mind? Why are they something that you wonder about? Make notes including phenomena that come to your mind and trust that you will know what to do with those notes as time goes by and you learn more and more.

After questions have been answered and students have been told once again that they can be successful in this class, the instructor will further build a structure for knowing. This can be done by stating that it is time to further build the language of theory development. This is followed by a discussion of conceptual frameworks, theory bases, phenomena, concepts, and constructs. It is important to present this discussion in a manner that helps students condense and recode previously acquired knowledge. It also helps them integrate newly learned information with past learning. Examples and extensive discussion of the relationship among concepts, phenomena, and constructs is necessary. It often helps students to understand these relationships by talking about the need to "chunk" information in order to be able to handle it. For example,

We form concepts by linking factors all of the time. This is because we can only keep a limited amount of unassociated information in our minds at one time. Memory learning theory says that we can only keep seven, plus or minus two pieces of information at a time. Thus, we associate information in order to handle it. An example in everyday life is the telephone number. It contains five pieces of information. There is a prefix (e.g., 665) that is followed by four individual numbers (e.g., 665-5703). We tend to link the three numbers in the prefix, thus end up with only one piece of information. However as the factors are linked and become one piece of information we lose sight of the individual factors in the "clump of information." Thus, we have to explore the whole in order to understand the parts.

Common examples that can be used here are the concepts "classroom" or "car." Several factors have been linked together in either case. To fully know whether something is a classroom or car, one must explore the parts. Common examples from clinical practice are pain and anxiety. The factors that make up these concepts are linked together in such a way that nurses often have difficulty articulating specifically what is meant by either concept. This, of course creates trouble for us when we try to communicate with one another, when we try to specify what we mean, and when we try to predict or plan care. Thus, the factors must be specified. Students can be reminded repeatedly, and under different circumstances, that this is what they are doing in this class. They are going to identify phenomena, develop concepts and constructs, and articulate relationships among phenomena and concepts so that they can initiate a model for professional practice that can be scientifically built, tested, and refined.

It is important to provide sufficient time for questions and discussion at regular intervals. Students often have difficulty distinguishing among concepts, constructs, and phenomena. Reinforcement for asking questions can be handled by simple statements such as, "That's a very good question. Let me see how I can say this in a slightly different way." This type of statement not only reinforces the student for taking risks needed to ask questions, but also for trying to categorize and consolidate knowledge. The instructor can use every question as an opportunity to relate past learning to current learning. Clinical examples help at this point. After a general discussion of the language, including defining conceptual framework, theory bases, concepts, phenomena, functional relationships, and constructs, a more personal discussion helps the student consolidate and internalize new knowledge. This can be done by using theories such as Kuebler-Ross, Maslow, or Selye as examples. Concepts such as pain, anxiety, or depression provide a common base for discussion on concepts, phenomena functional relationships, and constructs.

This session can be summarized by briefly restating the goals for the session with particular emphasis on the building of a new language and consolidation of past learning and new knowledge.

IV Session 3 Supplement: Slides Used to Facilitate Learning

Slide 21: Characteristics of a Theory Base

1. Phenomena are identified
2. Contains constructs
3. Explains relationships
4. Is testable
5. Is self-correcting
6. Predictions can be made based on relationships among phenomena

Slide 22: Characteristics of a Conceptual Framework

1. Is a matrix of concepts
2. Describes area of study
3. Does not explain relationships

4. Usually does not identify phenomena
5. Is not testable

Slide 23: Simple Definitions

a. Phenomenon: a fact, occurrence, circumstance observed or observable.
b. Concept: a general notion or idea, an idea formed by mentally combining all the characteristics into a particular, an abstract idea drawn from generalizing specifics.
c. Construct: formed by putting together the parts. It fulfills certain conditions. It specifies the concept.

Slide 24: Relationships among Phenomena, Concepts and Constructs

(Please see Figure 9.1, Chapter 9)

Session 4: Levels of Theory Development: Deductive, Inductive, and Retroductive Processes

I Learning Activities

A. Purpose The purpose of this session is to further develop a meta-language base for theory development. The focus is on the four levels of theory development as described by Dickoff, James, and Weidenbach. Deductive, inductive, and retroductive methods of theory development are also explored.

B. Lecture Content

1. Review content covered the previous week.
2. Restate the relationship between past learning and course objectives.
3. Review the objectives for this session in respect to past learning.
4. Compare a theory base for a practice discipline and a theory base for a non-practice discipline.
5. Discuss the four levels of theory as defined by Dickoff, James, and Weidenbach.
6. Discuss the relationships among the four levels of theory, the language of theory development, and the nursing process.
7. Discuss the inductive, deductive, and retroductive methods of reasoning and theory development.

II Instructor Preparation

A. Objectives for Instructor . When teaching this session the instructor will:

1. Maintain and direct the act of learning.:
2. Sequence new knowledge

3. Facilitate students' acquisition and integration of new knowledge.
4. Facilitate students' identification with the nursing profession and professional goals.
5. Pace reinforcements

III Application To Course

When using Bruner's discovery-learning model, the emphasis is always on learning. Teaching strategies and techniques are merely a means to the end goal of learning.

Start the class with a statement of the goals for this session. Identifying goals provides a structure for students' learning process; goal statements should conceptually incorporate the instructor's objectives, yet focus on students' learning. Goals for this session might include:

1. Review of past learning.
2. Continued development of meta-language for theory development.
3. Clarification of questions from last session.

As in the previous sessions, a brief restatement of the expected outcome of the course and the expected process for outcome achievement is a good starting place. This is followed by an invitation to discuss any issues addressed previously, to challenge any comments, and explore alternative perspectives. Positive reinforcement for exploratory behaviors is important. After questions have been exhausted, a summary of the sequence in learning helps to move the student to the next stage of learning. Acquisition of more knowledge is best done when the student is able to understand how the "to be acquired information" relates to past learning. For example, the following statement will help summarize previous classes while simultaneously moving toward new learning. This is a strategy for sequencing knowledge:

> *We have talked briefly about why we need to have a common knowledge base in nursing, and how nursing knowledge relates to theory building. We've also discussed how we acquire knowledge and the four ways we categorize everything that we know (tenacity, expert, a priori, and the scientific method). We discussed the pros and cons of each method, and why we continue to use knowledge acquired by tenacity and from the expert or authority. We've also talked about the relationship between the a priori method and the nursing process as commonly practiced.*
>
> *Since our goal in this class is to work toward building knowledge using the scientific method, we have started to develop a language for theory development. Today we will go one step further and talk about the various levels of theory development.*

This approach will lead into a discussion of how a theory for a practice profession differs from that of the basic sciences and to the four levels of theory development as described by Dickoff, James, and Weidenbach. The relationship between the goal content, explicit purpose, prescriptions, and survey list is Level IV and the ANA Social Policy Statement provides a base of reference for students' own conceptualization.

A technique for sequencing learning and structuring knowledge is to discuss the four levels of theory development and relate this discussion to isolation and identifying phenomena of nursing (i.e. human responses, not the problem itself), relating those phenomena, making predictions, and defining prescriptions, and the expected outcomes of the course. This discussion is linked to a discussion of the ANA Social Policy Statement to help the student transform and evaluate acquired knowledge within the context of knowledge specific to the nursing profession (see Session 4 Supplement).

The relationship between inductive, deductive, and retroductive reasoning and theory development is then covered. Students are encouraged to use an inductive process, since the aim is to aggregate clinical practice in order to isolate and identify phenomena and concepts that are common among a group of clients and to describe the relationships among these factors. This is similar to Levels I and II in theory development. When students use a deductive method, they are assuming that phenomena have been isolated and identified (i.e. Level I has been completed). Often, however, these phenomena have been isolated within the context of a medical model or philosophical base, rather than a nursing base of reference. Students are advised that success in this course is related to discovery of phenomena that are common among man and to consideration of how those phenomena vary across the sample selected. They are also told that they will discover that the variance across the sample will help explain some of the differences among the subjects studied.

As students learn to isolate and identify phenomena unique to nursing, they gain a stronger sense of identification with the profession. Reinforcement is important in order to maintain learning, since nurses have often isolated and related such phenomena (e.g., nurse practice models), but are rarely reinforced for their observations. Reinforcement also motivates the student in continuing exploratory behaviors.

Summarize the session by briefly restating what was presented in this session and how it relates to learning from the previous session. This will help the student transform knowledge, economize energies, and use effective powers.

Session IV Supplement: Slides Used to Facilitate Learning

Slide 25: Inductive Reasoning

The conclusion is supported by the premises but doesn't necessarily follow from the premises. Example:

1. this animal is a dog,
2. this animal has four legs,
3. therefore, all four legged animals are dogs.

Slide 26: Deductive Reasoning

The conclusion is drawn form a set of premises which contain no more information than the premises take collectively. Example:

1. all dogs are animals,
2. this is a dog,
3. therefore, this is an animal.

Slide 27: The Inductive Process for Theory Development

Phenomena→similarities→relationships→literature→research

Slide 28: The Deductive Process for Theory Development

Relationships→literature→relationships→research

Slide 29: The Retroductive Process for Theory Development

1. Combination of inductive and deductive reasoning
2. A surprising or unexplained event occurs
3. A theory, idea, or analogy is borrowed to explain event
4. Result is a combination that is a new explanation or theory

Slide 30: Theory Development Definitions

1. Theory: A current group of general propositions used as principles of explanation for a class of phenomena.
2. Development: The act of being developed; to be advanced or expanded to a more complex or complete form.
3. Theory Development: The advancement and expansion of a class of phenomena to an ever-higher, more complex form.

Slide 31: Theory Development: Dickoff, James, and Wiedenbach (1968)

	Level	Goal
I	Factor Isolating	Identify and name phenomena
II	Factor Relating	Describe relationships between/among phenomena
III	Situation Relating	Predict outcomes based on relationships
IV	Situation Producing	Define interventions given the functional relationship

Slide 32: Relationship between the Nursing Process, Theory Development Language, and the Levels of Theory Development

<table>
<tr><td colspan="4">NURSING PROCESS</td></tr>
<tr><td>ASSESSMENT
•Observations
•Data collection</td><td>DIAGNOSIS
•Interpretation
•Analysis</td><td>PLAN
•Goals
•Strategies</td><td>IMPLEMENT
CARING</td></tr>
<tr><td colspan="4">THEORY DEVELOPMENT LANGUAGE</td></tr>
<tr><td>PHENOMENA
•Identify
•Label</td><td>CONCEPT
FORMATION
•Explain
•Articulate relationships</td><td colspan="2">CONSTRUCTS
•Describe
•Predict outcomes
•Prescribe interventions</td></tr>
<tr><td colspan="4">LEVEL OF THEORY</td></tr>
<tr><td>1. FACTOR
ISOLATING</td><td>2. FACTOR
RELATING</td><td>3.SITUATION
RELATING</td><td>4.SITUATION
PRODUCING</td></tr>
</table>

SESSION 5:
REINFORCEMENT OF LEARNING PROCESS

I. Learning Activities

A. Purpose: To provide the student with an opportunity to evaluate the status of knowledge acquisition, integration, and consolidation and to be reinforced for this knowledge.

B. Lecture Content: Test students for understanding of major concepts presented in class to date. These include (see Session 5 Supplement):

1. Definitions and examples of language (concepts, phenomena, construct, theory, conceptual framework).
2. Levels of theory development.
3. Need for nursing theory.

II Instructor Preparation

A. Objectives for Instructor When teaching this session the instructor will:

1. Use quiz as means to "guide discovery."
2. Provide feedback to students as soon as possible.
3. Reinforce positive learning and creativity of students.
4. Minimize negative reinforcements.
5. Encourage students' further exploration, creativity.

B. Instructor's Notes It is important that reinforcement is given at a time and place where students can use the knowledge for corrective purposes, if necessary. According to Bruner, the effectiveness of new knowledge depends on:

1. Where and when the learner will be able to put the corrective information to work.
2. The conditions under which corrective information can be used by the learner.
3. The form in which correction is received by the learner.

III. Application to Course

Students need reassurance that they have acquired the knowledge expected for course completion; instructors need to know whether students have acquired and integrated conceptual knowledge necessary to proceed to the next stage of learning. Therefore, there are two purposes to giving the quiz during this session. The first purpose for the quiz is to provide the student (and instructor) with information about the student's current knowledge base (i.e. had she been able to acquire, integrate, and consolidate knowledge necessary to go the next stage of learning). This information can help the student and instructor to further structure the learning process to maximize the learning. The second purpose of the quiz is to reinforce the learning that has taken place.

Instructor comments that reinforce learning that has occurred and minimize erroneous learning or lack of learning are most helpful. Encouragement to keep trying and reassurance that successful course completion is possible motivates students to continue to work toward course goals. It is necessary to pace these reinforcements in order to maintain and further direct the act of learning. It is important to remember that students will have difficulty with all aspects of the act of learning–acquisition of learning, transformation of knowledge, and evaluation of knowledge acquired–if they are asked to assimilate new information (attend to new information in class) before they have been reinforced for past learning and have had an opportunity to participate in corrective learning. In this regard, feedback on the quiz should be done as soon as possible. Thus, it is important to pace reinforcements for learning and to provide feedback as soon as possible.

SESSION 6: SUMMARIZE LEARNING AND AGGREGATION OF CASES

I. Learning Activities

A. Purpose: This session is designed to consolidate the first phase of the course by:

1. Reviewing content included in the quiz,
2. Clarifying unanswered questions, and
3. Linking all prior sessions to the next phase of the course (Unit 2).

In this respect, emphasis will be placed on helping students with any corrective learning necessary. A secondary focus of this session is movement into the second stage of the course: case aggregation and synthesis of nursing knowledge.

B. Lecture Content

1. Review quiz, clarify issues, answer questions.
2. Discuss relationship between first phase of course, upcoming phase, and final phase.
3. Review overall process for class; restate outcome objectives.
4. Review requirements for paper.
5. Present examples of aggregation process; identify phenomena, concepts, and constructs; and give examples of four levels of theory.
6. Review what is needed for success in writing the paper and in group work.

II. Instructor Preparation

A. Objectives for Instructor When teaching this session the instructor will:

1. Maintain and direct the act of learning.
2. Provide safe environment for discovery learning process.
3. Facilitate transformation and evaluation of knowledge.

4. Using discovery learning process, help students with the transition from Unit 1 to Unit 2.
5. Set stage for student transition to Unit 3.

B. Instructor's Notes Bruner emphasizes the need to break the content into small manageable units and to sequence learning around those units. Sequencing of knowledge helps students to learn and to evaluate the learning process. It also helps students synthesize or recode what has been learned. Recoding and transformation of knowledge is necessary if students are to be able to recall and use newly acquired knowledge. Unit 1 focused on the acquisition of new knowledge with some consideration for evaluating, analyzing, transforming, and recoding old knowledge. Unit 2 focuses on the synthesis of all knowledge obtained. Unit 3 expands on this cognitive domain (Bloom, 1956).

The structuring of knowledge is essential if students are going to condense or consolidate knowledge. That is, movement from the enactive mode to the iconic mode helps students integrate and consolidate knowledge. Integration and consolidation are prerequisite to synthesis of knowledge. The instructor's teaching responsibility lies in helping students economize and use effective powers so that synthesis can occur.

III. Application to Course

The instructor starts with a statement regarding the goals for the session. These goals will reflect the need to consolidate learning from Unit 1 as well as the movement into Unit 2. Following the goals statement, the instructor moves immediately into corrective teaching. This is done through didactic lecturing and a question and answer session.

The content for didactic lecturing aimed at corrective teaching will be determined based on an evaluation of the quizzes as a whole. While some students might need individual assistance (and will have been encouraged to seek such help through comments on their quizzes), the instructor will want to address issues that still seem to be unclear for the group as a whole. This lecture, followed by a question and answer period, maintains and directs the act of learning while facilitating transformation and evaluation of acquired knowledge. The instructor might find it helpful to review the model (see Session 1 Supplement, Slide 7) that illustrates the process to be used in this course. Relating the levels of theory to the steps in the process is helpful.

As the instructor determines that students are ready to move into the next stage of discovery learning (Unit 2 of this course), a statement to this effect will direct the learning. Specific examples demonstrating the synthesis process of others motivates students to further explore their own clinical practice. This can be done by referring to Session 6 Supplement, the Teddy Bear Method, or by using your own aggregation-synthesis processes for knowledge building. Personalization of the process can be achieved by asking students to share a set of clinical cases. These cases can be aggregated and synthesized by the students as a group during class time. During the synthesis process, students are encouraged to describe subjects that spring to their mind and not to be concerned about the commonalities amongst these subjects. After the data are recorded on the blackboard, the instructor can ask the students to look for commonalities, noting that sometimes there will be commonalities that exist, but vary, among the subjects. Use an example (e.g., behaviors in response to the nurse, feelings of loss of control, or availability of support) to initiate exploration on the part of the students. Following discoveries of similarities, students are encouraged to explore differences and to hypothesize why the differences exist. Competing hypotheses are encouraged. Functional relationships are discussed, with potential for prediction models. Alternative interventions follow, based on the functional relationships among the concepts. This process can be repeated until the students indicated that they have internalized the process and are ready to explore and synthesize their own clinical and academic knowledge bases.

Once students have internalized the process, the instructor can move to the next phase of internalizing knowledge—helping the student personalize and "own" the knowledge. In this respect, two techniques are suggested. First, teach students to "own" their ideas, to be proud of them, and to recognize them as unique, important thoughts. This can be facilitated with a general comment such as,

> *Your ideas are very important; you know what nursing is about. You have unique thoughts that need to be protected and valued. Therefore, I want each and every one of you to copyright your paper before you turn it in to me. In fact, I believe that this is so important that I will not read your paper until you have recognized your ideas (symbolically) by copyrighting your paper.*

These comments should be followed by teaching students how to copyright their papers.

Another technique used to help students to "own and personalize" knowledge is to teach them to reference one another when appropriate. In this respect, since their paper is an aggregation of what they know, not what others think, they should be told that they might possibly write the entire paper without any references. On the other hand, as they discuss their cases with their colleagues, they might find that a comment or observation from a colleague, staff nurse, friend, or instructor had resulted in that "aha, now I know" experience. In this case, that particular individual should be on their reference list. It is important to emphasize that nurses need to learn how to value their own thoughts and how to value and give credit to thoughts of their colleagues.

Finally, the instructor can help the student to internalize learning and to further direct the learning process by listing factors that will help the student be successful in this process (see Section 6 Supplement). It is important at this point to reinforce the students' knowledge, both concrete and intuitive, so that they will value their own contribution to the profession and internalize the profession as an autonomous unique discipline.

The session can be summarized by restating the goal for this phase of the course: an inductive exploration, analysis, and synthesis of clinical practice in order to identify commonalities and explain differences among clients. Techniques to motivate students are helpful in activating, maintaining, and directing the act of learning.

IV Session 6 Supplement

A. The Teddy Bear Method (*AJN* October 1981, p. 1831).

This brief report provides an example of how nurses develop nurse practice models through inductive processes, but don't specify the concept in the model nor the functional relationships among the concepts.

Let's think about a group of nurses sitting in the conference room talking about little Billy who cried and kicked when they inserted the intravenous needle.

"Boy," said one nurse, "Was he strong! It took four of us to hold him down." "Yeah," said another, "He wouldn't mind no matter what we said." A third nurse, named Jane replied, "Well, he was just afraid. I don't think that you should hold him down." "What are we supposed to do? Let him go without the IV? He needs it! That's what he's here for!" Jane responds, "No, let him sit up when you're starting his IV, give him more control."

Now another nurse joins in, "Well, I've found that you can get those IVs started without trouble if you let the kids hold their teddy bear while you do it. In fact, they almost help you if you let them. That is, if Teddy has an IV that we (the kids and I) have started together."

From this point, the nurses might very well begin to aggregate their experiences. If they developed a chart illustrating their clinical experiences, it might look like Slide 33. The instructor should inform the class that this exercise is in reality the first level of theory development.

The second level of theory development is factor relating or defining functional relationships. To clarify this area the instructor can use examples such as those shown in Slides 34-37. Plotting the phenomena also helps the students see relationships.

Once the students can conceptualize some of the functional relationships, the instructor can move into a discussion about their long-range goals for care. For example, if they are interested in increasing cooperation (for the nurse's benefit), then predictions could be made based on this view. On the other hand, if the students are interested in the long-range goals as defined by the profession (i.e., growth, health, development, adaptation), then the primary concern (using the earlier example) is decreasing the child's anxiety rather than increasing cooperation. While there appears to be a relationship between these two, case analyses (Slide 33) show that there are a few children who cooperate, but continue to have high anxiety. Here, it helps students to integrate all knowledge if the instructor talks briefly about variance across the cases, and then shows that the variance might be explained by age groups. In this sample, those under 2 to 2 ½ years old are somewhat different than those over this age.

Once factor analyses are complete and there is an understanding of the goal content for the theory, the students can begin to consider competing hypotheses and to conceptualize prescriptions for care. (Slides 33-37 can easily be used to demonstrate competing hypotheses.)

During this process, students should read the article and identify concepts, functional relationships, predictions, and prescriptions embedded in this article. This exercise helps students to internalize the process, gain a sense of the uniqueness of nursing theory, and recognize the potential for theory development by aggregating their own practice.

*This discussion is based on the article "Teddy Bears are for More than Hugging." *AJN* October 1981, p 1831.

Slides Used to Facilitate Learning

Slide 33: Factor Isolating

Age	3	2	4	3	4	5	2	2	2 1/2
Venipuncture	Y	Y	Y	Y	Y	Y	Y	Y	Y
Teddy	Y	N	N	Y	Y	Y	Y	Y	Y
Parent support	Y	N	N	Y	N	N	N	N	Y
Sit upright	Y	N	Y	Y	Y	Y	Y	N	N
Fear	L	H	H	L	M	L	H	L	L
Restraint	N	Y	N	N	N	N	Y	Y	Y

Key: L=low, M=moderate, H=high

Slide 34: Factor Relating: Parent Support and Fear

Fear	Parent Support (Yes)	Parent Support (No)
H	0	3
M	0	1
L	4	1

Observation: ↑support→↓fear
↓support→↑fear

Slide 35 Factor Relating: Teddy and Fear

Fear	Teddy (Yes)	Teddy (No)
H	1	2
M	1	0
L	5	0

Observation: With Teddy→↓fear; Without Teddy→↑fear

Slide 36: Factor Relating: Restraint and Fear

Fear	Restraint (Yes)	Restraint (No)
H	2	1
M	0	1
L	2	3

Observation: No clear relationship

Slide 37: Factor Relating: Restraint and Cooperation

Cooperation	**Restraint (Yes)**	**Restraint (No)**
H	2	1
M	0	1
L	2	3

Observation: No clear relationship

Guidelines for Student Papers

Purpose

This paper is designed to help students learn how to systematically identify, label, and discuss phenomena. You will start with a single case and then aggregate data among clients.

Process

A. Select 3-4 cases from your past clinical experiences. Using the following questions as a guide, analyze each case.

1. What are the phenomena?
2. How do the phenomena relate?
3. What can I call this functional relationship among the phenomena?

B. Aggregate the information obtained in the first step and consider:

1. How are the cases alike?
2. How are the cases different?
3. Speculate on why the similarities and differences exist.
4. How would the nursing care your clients received be supported or changed based on your present analysis and synthesis of these cases?
5. List references.

Scholarship

Plan to prepare your paper in a scholarly manner, including typing of final draft (spelling, grammatical, and other corrections are done *before* the final draft). Use APA format, and ask your instructor if you have any questions.

SESSIONS 7 AND 8: FACILITATING THE AGGREGATION AND SYNTHESIS OF CLINICAL PRACTICE

I Learning Activities

A. Purpose: These two sessions are designed to further facilitate the aggregation and synthesis process. Emphasis is placed on providing a safe environment and providing necessary time for exploration of cases to discover phenomena and functional relationships.

B. Lecture Content

1. Restatement of the goal for this phase of the course.
2. Restatement of the process that the student will use for goal achievement.
3. Discussion regarding references/literature.
4. Practice clinical case aggregation, synthesis, discovery of phenomena (isolation and identification), functional relationships among phenomena/concepts, hypotheses, competing hypotheses, potential research questions, and potential nursing interventions.

II Instructor Preparation

A. Objectives for Instructor. When teaching this session the instructor will:

1. Continue to motivate students to aggregate and synthesize knowledge acquired from formal and informal learning experiences.
2. Continue to direct the discovery learning process.
3. Reinforce evidence of learning and exploring.
4. Create safe environment needed for exploratory behaviors.
5. Provide time for creative thinking.

B. Instructor's Notes. Bruner (1967) stated that creative thinking requires that students be given sufficient time to explore the *possible*. He argues that it is important to provide structured time for this purpose, and to guide the discovery process during this time. Wittrock (1966) stated that a sequence of verbal materials and some practice at discovery is better than an equal amount of time devoted only to practice. In other words, learning by discovery may best be achieved by *guided* discovery.

III Application to the Course

Guided discovery is the primary purpose of this session. To maintain and further direct the act of learning initiated in the previous session, a known theorist is used as an example. The Kuebler-Ross conceptual model on Death and Dying provides an excellent framework to practice from since she has both described her process in developing this model and has also clearly described the model itself.

Once students have had an opportunity to work together analyzing deductively a theory or conceptual model, they will have a better understanding of the components to be identified and related. Then it is time for them to begin to aggregate their own cases. During this session students are further assisted in aggregating their clinical cases, identifying commonalities, and explaining differences among the cases. Students are asked to describe individual cases, describe how the data in the cases relate, and then how the data among the cases relate. They are also encouraged to label the functional relationships discovered among the phenomena and concepts across cases.

Students are told that they can be dismissed from class when they feel that they are ready to write their paper. They are reminded that the papers are to be written in a scholarly manner and that they are capable of high-quality scholarship. They are also reminded that their thoughts are important and that they need to protect them with a copyright. Students are encouraged to use their time efficiently and to seek assistance from the instructor as needed. They are reminded that there are no dumb questions; instead all questions are basic to the students learning process. (Discovery-learning requires that the instructor teach from the students state of learning, reinforce what has been learned, and build on that state.) Papers are to be turned in by the due date.

IV Instructor's Preparation Before Next Class

Putting instructor comments on the papers is an essential aspect of reinforcement and direction of learning. When students have achieved the assignment, positive reinforcement is warranted. When students have been partially successful, the instructor needs to make comments that will *further motivate* the student to take risks necessary to practice discovery learning. Students often have difficulty identifying functional relationships among the phenomena. Therefore, comments that will be helpful might follow these lines: *"I wonder how...relates to...," or "Isn't it interesting that several of your clients..."*

While the tables (see Teddy Bear Method, Session 6 Supplement) help students to identify phenomena and concepts, students still have difficulty noting functional relationships. Students also have difficulty moving into an objective mode of thinking. Often they will defend their nursing care from a tenacity viewpoint rather than critique it from an a priori perspective. Reinforcement for learning and taking risks helps the student continue to risk being open and using exploratory behaviors.

SESSIONS 9 AND 10: AGGREGATION AND SYNTHESIS

I LEARNING ACTIVITIES

A. Purpose

These two sessions are designed to further direct the act of discovery learning. Emphasis is placed on consolidating learning from Units 1 and 2 and reinforcement for movement into the last phase of the course. The expected outcome of this phase of the course is further aggregation and synthesis of knowledge resulting in the development of a model for the practice of nursing. This model will demonstrate functional relationships among factors and provide a base for predictions and prescriptions. Students will be expected to identify research questions based on their model.

B. Lecture Content

1. Statement of the goals for this phase (unit) of the course.
2. Review of the process used to arrive at the point of learning currently experienced.
3. Discussion of the process that will be used to successfully complete this phase of the course.
4. Reinforcement for learning.

II Instructor's Preparation

A. Objectives for Instructor: When teaching this session the instructor will:

1. Reinforce learning that was demonstrated in papers.
2. Direct the learning necessary to achieve course goals.
3. Motivate students to use discovery learning as both an end and as a means to an end.
4. Relate the process of discovery learning to the scientific process.
5. Reinforce working together as a group and using group process to achieve expected outcome.

B. Instructor's Notes Dewey (1938) described discovery learning as both a means and an end. Students who benefit the most from using the discovery learning process are those who can achieve their goals using this process and, at the same time, learn a way of thinking that can be used in future problem-solving situations. Since discovery learning promotes analytical thinking (as compared to reciting or comprehending acquired knowledge), the instructor must keep learning as the focus of the process, not teaching. Directing and maintaining learning is the primary role of the faculty. This requires that the content be personalized and the student be motivated to spend the energy necessary to practice discovery learning. Practice with guided discovery is important at this point in the process.

III Application to the Course

The first session can be started with a general statement about the papers. General statements that I have used include, *"Thank you for sharing such fine thoughts with me. I really enjoyed your papers. I know that nursing will move forward with such fine minds working for the profession."* These comments are general in nature, reinforce the learning demonstrated in the papers, reinforce the students' identification with the profession and owning responsibility for the profession, as well as set the stage for further work. These comments can lead the instructor into initiating the final phase of the course. This can be done by commenting that the papers demonstrate that the students have learned a great deal, have aggregated knowledge, and have begun to synthesize their knowledge, and now it is time to move into the last phase of the course: group aggregation and synthesis. (These comments are also designed to reinforce the learning demonstrated in the papers, thus maintaining the act of learning while setting the stage for further directing the discovery learning process.)

Goals for the session can be stated to direct the learning process for the remainder of the course (see Sessions 9 and 10 Supplement). As always, students should be given an opportunity to ask **questions** about their papers. First, however, the instructor needs to return them for the students' review of comments. As the papers are being distributed, it helps to tell the students that there are many comments on their papers. This is because the instructor is hoping to help the student go to the next level of thinking, not because there is anything wrong with the way they have been thinking. Further comments regarding the difference between critiquing and criticizing also helps student understand that the goal is to facilitate the student to continue to explore and synthesize. A statement to the effect that *learning how to use the discovery learning method is the most important aspect of this course* helps students focus on continuing exploratory behaviors, rather than assuming that the paper is an end in itself.

After students have had an opportunity to review the comments, questions regarding the papers are entertained and answered. If the questions are related to an individual's isolated concerns, the faculty can ask the student to either see her after class, or make an appointment to discuss the paper. If the questions raised are common to the class process, they are answered as completely as possible. This stage in this session provides the instructor an opportunity to discuss issues that were identified during the grading of papers. For example, if several students demonstrated (in their papers) that they need assistance understanding issues such as functional relationships, the nurse-client interpersonal relationship, health as a process–not just a state, or holistic health–not just biophysical health, then this is the time for the faculty to address these issues. This corrective learning is necessary if students are to be expected to aggregate and synthesize the work of several other students.

It is important that students are clear about the goals of the course if they are to achieve those goals. In this case, the goals of the course include the development of a nursing practice model using an inductive approach. This model (since it is for the practice of nursing) must be developed within the context of the philosophy of nursing and with the long-range goals of nursing in mind. Students can be reminded that they might want to review the ANA Social Policy Statement if they have any questions regarding these issues.

As the instructor initiates the process that students will use in the final phase, she can use the guidelines for the group process that are included in the syllabus as means of directing learning (see Sessions 9 and 10 Supplement). A discussion of the guidelines, coupled with a discussion of the evaluation form for the presentation will make clear the expected outcome of the next two sessions. The instructor can use examples of how students might aggregate several papers and, based on a synthesis of these papers, develop a nursing model. Models developed by other students can be used as illustrations.

Students are informed that they will use the same inductive discovery approach for the group process that they used for their papers. There are few additions that need to be pointed out. These relate to aggregating and synthesizing a group of three to five "groups of clients" as opposed to aggregating three or four cases. That is, now students will be in the second stage of aggregating and synthesizing, rather than the first (as with their papers). Another difference is that students will now go the literature to learn what has been written about the concepts and functional relationships that they "have discovered." A third addition is that they will now develop a model to demonstrate the functional relationships among their concepts; they will also identify research questions related to those relationships. Examples of each of these additions can be provided using a model drawn from the literature (e.g., the APAM Model (Erickson and Swain, 1982)) or previous student models.

After completing a discussion of the expected process, questions are entertained. Following this, students are told that they will soon be grouped by the concepts and functional relationships reported in their papers. After this occurs, they are grouped together to begin their aggregation and synthesis process. They are told that the instructor will be available (in the classroom or office) for their questions, and that they should feel very free in seeking assistance. They are encouraged to work as a group first to identify group member tasks, their model, and their research questions. Most students are able to complete this phase of the course without difficulty. However, most also perceive the need to share their "dis-coveries" with the instructor to validate that they have made the "right discoveries." Positive reinforcement is essential if the students are to continue to explore and make additional discoveries. Comments regarding the value of their work, coupled with comments such as, "I wonder what else you are going to find!" helps motivate and direct additional learning.

The second session designated for this activity is an informal class session. Groups of students can use this time to work directly with the instructor, as well as use it to work with one another. Class time is provided for this work based on Bruner's argument that discovery learning requires time for thinking. If discovery learning is valued and expected, then students need to have this validated by giving them time to think and explore. In addition to class time, students are expected to spend about two hours of preparation for every hour of class time. In fact, many students have stated that they spend more time than this, but enjoyed the learning process and, therefore, felt that it was a good use of their time. Few students have complained about the time spent on the course. Most have indicated that the course was very valuable and that all students should be required to take it.

SESSIONS 9 AND 10 SUPPLEMENT

I. CLASS GOALS

1) Review and discuss the papers.
2) Consider:
    a) The next phase of the course.
    b) The group process guidelines.
    c) The group summary.
    d) The group model.

3) Discuss the timeline and format for presentations.
4) Discuss any unfinished business, answer questions.

II GUIDELINES FOR GROUP PRESENTATION

A. Purpose

This project is designed to help students learn how to consider similarities and differences among cases and identify research problems based on these similarities and differences. Functional relationships will be noted and demonstrated in a model for practice. Students will work in groups to develop research problems from their clinical aggregation and synthesis process. They will present their finding to the group on a predetermined date. Guidelines for the process are below.

B. Process

1. Identify tasks to be accomplished by group.
2. Using group theory, establish functional roles for group members.
3. Compile aggregated clinical cases and synthesize your knowledge. Identify similarities and differences among the cases. Use the guidelines for student papers to assist you. Identify competing hypotheses and explain variance among cases. Consider the implications for nursing practice.
4. Develop research questions based on the compilation of your clinical cases.
5. Do a literature search to determine what others have said and learned about your research questions.
6. Revise your questions as appropriate.
7. Develop an outline and model for your presentation. The presentation should include: a description of similarities and differences in aggregated cases, a theoretical explanation for both similarities and differences including concepts identified, and a statement of at least one research problem based on the above. Students provide research references related to their findings.
8. Guidelines for group summary can be used to guide the presentation.
9. Evaluation of the presentation includes consideration of professional appearance and composure.

C. Group Summary

The group summary is to be prepared in a scholarly manner using the following format:

1. Introduction of members and title of presentation.
2. Brief summary from each individual regarding observations about phenomena, concepts, constructs, and functional relationships.

3. Brief summary of group consensus about concepts and all competing hypotheses that have emerged. Explain variance among the cases. (Model is shown at this point.)
4. Future research questions to be addressed.
5. References and bibliography.

SESSIONS 11-14: GROUP PRESENTATIONS

I Learning Activities

A. Purpose

These sessions are designed to illustrate how the discovery learning method is a means as well as an end to goal achievement. As student groups present their findings to their colleagues, the emphasis is placed on the findings, not the process. Comparison of presentations in respect to identification of common concepts, noting functional relationships and suggesting nursing actions and future research questions, provides activation and motivation for the students' future learning.

B. Lecture Content

1. Student presentations with question/answer sessions.
2. Faculty summary statement at the end.

II Instructor Preparation

C. Objectives for Instructor: When teaching this session the instructor will:

1. Motivate students to use discovery learning as a means to problem-solve.
2. Help students consolidate/condense knowledge.
3. Help students develop stronger identity with profession.
4. Encourage students to reinforce and assist one another in future learning and explorations.
5. Help students terminate course without terminating learning experiences.
6. Help students learn from one another.

III Application to Course

Throughout this course, your primary goals have been to teach students how to think analytically, learn, have fun learning, be curious, be aware of being aware, use discovery techniques for learning, value nursing knowledge, and work harmoniously with colleagues. Now you want to facilitate retention of their newly learned knowledge and skills and the application of knowledge to future experiences (Snelbecker, 1974). In addition, it is time to help students end their experiences with this particular group of colleagues without experiencing let-down. Therefore, it is important to consider all the techniques suggested in General Methods for Teaching (Addendum). You will need to help students synthesize all practice models as a final experience. Point out the joy of learning and discovering (see Direction techniques), reinforce the work that has been done over the term, their skills as "budding scientists," and their maturity in self-analysis that has occurred as they have explored and evaluated their own nursing care.

Encourage them to use these skills in other settings, to remember that they know how to learn and be aware, and to work with colleagues on *knowing (not just doing).* Encourage them to continue to think about their research questions, to gather more data, to read the literature. Reinforce that there is *no single truth, only new knowledge.* Continue to challenge their thoughts (not criticize, but encourage deeper thought) while you simultaneously reinforce the work that is presented.

Provide specific comments on how they have performed and suggestions for the future (see student presentation evaluation form). Encourage classmates to evaluate their colleagues thoroughly and thoughtfully. It often helps to discuss the difference between critiquing and criticizing and to offer a few techniques for critiquing. In short, this is the time to provide mentorship by directing the students' future behaviors.

SESSIONS 11-14 SUPPLEMENT

STUDENT PRESENTATION EVALUATION FORM

Criteria	Ranking low----------------------------------high				
The group utilized group theory by specifying tasks for members	1	2	3	4	5
Members presented their aggregated findings as individuals	1	2	3	4	5
The group presented its findings as a group	1	2	3	4	5
Competing hypotheses were identified	1	2	3	4	5
Variance was explained	1	2	3	4	5
Implications for nursing were addressed	1	2	3	4	5
Appropriate literature was presented	1	2	3	4	5
Research questions were identified	1	2	3	4	5
Professional appearance/composure	1	2	3	4	5
Overall quality of presentation	1	2	3	4	5

Comments:

Group members:

Synopsis of Appendix D

I. COMPONENTS OF BRUNER'S MODEL FOR DISCOVERY LEARNING

A Predisposition toward learning

1. Act of learning
   a. Acquisition of knowledge
   b. Transformation of knowledge
   c. Evaluation of knowledge acquired
2. Motivation: intrinsic versus extrinsic factors
3. Cognitive facilitators
   a. Activation
   b. Maintenance
   c. Direction

B Structure of learning

4. Mode of representation
   a. Enactive
   b. Iconical
   c. Symbolic
5. Economy
6. Effective powers

C Sequencing of knowledge

D Nature and pacing of reinforcements

II. ADVANTAGES TO DISCOVERY LEARNING

Bruner states that his model helps students focus on learning how to think rather than focusing on what the teacher expects from the student. He argues that the evaluation process has the following advantages:

1. Breaks learning into small parts that can then be synthesized into a greater whole.
2. Helps students internalize knowledge and rewards which ultimately results in a decreased competition among the group.
3. Mastery itself–rather than the teacher's feedback–becomes the reward.

Snellbecker states that Bruner's discovery model for teaching and learning has the following advantages:

1. It increases intellectual capabilities.
2. It produces intrinsic rather than extrinsic rewards.
3. It teaches the value of working to learn.
4. It teaches strategies for making future discoveries.
5. It aids retention and retrieval of information.

III. GUIDELINES EXTRAPOLATED FROM BRUNER'S MODEL FOR DISCOVERY-LEARNING

1. Meet learning preconditions.
2. Decrease competition; facilitate cooperation.
3. Break content into small units and sequence learning of content.
4. Facilitate "chunking" of information.
5. Personalize knowledge.
6. Encourage intuition.
7. Facilitate identification and labeling of intuitive knowledge.
8. Stress difference between inductive and deductive learning.
9. Resolve conflict between intrinsic and extrinsic problem-solving.
10. Pace positive reinforcements.
11. Minimize negative reinforcements.
12. Guide discovery.
13. Teach discovery as a means *and* end for learning.
14. Encourage curiosity, being aware of being aware.

IV. GENERAL METHODS FOR TEACHING

A. Predisposition toward learning

1. Act of learning

a) Acquisition of knowledge:

i. Pace.

ii Teach in units.

iii Chunk information.

b)Transformation of knowledge and discrimination of information:

i Personalize.

ii Present knowledge in several ways; use Piagetian levels of cognition.

c) Evaluation of knowledge acquired:

i) Use Bloom for objectives and evaluation of knowledge acquisition.

ii) Break content/process into small units to evaluate.

3. Motivation: intrinsic versus extrinsic factors

a) Reinforce past learning.

b) Encourage "labeling" intuition.

c) Encourage curiosity.

d) Focus on learning, not teaching.

e) Reinforce discovery, discount failure.

f) Encourage student to be curious, to wonder.

g) Learn to be aware of being aware, to allow themselves the pleasure of discovery.

4. **Cognitive facilitators:**

a) Activation:

i Stimulate curiosity.

ii Provide security for exploratory behaviors.

b) Examples of activation statements:

i. I wonder what you will discover as you aggregate and synthesize you knowledge?

ii. I wonder when you will become aware of being aware.

iii. You are becoming scientists—I think you'll find it fun.

iv. This might be very scary at first, but you will soon discover that it is fun.

v. There are no failures, only discoveries.

vi. You have faculty who can help you when you want help.

vii. Your faculty is here to help you on your path of discovery.

c) Maintenance:

i. Critique, don't criticize.

ii. Support, don't ridicule.

iii. Maximize strengths and knowledge, diminish errors; for example, class activities, didactic lectures, faculty model the process with own and student experiences, class assignments, quiz, paper, group presentations.

d) Pacing of reinforcement statements: *Now I know what budding scientists look like. Thank you for a delightful weekend of reading; your ideas are great.*

e) Direction:

i. Challenge, don't threaten.

ii. Encourage students to believe in themselves, their ideas.

iii. Specify nursing goals as profession, not personal goals as individuals.

iv. Encourage students to think about and believe in nursing.

v. Use models to show relationships of nursing to other professions.

vi. Encourage students to be curious, to explore, and wonder.

vii. Encourage students to think about past learning, reframe past learning. (use "file cabinets in mind" as an example).

viii. Encourage students to talk with one another, with staff nurses, with faculty.
viv. Encourage students to explore.
x. Be clear with students about expectations for course completion; restate expectations: *You will recode some of your past learning as you make new discoveries. You have good ideas; protect them with a copyright. You have opened the door to discovery—enjoy knowing what you know, and enjoy discovering what you know. Have fun learning and discovering what you know and who you are. As your self-confidence grows, your insights will grow. As we draw closure to this part of the journey in discovery, know that you can continue to enjoy discovering nursing, and yourself as a person and nurse.*

B. Structuring knowledge (mode of representation):

1) Enactive: use concrete examples such as anatomy and physiology; Kuebler-Ross, Selye, Maslow, Erikson.
   a) Iconical: graphic presentation shows relationships.
   b) Symbolic: use alpha-numeric presentations and measurements:
2) Economy (amount of information that can be juggled at one time).
   a) Discuss memory learning theory regarding chunking information.
   b) Group and chunk information and build associations with pieces of information.
3) Effective powers: condense and recode information for comprehension.

INDEX

INDEX

INDEX

INDEX

W

www.ingramcontent.com/pod-product-compliance
Lightning Source LLC
Chambersburg PA
CBHW081102170526
45165CB00008B/2301

* 9 7 8 1 4 5 1 5 1 1 7 3 4 *